Mosby's

Comprehensive Review
of
RADIOGRAPHY

THE COMPLETE STUDY GUIDE AND CAREER PLANNER

left hand generator rule =

    thumb = motion of conductor
    index finger = direction of magnetic field
    middle finger = flow of induced current

Comprehensive Review
of
RADIOGRAPHY
THE COMPLETE STUDY GUIDE AND CAREER PLANNER

THIRD EDITION

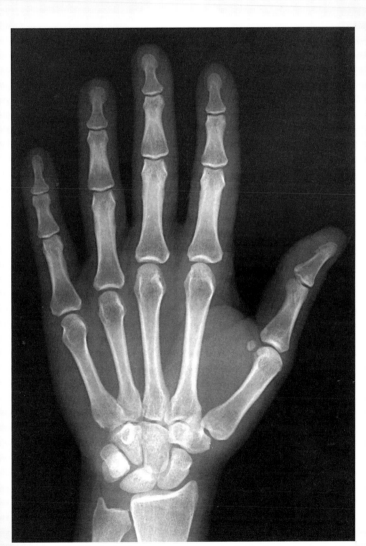

William J. Callaway, BA, RT(R)

Chair, Allied Health Division
Director, Associate Degree
    Radiography Program
Lincoln Land Community College
Springfield, Illinois

with 131 illustrations

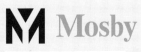

Mosby

An Affiliate of Elsevier

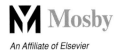

Acquisitions Editor: Jeanne Wilke
Developmental Editor: Jennifer Moorhead
Project Manager: Linda McKinley
Production Editor: Judy Ahlers
Designer: Julia Dummitt
Cover Art: Julia Dummitt

NOTICE

Pharmacology is an ever-changing field. Standard safety precautions must be followed, but as new research and clinical experience broaden our knowledge, changes in treatment and drug therapy may become necessary or appropriate. Readers are advised to check the most current product information provided by the manufacturer of each drug to be administered to verify the recommended dose, the method and duration of administration, and contraindications. It is the responsibility of the licensed prescriber, relying on experience and knowledge of the patient, to determine dosages and the best treatment for each individual patient. Neither the Publisher nor the editor assumes any liability for any injury and/or damage to persons or property arising from this publication.

Permissions may be sought directly from Elsevier's Health Sciences Rights Department in Philadelphia, USA: phone: (+1)215-238-7869, fax: (+1)215-238-2239, email: healthpermissions@elsevier.com. You may also complete your request on-line via the Elsevier Science homepage (http://www.elsevier.com), by selecting 'Customer Support' and then 'Obtaining Permissions'.

Quotations from SUCCESSORIES are used with permission and published by Celex Group, Inc/ Celebrating Excellence, all rights reserved.

Mosby, Inc.
An Affiliate of Elsevier
11830 Westline Industrial Drive
St. Louis, Missouri 63146

Printed in China

Library of Congress Cataloging in Publication Data

Callaway, William J. (William Joseph)
    Mosby's comprehensive review of radiography : the complete study guide and career
    planner / William J. Callaway. —3rd ed.
        p. ; cm.
    Includes bibliographical references.
    ISBN 0-323-01839-4
    1. Radiography, Medical—Outlines, syllabi, etc. 2. Radiography,
Medical—Examinations, questions, etc. 3. Radiography, Medical—Vocational guidance.
    I. Title: Comprehensive review of radiography.   II. Title.
        [DNLM: 1. Technology, Radiologic—Examination Questions. 2.
Radiography—Examination Questions. WN 18.2 C156m 2002]
    RC78.17 .C35 2002
    616.07'572'076–dc21   2001058738

04   05   06   GW/MV   9   8   7   6   5   4

About the Author

William J. Callaway, BA, RT(R), has been involved in radiography education for more than 25 years, directing both hospital-sponsored and associate degree programs. He is coauthor of *Introduction to Radiologic Technology*, also published by Mosby, and has had articles published in state and national radiologic technology journals.

He speaks extensively to students, educators, and practicing technologists at international, national, state, and local radiologic technology meetings. His presentations include "Face to Face with Moments of Truth," "Survival in the Dysfunctional Workplace," "Practical Physics for the Radiographer (and You Thought Physics Had to Be Boring!)," "Just Do Something—The You-Shaped Piece of the Puzzle," "Motivation's Greatest Hits," and "Hey, I Have a Life Away From Here Too, You Know!"

Mr. Callaway also has an extensive background in staff development and has served as a management and quality service consultant for health care institutions all over the United States. He has coauthored a quality customer service guide for radiology and has presented more than 500 workshops on management, customer service, and communications in health care.

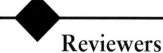

Reviewers

Debra Caldwell, MA, RT(R)(QM)(CV)
Radiologic Technology Program Director
York Technical College
Rock Hill, South Carolina

Gerald Graddy, MS, RT(R)
Radiography Program
Jackson State Community College
Jackson, Tennessee

John Skinner, MEd, MSA, BA, RT(R)
Radiography Program Director
Mid Michigan Community College
Harrison, Michigan

Bonnie Tobias, MSA, RT(R)(M)(QM)
Radiographer Program Director
Henry Ford Community College
Dearborn, Michigan

The third edition of this book is dedicated to my wife, Karen,
our children, Amy, Adam, Cara, David, and Kim,
and our grandchildren, Alex, Kailin, and Mariah.

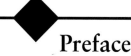

Preface

CONTENT AND ORGANIZATION

Mosby's Comprehensive Review of Radiography is designed for use by students as a study guide throughout their radiography education and as a review book as they prepare to take the Registry examination. Part I offers a comprehensive review, in outline form, of the five major content areas covered on the ARRT exam in radiography. Each content review is followed by a set of 100 questions related specifically to that area. After students have reviewed all five subject areas, they are ready to take the three 200-question challenge tests printed in the text. Answers and rationales to the review questions and challenge tests are provided in an appendix. To further prepare students for the ARRT exam, Part I offers instruction in the most effective way to schedule and use review time, explores strategies for answering multiple-choice questions, and provides information on the test application procedure.

Unlike other review books, *Mosby's Comprehensive Review of Radiography* also serves students as a career planner. Part II, Preparation for Employment, offers examples of real resumes and cover letters and other important information on preparation for employment. Part III, Continuing Education Opportunities, instructs students in how to fulfill requirements for certification renewal and offers advice on advancing in the field of radiologic technology. No other book provides this valuable information to help students make the transition to their careers as practicing radiographers.

NEW CONTENT AND FEATURES

New content reflects the latest changes to the ARRT exam. The list of conventional terminology, abbreviations, and formats adopted by the ARRT has been revised. New ARRT coverage of computed radiography and handling of biohazardous materials is reviewed in Chapter 4, *Review of Image Production and Evaluation,* and in Chapter 6, *Review of Patient Care and Management,* respectively. Enhancements to existing features include the addition of a third 200-question test in Chapter 7 and new career preparation content in Chapter 10 that covers basic financial planning, especially as it applies to salary and benefit negotiation.

An exciting new feature of this edition is the accompanying CD-ROM, designed to simulate the computer-based exam now administered by the ARRT. This study and review tool contains more than 1150 questions—all different from the 1100 questions in the text and all relevant to preparation for the ARRT examination. The student can work in tutorial mode, answering hundreds of multiple-choice questions for each content area, sectioned according to the ARRT content specifications. Rationales and study tips provide immediate feedback, and questions can be bookmarked for later reference. In test mode, an unlimited number of randomly generated, 200-question multiple-choice exams are available. The rationales and study tips for each question can be accessed when reviewing the results of a completed exam.

HOW TO USE

Care has been taken to create questions that cover the primary information taught in radiography programs and that are therefore relevant to the ARRT exam. This philosophy, coupled with the outline form, helps students optimize study time. The questions, however, are not easy. They are designed to stimulate critical thinking so that the reader's understanding of the material is truly tested. Students who have difficulty understanding an answer are advised to return to the study guide for additional review. This text should not be viewed as a substitute for a textbook or coursework that comprehensively covers a subject area. Additional reference to a course text may be necessary for some students. A final note on the use of this guide: Variation in the details of test content will occur across certification exams. Therefore inclusion of specific information in this guide does not guarantee that it will be tested, and the exclusion of certain information is not meant to suggest its absence from the exam. The ARRT does not review, evaluate, or endorse publications. Permission to reproduce copyrighted materials within this publication should not be construed as an endorsement of the publication by the ARRT.

Acknowledgments

Mosby once again assembled a great team to bring this project to fruition. Special acknowledgment goes to Jeanne Wilke for her continued support of this text. Jennifer Moorhead expertly guided the manuscript development and moved it smoothly through its revision. Given the talents of the entire Mosby staff, any errors or omissions from this book are solely mine.

Finally, I extend my thanks to the hundreds of educators and thousands of students who have used this text and given it their overwhelming support.

William J. Callaway

Contents

Mosby's

Comprehensive Review
of
RADIOGRAPHY

THE COMPLETE STUDY GUIDE AND CAREER PLANNER

PART I

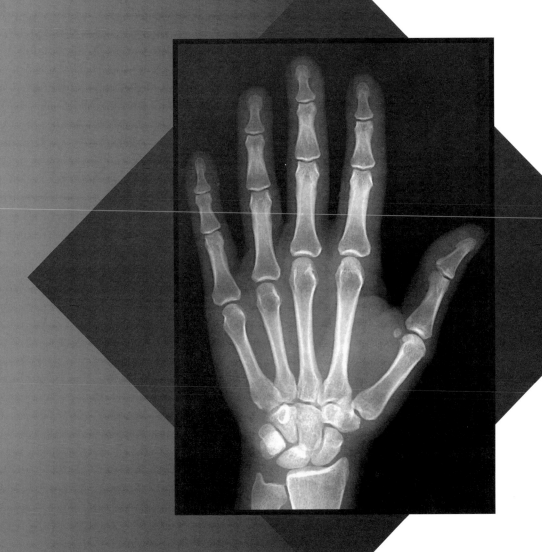

Review

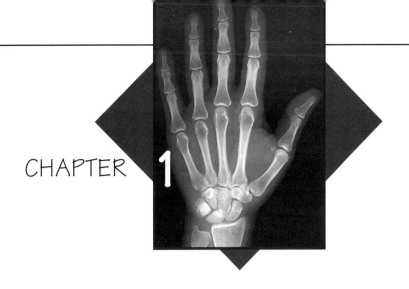

CHAPTER 1

Preparation for Review

WELCOME TO YOUR STUDY GUIDE AND CAREER PLANNER!

The future belongs to those who believe in the beauty of their dreams.

Congratulations on acquiring the most complete study guide available to prepare for radiography classes throughout the educational program and the radiography examination. By reviewing the major subject areas contained in Part I of this guide, answering and studying the exam questions, and understanding the skills involved in various areas of radiography, you will be well on the way to achieving the goal of excelling in class and passing the radiography exam.

However, passing the courses and the examination is only one of several steps in building your new career. As you look toward graduation, you are probably contemplating your transition into the work environment or considering further education. In addition to thoroughly preparing you for the exam, this book helps you develop your career goals. In Part II, *Preparation for Employment,* you will have an opportunity to describe the events that have been rewarding and motivating during your education. This activity will enable you to set goals for establishing your practice of medical radiography and plan for either immediate employment or continued education.

The most important tools that are used during the transition into the workforce are the resume and the interview, each of which is covered in separate chapters to thoroughly prepare you for marketing yourself in today's ever-changing health care environment. So that you may be fully aware of your role as an entry-level radiographer, a complete chapter has been dedicated to helping you anticipate employer expectations for your first postgraduate job.

The competitive, and at times chaotic, nature of health care delivery requires that you understand these expectations well before you write your first resume or have your first interview. The goal of presenting this information is to ease the transition from student to entry-level radiographer.

Because the American Registry of Radiologic Technologists (ARRT) requires proof of continuing education for recertification, an entire chapter describes the process of acquiring continuing education credits in a manner that complies with ARRT regulations. Part III also provides information about the content specifications of and the requirements to take the ARRT's advanced-level examinations in mammography, computed tomography (CT), magnetic resonance imaging (MRI), cardiovascular-interventional radiography, quality management, sonography, vascular sonography, and bone densitometry.

Increasing numbers of radiographers are choosing to further their education by pursuing diagnostic medical sonography, nuclear medicine technology, and radiation therapy technology, or higher academic degrees. One of the most common questions asked by radiography students is about the location of these educational programs and degrees. Chapter 15 provides information about how to obtain the most current information relating to these important career goals. It also provides a sample letter that can be used to request information.

PRIORITIZING SUBJECTS AND SCHEDULING STUDY TIME
Determining the Length of Review

As you begin the exciting task of planning your review for the ARRT exam, you may wish to take a few moments to think about the study habits you will want to use. It is never too early to begin studying for the examination. Because you may take the exam immediately after graduation, you will probably want to begin your review very soon. If you are also using this text as a study guide throughout your radiography program, you are already becoming familiar with the topics and use of the book. Most radiography educators would prefer that their students begin a well-thought-out review approximately 6 months before taking the exam. Not all students will require that much time to prepare adequately; those who are better able to retain the material they have already learned may complete their review more quickly.

Another factor that can greatly influence how far in advance you should begin studying is the amount of time you have available. In all likelihood, you are beginning to review while still taking other courses in your educational program. Those courses must be given a high priority as you begin budgeting your time. It does little good to review for the certification exam only to find that you are hopelessly behind in another required course. In addition, you may have employment obligations that take up a considerable amount of time or marriage and family commitments that must not be allowed to falter while preparing for the exam.

Use the 6-month preparation time as a guide. If you need to begin reviewing earlier, then do so. However, begin reviewing at least 6 months before the exam. If you finish your review sooner, you can either stop reviewing or go back over the material in less detail one more time. If you wait too long to begin reviewing—only 4 or 5 months ahead of time—you may find yourself with insufficient time to go over the material thoroughly, consequently needing to postpone your examination date.

Before you begin budgeting your review time, consider the suggestions and encouragement provided by your instructors, who probably have several years' experience in working with students about to prepare for the exam. Their wisdom and suggestions should be taken seriously. If you follow the routine they suggest, as well as the guidelines contained in this review book, you should be more than adequately prepared to pass the exam. Remember, however, that managing the quality and quantity of your review time is ultimately up to you. Now that you have successfully reached this point in your educational program, you should use your energy, time, and skills wisely during these final months of preparation. Just as with running a race, finish strong.

Scheduling Your Study Time

Next, go through the process of planning your study time and evaluating your commitments so that you may set goals for reviewing all of the material. Browse through Chapters 2 through 6 and briefly refresh your memory about the topics. Are there large amounts of information that you can't seem to recall? Is there information there that you have never seen before? Does most of it look familiar, and is it fairly easy to recall?

Try answering a few of the exam questions after each section and sample some of the questions from the comprehensive exams in Chapter 7. Were you able to answer the questions easily? Do you feel confident about your answers, or were they educated guesses? How many did you get correct compared with the number you missed? Are there specific subject areas in which you feel particularly strong or weak? Will you need to spend more time studying one area than another? All of these questions need to be answered as you attempt to budget your review time.

Pause now to consider each of them carefully.

If you are already using some form of daily, weekly, or monthly calendar to plan your study time, you simply need to decide where within your study schedule to include your review. If you have not been using a calendar to budget your time, this is a great time to start. It is not necessary to purchase an expensive time planner. Most students use a calendar with squares large enough to write in times and planned activities. Figure 1-1 is an example of a simple calendar that is being used to budget time for current classes and for review.

The importance of writing study time on a calendar cannot be overemphasized. You are much more likely to adhere to a study schedule if you have thought it through, written it down, and posted it where you see it daily. It is highly recommended that once you plan your review time, you make a copy of your calendar and give it to your instructor. Educators can be powerful motivators by occasionally reminding a student of a written commitment to review. Filling in a calendar in this way is also a form of establishing a written contract with yourself. In so doing, you recognize that only *you* are ultimately responsible for covering the review material.

When setting up a review calendar, it is most important to be regular and consistent. Be certain that you are setting aside specific time to review on a regular basis. Don't save review for those times when you have nothing else to do. State your commitment in terms such as the following: "I will review physics every Thursday evening for the next 8 weeks for approximately 2 hours each time." This contract with yourself describes the activity, the time commitment, and the subject involved. Avoid entries such as, "I will study physics 4 times this month." There is little commitment to that statement, and the ambiguous goal it sets forth is not likely to be accomplished.

As an adult learner, you have probably developed an awareness of your strengths and weaknesses relative to time management and commitment to studies. Whatever your self-appraisal, the fact that you are using this book suggests that you are a successful student with the capability to manage your time effectively. You should now spend some

Sunday	Monday	Tuesday	Wednesday	Thursday	Friday	Saturday
				1 10:00 Advanced Positioning 1:00 Pathology Class	2 7:30 Clinical Education 7:00 Review: Radiation Biol	3 No Study Day
4 7:00 Review: Radiation Biol	5 7:30 Clinical Education	6 10:00 Advanced Positioning 1:00 Pathology Class	7 7:30 Clinical Education	8 10:00 Advanced Positioning 1:00 Pathology Class	9 7:30 Clinical Education 7:00 Review: Physics	10 No Study Day
11 7:00 Review: Physics	12 7:30 Clinical Education	13 10:00 Advanced Positioning 1:00 Pathology Class	14 7:30 Clinical Education	15 10:00 Advanced Positioning 1:00 Pathology Class	16 7:30 Clinical Education 7:00 Review: Quality Control	17 No Study Day
18 7:00 Review: Quality Control	19 7:30 Clinical Education	20 10:00 Advanced Positioning 1:00 Pathology Class	21 7:30 Clinical Education	22 10:00 Advanced Positioning 1:00 Pathology Class	23 7:30 Clinical Education 7:00 Review: Image Intensifier	24 No Study Day
25 7:00 Review: Image Intensifier	26 7:30 Clinical Education	27 10:00 Advanced Positioning 1:00 Pathology Class	28 7:30 Clinical Education	29 10:00 Advanced Positioning 1:00 Pathology Class	30 7:30 Clinical Education 7:00 Review: Skull Anatomy	

Figure 1-1 Calendar for scheduling study time.

time applying your scheduling and time management skills to the planning of your review.

Keep in mind that if you are allotting at least 6 months to prepare for the exam, you should have plenty of time to cover all of the material and take and review the exams in this book. Again, if you will do all of the expected regular studies and review, you should have little difficulty on the exam. It is hoped that by the time you take the exam, you will regard it as just another quiz.

Planning the Review Process

If one advances confidently in the direction of

their dreams and endeavors to lead a life which

they have imagined, they will meet with a success

unexpected in common hours.

HENRY DAVID THOREAU

It is now time to turn your attention to the actual review process. Look through the chapters containing the review

material if you have not already done so. In the following space provided, make a list of those subject areas in which you feel particularly strong or weak. By listing the subject areas in this way, you will be able to prioritize the material that you need to cover. A common mistake made by second-year radiography students who are preparing for the exam is reviewing the easiest material first. This is the opposite of what you should do.

Strong Subjects

_____

_____

_____

_____

_____

_____

Weak Subjects

_____

_____

_____

_____

_____

_____

Look again at the entries you made. Transfer these subjects to the spaces that follow, ranking the weakest subjects first. Then progress, in order, to the subjects in which you are strongest.

Priority of Studies, Weakest to Strongest

I need to study the following subjects in this order:

1. _____
2. _____
3. _____
4. _____
5. _____
6. _____
7. _____
8. _____
9. _____
10. _____
11. _____
12. _____

This second prioritizing exercise helps identify what you must study first. The rationale for studying more difficult content first is twofold: (1) the more difficult material is going to require more time, which you will have in greater supply at the beginning of the 6-month period than at the end; (2) if you have had serious difficulty with some of the subject areas and you study those first, you will have additional time to seek explanation from your instructors

and to read the material again. Save the subjects with which you are the most comfortable for last. They will require the least amount of study and should your time become limited, reviewing them quickly will not be as detrimental.

The time you spend now on planning a study calendar and prioritizing your study needs will pay great dividends as you begin the review process. Such planning should allow you to proceed more efficiently and dedicate more time to studying. If you are not filling in a calendar or prioritizing your study needs as you read this chapter, take the time right now to select a day and time when you will reread Chapter 1 and follow the directions for time management and prioritizing.

_____ I have completed my planner calendar and prioritized my subjects areas for study.

_____ I will complete my planner calendar and prioritize my subject areas for study on _____ (day), _____ (date) _____ at AM/PM.

Now that you have established your priorities or made an appointment with yourself to plan your calendar, you have set your first goal for reviewing and passing the certification exam. What is even more exciting is that you have taken the initial step toward your first radiography job or continued education. Be sure to congratulate yourself on accomplishing this task, and then finish reading this chapter.

Before discussing study habits, let's address concerns that many second-year students develop in response to feedback from others who have recently taken the exam. You may have been told to give little attention to certain subject areas because they did not appear on the exam. You may hear that the exam was particularly easy and may be advised not to worry about it. Although some may scoff at your calendar planning and the amount of time you choose to spend reviewing, others may feel that you are not spending enough time preparing. If you are in this position, all of the suggestions, hints, and guidelines may become confusing. Again, you should refer to the suggestions made by your instructors and those contained in this study guide.

Be aware that a person's ability to recall material from an examination can decrease significantly with the passage of time. Although individuals who are providing you with feedback about the exam have good intentions, the reliability of their memory of the exam items is questionable. In addition, because of the size of the item bank for the exam, the questions vary each time the exam is administered. Even if the individuals to whom you are speaking are accurate in their recall of the exam content, you will not be taking the same exam. Each radiography exam is different from the preceding exam.

Discussing the exam with your classmates immediately after you complete it may prove interesting. You will be surprised to find, even 2 to 3 hours after completing the examination, how rapidly recall of specific exam content has declined. In fact, many students taking the exam become anxious immediately after the exam as they hear others referring to questions that they can't recall. A bystander overhearing such a conversation could incorrectly conclude that each student had taken a different exam. When speaking with individuals who have taken the exam in recent months, you may also be surprised to hear comments such as, "There was almost no positioning on the exam" or "My goodness, it was all physics!" Actually, the radiography exam adheres to content specifications that are included in this chapter. In most cases, when individuals think one category had significantly more questions than another category that had almost none, it is a reflection of their command of the category's content or of their preparation for the exam.

Greet such advice with friendly skepticism. By choosing to ignore advice from even the most well-intentioned person who has recently taken the exam and following the study routine that you are planning under the guidance of your instructors and this book, you will guarantee that you are the one controlling the exam outcome and can be assured that you are undertaking the best preparation for the exam.

STUDY HABITS

Study habits mirror the individuality of each student. Some students prefer to study alone. They may read small sections of a chapter at a time, pausing to reflect on the content and taking additional notes if necessary, or they may recite the material aloud. Others choose to read over a section or an entire chapter many times, reviewing the material to facilitate their recall. Some students find it helpful to study in groups, taking turns quizzing one another and answering practice questions.

By now, you probably have formed your own set of effective study habits. In using this book to prepare for the exam, you should consider every suggestion that may improve your method of study. Do not, however, greatly alter study habits that have proven successful. Also, keep in mind that as you review for the exam, you should not be learning new material. By definition a *review* should be a revisiting of material that you have already learned and learned well.

A few reminders about study habits or study conditions are now in order. Remember to choose your most difficult subjects to study first. You have already listed these in the previous section. When you study, be sure you have time set aside during which you can be quiet with no interruptions. For some, soft music in the background can aid study, whereas others prefer silence. Other types of music, as well as television, simply interfere with concentration. Although you should be comfortable while studying, you should not be too comfortable. It is particularly important to remain upright.

Take regular but infrequent breaks. Be sure that you have adequate lighting and the room temperature is controllable and comfortable. Arrange the study conditions so that you can focus all of your attention on what you are doing. Regardless of the study method used, quiet concentration is of utmost importance. You may wish to reinforce your learning by reciting the material aloud—a practice that requires a fairly isolated and distraction-free study setting. In addition, study at the time of day when your mind is most alert. Some students prefer to study early in the morning, whereas others have found that they study better later in the afternoon or early evening. Cramming late at night or into the early hours of the morning is ineffective for most individuals. Besides, if review is a priority, you will want to assign it a place of importance in your schedule.

EXAM SPECIFICATIONS

Although the exam specifications for the ARRT radiography examination (Table 1-1) do not divulge specific questions, they do give the reader the outline from which the exam is constructed. In addition, the approximate number of questions in each category is listed to allow you to see the relative importance placed on the different subject areas.

You may wonder why these particular categories were selected for the exam and are weighted in this way. The ARRT periodically performs an extensive study called a *task analysis*. The resulting task inventory (see Chapter 13) for radiographers lists all of the specific skills required of an entry-level radiographer.

The skills in the task inventory should coincide with the terminal competencies of all approved educational programs. It is from this task inventory that the categories for the exam are constructed and the relative importance of each is weighted. The review of the major categories on the exam is covered in the next five chapters.

Analysis of Category Components

An approximate number of questions for each of the major subject areas is shown in the detailed listing that follows.* The percentages of subcategory content within the major areas are general guidelines and may vary to a certain extent with each exam administration.

Radiation Protection (30 questions)

A. Patient protection (12 questions)
  1. Biologic effects of radiation
    a. Dose-effect relationships
    b. Long-term effects
      (1) Cancer (including leukemia)
      (2) Cataracts
      (3) Life span shortening

---

*From *Examinee handbook,* St Paul, 2001, The American Registry of Radiologic Technologists.

    c. Somatic effects
      (1) Embryonic and fetal effects
      (2) Bone marrow
      (3) Thyroid
      (4) Skin
    d. Genetic effects
    e. Relative tissue radiosensitivities
  2. Minimization of patient exposure
    a. Exposure factors
      (1) kVp
      (2) mAs
      (3) Single-phase, three-phase, and high-frequency generators
    b. Shielding
      (1) Rationale for use
      (2) Types of protective devices
      (3) Placement of protective devices
    c. Beam restriction
      (1) Purpose of primary beam restriction
      (2) Effect on secondary (scatter) radiation
      (3) Types (collimators, cones, and aperture diaphragms)
    d. Filtration
      (1) Effect on skin and organ exposure
      (2) Effect on average beam energy
      (3) National Council on Radiation Protection (NCRP) recommendations
    e. Patient positioning
    f. Film, screens, and film-screen combinations
    g. Grids and air gap techniques
    h. Automatic exposure control
B. Personnel protection (9 questions)
  1. Sources of radiation exposure
    a. Exposure to primary x-ray beam
    b. Secondary radiation
    c. Scatter
    d. Leakage
  2. Basic methods of protection

    a. Time
    b. Distance
    c. Shielding
  3. NCRP recommendations for protective devices
  4. Special considerations
    a. Portable (mobile) units
    b. Fluoroscopy
      (1) Protective drapes
      (2) Protective Bucky slot cover
      (3) Cumulative timer
    c. Guidelines for fluoroscopy and portable units (NCRP, Code of Federal Regulations [CFR]-21)
C. Radiation exposure and monitoring (9 questions)
  1. Basic properties of radiation
  2. Units of measurement
    a. Rad (gray)
    b. Rem (sievert)
    c. Roentgen (coulomb/kg)
  3. Dosimeters (types, proper use)
  4. NCRP recommendations for personnel monitoring
    a. ALARA (as low as reasonably achievable—radiation exposure) and dose equivalent limits
    b. Evaluation of cumulative dose records
    c. Maintenance of cumulative dose records

Equipment Operation and Maintenance (30 questions)

A. Radiographic equipment (21 questions)
  1. Components of basic radiographic unit
    a. Operating console
    b. X-ray tube
      (1) Tube construction
      (2) Warm-up procedures
    c. Automatic exposure control
      (1) Radiation detectors
      (2) Backup timer
    d. Manual exposure control
    e. Beam restriction devices
  2. X-ray generator, transformers, and rectification system
    a. Basic principles
    b. Phase, pulse, and frequency
  3. Fluoroscopic unit
    a. Image intensifier
    b. Viewing systems
    c. Recording systems
    d. Automatic brightness control
  4. Digital/electronic imaging units
    a. Digital fluoroscopy
    b. Computed radiography
    c. Digital radiography
  5. Types of units
    a. Stationary
    b. Portable (mobile)
    c. Specialized or dedicated units

B. Evaluation of radiographic equipment and accessories (9 questions)
1. Equipment calibration
   a. kVp
   b. mA
   c. Time
2. Beam restriction
   a. Light field to radiation field alignment
   b. Central ray alignment
3. Recognition of malfunctions
4. Screens and cassettes
   a. Construction
   b. Handling
   c. Artifacts
   d. Maintenance
5. Shielding accessories (e.g., lead apron testing)

Image Production and Evaluation (50 questions)

A. Selection of technical factors (26 questions)
1. Density
   a. mAs
   b. kVp
   c. Distance
   d. Film-screen combinations
   e. Grids
   f. Filtration
   g. Beam restriction
   h. Anatomic and pathologic factors
   i. Anode heel effect
2. Contrast
   a. kVp
   b. Beam restriction
   c. Grids
   d. Filtration
   e. Anatomic and pathologic factors
3. Recorded detail
   a. Object-to-image distance (OID)
   b. Source-to-image distance (SID)
   c. Focal spot size
   d. Film-screen combinations
   e. Motion
4. Distortion
   a. Size
   b. Shape
5. Film, screen, and grid selection
   a. Film characteristics
      (1) Film contrast
      (2) Film latitude
      (3) Exposure latitude
   b. Film-screen combinations
      (1) Phosphor type
      (2) Relative screen speed
      (3) Single versus double film-screen system
   c. Conversion factors for grids

6. Technique charts
   a. Caliper measurement
   b. Fixed versus variable kVp
   c. Anatomic considerations
      (1) Tissue density
      (2) Part thickness
   d. Special considerations (e.g., casts, pathologic conditions, pediatrics, contrast media)
   e. Automatic exposure control
7. Manual versus automatic exposure
   a. Effects of changing exposure factors on radiographic quality
   b. Selection of detector
   c. Alignment of part to detector

B. Image processing and quality assurance (12 questions)
1. Film storage
   a. Pressure artifacts
   b. Fog (e.g., age, chemical, radiation, temperature, safelight)
2. Cassette loading
   a. Matching film and screens
   b. Film-handling artifacts (e.g., static, crinkle marks, fog)
3. Image identification
   a. Methods (e.g., photographic, radiographic)
   b. Legal considerations (e.g., patient data, examination data)
4. Automatic film processor
   a. Processor chemistry
   b. Components and systems
      (1) Transport
      (2) Replenishment
      (3) Temperature regulation
      (4) Recirculation
      (5) Dryer
   c. Maintenance
      (1) Start-up and shutdown procedure
      (2) Removal and cleaning of crossover assembly
      (3) Sensitometric monitoring
   d. System malfunction
      (1) Observable effects (e.g., artifacts, fluctuations in density, contrast, fog)
      (2) Possible causes of malfunctions (e.g., improper temperature, roller alignment, replenishment, water flow; contamination)
   e. Processing digital/electronic images

C. Evaluation of images (12 questions)
1. Criteria for diagnostic quality radiographs
   a. Density
   b. Contrast
   c. Recorded detail
   d. Distortion
   e. Artifacts
   f. Grid alignment

g. Proper demonstration of anatomic structure

h. Identification markers (e.g., anatomic, patient, date)

2. Causes of poor image quality

a. Technical factors (e.g., kVp, mAs, distance, filtration, film-screen combination, grids)

b. Positioning (e.g., OID, SID, tube-part-image receptor alignment)

c. Patient considerations (e.g., pathologic conditions, motion)

d. Processing (e.g., fog, contamination, temperature)

e. Artifacts

3. Improvement of suboptimal image

Radiographic Procedures (60 questions)

A. General procedural considerations (6 questions)

1. Explanation of procedures (e.g., removal of radiopaque objects, patient preparation)

2. Positioning terminology

3. Patient respiration and motion control

a. Instructions for examination

b. Effect on radiographic quality

c. Adapting to patient's cooperative ability (e.g., mA and time adjustments)

d. Immobilization devices and techniques

4. Technique and positioning variations (e.g., for trauma or age-specific patients, adapting to patient's body habitus)

B. Specific imaging procedures (54 questions, including positioning, technical factors, anatomy, physiology, and pathology)

1. Thorax (6 questions)

a. Chest

b. Ribs

c. Sternum

2. Abdomen and gastrointestinal (GI) studies (10 questions)

a. Abdomen

b. Esophagus

c. Swallowing dysfunction study

d. Upper GI series

e. Small bowel series

f. Barium enema: single-contrast

g. Barium enema: double-contrast

h. Operative cholangiography

i. T-tube cholangiography

j. Cholecystography

k. Endoscopic retrograde cholangiopancreatography (ERCP)

3. Urologic studies (4 questions)

a. Cystography

b. Cystourethrography

c. Intravenous (IV) urography

d. Retrograde urography

e. Retrograde urethrography

4. Extremities (16 questions)

a. Toes

b. Foot

c. Os calcis

d. Ankle

e. Tibia, fibula

f. Knee

g. Patella

h. Femur

i. Fingers

j. Hand

k. Wrist

l. Forearm

m. Elbow

n. Humerus

o. Shoulder

p. Scapula

q. Clavicle

r. Acromioclavicular joints

s. Bone survey

t. Long bone measurement

u. Bone age

v. Soft tissue/foreign bodies

5. Spine and pelvis (8 questions)

a. Cervical spine

b. Thoracic spine

c. Scoliosis series

d. Lumbosacral spine

e. Sacrum

f. Sacroiliac joints

g. Coccyx

h. Pelvis

i. Hip

6. Head and neck (7 questions)

a. Skull

b. Facial bones

c. Mandible

d. Zygomatic arch

e. Temporomandibular joints

f. Nasal bones

g. Orbit

h. Paranasal sinuses

i. Soft tissue neck

7. Other (3 questions)

a. Conventional tomography

b. Arthrography

c. Myelography

d. Venography

Patient Care (30 questions)

A. Legal and professional responsibilities (6 questions)

1. Scheduling and sequencing examinations

2. Legal aspects of radiology
   a. Request to perform examination
   b. Patient rights (e.g., bill of rights, advance directives)
   c. Professional liability
   d. Verification and obtaining of informed consent
3. Patient identification (e.g., wristband, questioning)
4. Verification of requested examination
   a. Clarification of terminology
   b. Comparison of request to clinical indications (e.g., left arm injured, but right arm requested)
   c. Evaluation of need for additional projections
   d. Modification of routine projection

B. Patient education, safety, and comfort (4 questions)
1. Communication with patients
   a. Review of patient history (e.g., age specific, pregnancy status)
   b. Explanation of current procedure
   c. Response to inquiries about other imaging procedures (basic concepts of mammography, CT, MRI, sonography, nuclear medicine)
2. Assessment of patient condition (e.g., motor control, severity of injury, support equipment)
3. Proper body mechanics for patient transfer
4. Patient privacy, safety, and comfort

C. Infection control and prevention (6 questions)
1. Disinfection and cleaning
   a. Medical asepsis
   b. Sterile technique
2. Centers for Disease Control and Prevention (CDC) isolation procedures
   a. Transmission of infection
      (1) Contact
      (2) Airborne
      (3) Droplet
   b. Types of precautions
      (1) Standard precautions (formerly *universal precautions*)
      (2) Transmission-based precautions (additional precautions)
3. Handling and disposal of biohazardous materials

D. Patient monitoring (9 questions)
1. Routine monitoring
   a. Equipment (e.g., stethoscope, sphygmomanometer)
   b. Vital signs (e.g., blood pressure, pulse, respiration, temperature)
   c. Physical signs and symptoms
   d. Documentation
2. Support equipment (e.g., IV tubes, chest tubes, catheters)
3. Common medical emergencies (e.g., seizure, cardiac arrest, loss of consciousness, bleeding)
4. Management of common medical emergencies (e.g., cardiopulmonary resuscitation, hemostasis)

E. Contrast media (5 questions)
1. Types and properties (e.g., iodinated, water soluble, barium, ionic versus nonionic)
2. Appropriateness of contrast medium to exam and patient condition (e.g., perforated bowel, patient age, patient weight)
3. Contraindications
4. Patient education
   a. Verification and obtaining of informed consent
   b. Instructions regarding preparation, diet, and medications
   c. Postexamination instructions
5. Administration
   a. Routes (e.g., parenteral, topical, oral)
   b. Supplies (e.g., enema kits, needles)
6. Complications/reactions
   a. Local effects (e.g., extravasation/infiltration, phlebitis)
   b. Systemic effects
      (1) Mild (e.g., flushing, hives, nausea)
      (2) Severe (e.g., shock, hypotension)
   c. Radiographer's response and documentation

CONVENTIONS USED IN THE ARRT RADIOGRAPHY EXAMINATION

The ARRT uses a list of conventions in an attempt to standardize nomenclature used in the examination. The conventions include terminology, abbreviations, and formats specific to the field of radiography. Many of the conventions listed are already quite familiar to you, so their exclusion from this chapter will have no effect on your understanding of the terminology. Other conventions involve terminology changes and additions or deletions with which you may be unfamiliar.

If as you examine the following list, you find that certain terms you have learned in your educational program are slightly different from those used in the exam, don't conclude that your educational program was in error. This list is an attempt to standardize terminology for the purpose of exam construction. The primary conventions follow.*

Absorbed dose measured in *rads*—energy absorbed per unit mass of the radiated material

Accumulated dose: 5(N-18) obsolete formula because of changes enacted by the NCRP

Anode-to-film distance replaced by *SID (FFD)*

Apron thickness for fluoroscopy minimum thickness—0.5-mm lead equivalent, according to NCRP Report #102

Automatic exposure control alternative term for *photo timing*

*From *Educator's handbook*, St Paul, 1994, The American Registry of Radiologic Technologists.

Automatic positive beam limitation referred to as *automatic collimation* on the exam

Blur alternative term for loss of *recorded detail;* used when describing the effect of patient motion on the radiograph; synonymous with *motion*

Caldwell referred to as *PA (Caldwell) projection* on the exam

Capitellum referred to as *capitulum* on the exam

Centigrade abbreviated as C

#21-CFR (1992) 21 Code of Federal Regulations; sections covered on the exam

Contrast (radiographic contrast) the visible differences between any two selected areas of density levels within the radiographic image

Cycles per second measured in *hertz (Hz)*

Definition referred to as *recorded detail* on the exam

Density (radiographic density) the degree of blackening or opacity of an area in a radiograph, which is caused by an accumulation of black, metallic silver following exposure and processing of a film; equals log incident light intensity divided by transmitted light intensity

Detail referred to as *recorded detail* on the exam

Distortion the misrepresentation of the size or shape of a structure recorded in a radiographic image

Dose equivalent measured in *rems*—absorbed dose multiplied by a quality factor that accounts for the difference in biologic effectiveness of different types of radiation; used in questions involving radiation protection and personnel monitoring

Dose equivalent limits used to refer to radiation exposure limits for radiation workers; replaces the term *maximum permissible dose (MPD)*

Edge gradient term not used

Entrance skin exposure alternative term for *skin exposure*

Exposure amount of radiation; measured in *roentgens (R)*

Exposure in air term found in questions involving use of ionization chambers

Exposure factors mA, time, kVp, and distance

Exposure latitude the range of exposure factors that will produce a diagnostic radiograph

Film refers to *unexposed* film; radiograph—*exposed* film

Film contrast the inherent ability of the film emulsion to react to radiation and record a range of densities

Film latitude the inherent ability of the film to record a long range of density levels on the radiograph

Film latitude, film contrast dependent on the sensitometric properties of the film and the processing conditions; directly determined from the characteristic H and D curve

Focal film distance, or FFD referred to as *SID (FFD)* on the exam

Geometric sharpness referred to as *geometrically recorded detail* on the exam

Grid radius referred to as *grid focusing distance* on the exam

Grid technique conversion factors because of variations in the many textbooks, answers are given in ranges

Impulse timers not included on the exam

Ionic contrast media included on the exam

Law referred to as *modified lateral (Law) projection* on the exam

LD 50/30 not included on the exam

Lead glove thickness minimum thickness—0.25 mm, according to NCRP Report #102

Long-scale contrast term that is used when the differences between densities are slight (low contrast) but the total number of densities is increased

Loss of recorded detail if caused by patient motion, referred to as *blur* or *motion;* if caused by a large focal spot or intensifying screens, referred to as *unsharpness* or *poor recorded detail*

Lower contrast, higher contrast alternative terms for *decreased contrast* and *increased contrast*

Manual processing not included on the exam

Mechanical timers not included on the exam

NCRP Report #91 included on the exam

NCRP Report #102 included on the exam; replaces *NCRP Report #33*

NCRP Report #105 included on the exam; replaces *NCRP Report #48*

Nonionic contrast media included on the exam

Nonscreen technique not included on the exam

Object-to-film distance, or OFD referred to as *OID (OFD)* on the exam

Par speed screens not included on the exam

Part-film distance referred to as *OID (OFD)* on the exam

Penumbra term not used on the exam; referred to as *motion, blur,* or *unsharpness of recorded detail* depending on the cause

Position (radiographic position) a specific body position such as supine or prone; refers only to the patient's physical position

Projection (radiographic projection) the path of the central ray

Radiograph *exposed* film

Recorded detail the sharpness of the structural lines in the radiographic image

Remnant radiation referred to as *exit radiation* or *image-forming radiation* on the exam

Rhese referred to as *parietoorbital oblique (Rhese) projection* on the exam

Scale of contrast the number of visible densities or the number of shades of gray

Screen speed expressed using film-screen system numbers rather than names

Sharpness referred to as *recorded detail* on the exam

Sharpness of detail referred to as *recorded detail* on the exam

Short-scale contrast   term used when differences among densities are considerable (high contrast) but the total number of densities is reduced

SI units   sieverts, grays, becquerels; not used on the exam

Size distortion (magnification)   the enlargement of the recorded image compared with the actual size of the structure

Shape distortion   the misrepresentation of the shape of the structure (elongated or foreshortened) of the recorded image compared with the actual shape of the structure

Spinning top test   only the principle of the test is covered on the exam

Stenvers   referred to as *posterior profile (Stenvers) projection* on the exam

Subject contrast   the difference in the amount of radiation transmitted by a particular part as a result of the different absorption characteristics of the tissues and structures that the part consists of

Submento vertical   referred to as *submento vertical (full basal) projection* on the exam

Target-to-film distance   referred to as *SID (FFD)* on the exam

Technique   referred to as *exposure factors* or *technical factors* on the exam

Valve tubes   not included on the exam

View (radiographic view)   refers to the body part as seen by the image recording medium such as film; used only in discussion of a radiograph or image

Waters   referred to as *parietoacanthial (Waters) projection* on the exam

Wavelength   term used only in reference to comparisons of x rays, gamma rays, and other forms of radiation; referred to as *average photon energy* in other situations

YOU'RE ON YOUR WAY!

Using this first chapter as a planner, you are now ready to work toward one of the crowning achievements of your educational career. Do all that is expected and use your time and talents wisely. Do not allow external distractions to send you off course. It is time to plan and work for what is yet to come—passing the radiography examination and moving on to the next phase of your career. You have numerous human and material resources available to assist you, one of which you are reading. Use them all and go for it!

Success is a journey, not a destination.

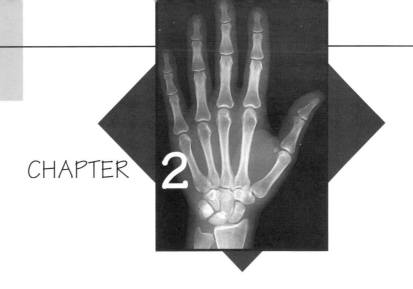

CHAPTER 2

Review of Radiation Protection

BASIC PRINCIPLES OF RADIATION PROTECTION

Responsibility for Radiation Protection

A. Radiographer is primarily responsible for protecting the patient from unnecessary exposure
  1. Best accomplished by avoiding repeat exposures
  2. Should use smallest amount of radiation that will produce a diagnostic radiograph
B. Radiologist and referring physician assume shared responsibility for radiation safety of the patient
  1. Best accomplished by consultation
  2. Should not order unnecessary exams
C. Safe use of radiation in diagnostic imaging to determine the extent of pathology or injury outweighs the risk involved

Ionizing Radiation

A. X-radiation exposure involves a transfer of energy through photon-tissue interactions
  1. Possesses the ability to remove electrons from atoms by a process called *ionization*
  2. Results of ionization in human cells
     a. Unstable atoms
     b. Free electrons
     c. Production of low-energy x rays
     d. Formation of new molecules harmful to the cell
     e. Cell damage may be exhibited as abnormal function or loss of function
B. General types of cell damage
  1. Somatic: damage to the cell itself
  2. Genetic: damage to cell's genetic code contained in the DNA

C. Sources of ionizing radiation
  1. Natural background radiation
     a. Contained in the environment
     b. Present since the formation of the universe
     c. Source of 82% of human exposure to radiation (annual effective dose equivalent per person of 295 mrem)
     d. Greatest source of exposure to humans: radon—55% (198 mrem annually)
     e. Second greatest source of natural background radiation: the human body—radioactive nuclides in tissues (carbon-14, potassium-40, strontium-90, and hydrogen-3)
     f. Terrestrial radiation from radioactive minerals such as uranium and radium; varies by geographic region
     g. Cosmic rays from the stars, partially shielded by earth's magnetic fields and atmosphere: annual absorbed dose equivalent of approximately 30 mrem; greater dose at higher elevations because of lower atmospheric shielding; dose equivalent during an airline flight—1 mrem per hour (depending on duration of flight and actual altitude achieved)
  2. Artificial radiation
     a. Made by humans
     b. Source of 18% of human exposure to radiation
     c. Annual effective dose equivalent of approximately 66 mrem: 54 mrem from diagnostic imaging procedures, 11 mrem from consumer products, 1 mrem from nuclear weapons testing and all other sources

PHOTON-TISSUE INTERACTIONS

A. Primary radiation: radiation exiting the x-ray tube

B. Exit radiation (image-producing radiation): x rays that emerge from the patient

C. Attenuation: absorption and scatter (loss of intensity) of the x-ray beam as it passes through the patient

D. Heterogeneous beam: x-ray beam that contains photons of many different energies

E. Most common photon-tissue interactions in diagnostic radiography: photoelectric and Compton's interactions

1. Photoelectric interaction (Figure 2-1)
   a. A photon absorption interaction
   b. Incoming x-ray photon strikes a *K*-shell electron
   c. Energy of x-ray photon is transferred to electron
   d. Electron is ejected from the *K* shell and is now called a *photoelectron*
   e. X-ray photon has deposited all of its energy and ceases to exist

f. Photon has been completely absorbed

g. Photoelectron may ionize or excite other atoms until it has deposited all of its energy

h. Hole in *K* shell is filled by electrons from outer shells, releasing energy that creates low-energy characteristic photons that are locally absorbed

i. Photoelectric interaction results in increased dose to the patient

j. Photoelectric interaction produces contrast in the radiograph because of the differential absorption of the incoming x-ray photons in the tissues

2. Compton's interaction (Figure 2-2)
   a. Also called *Compton's scattering* or *modified scattering*
   b. Incoming x-ray photon strikes a loosely bound, outer-shell electron
   c. Photon transfers part of its energy to the electron
   d. Electron is removed from orbit as a scattered electron, referred to as a *recoil electron*
   e. Ejected electrons may ionize other atoms or recombine with an ion needing an electron
   f. Photon scatters in another direction with less energy than before because of its encounter with the electron
   g. Scattered photon may interact with other outer-shell electrons, causing more ionization, or it may exit the patient
   h. Scattered photons emerging from the patient travel in very divergent paths
   i. Scattered photons may also be present in the room and expose the radiographer or radiologist

3. Coherent scatter (also known as *classical* or *Thompson's scatter*)
   a. Produced by low-energy x-ray photons

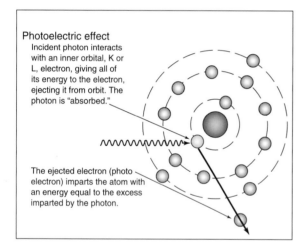

Photoelectric effect
Incident photon interacts with an inner orbital, K or L, electron, giving all of its energy to the electron, ejecting it from orbit. The photon is "absorbed."

The ejected electron (photo electron) imparts the atom with an energy equal to the excess imparted by the photon.

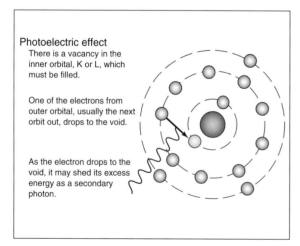

Photoelectric effect
There is a vacancy in the inner orbital, K or L, which must be filled.

One of the electrons from outer orbital, usually the next orbit out, drops to the void.

As the electron drops to the void, it may shed its excess energy as a secondary photon.

Figure 2-1 The photoelectric effect is responsible for total absorption of the incoming x-ray photon.

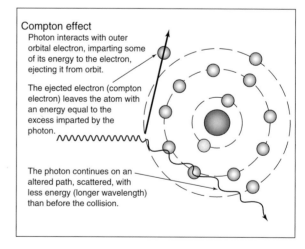

Compton effect
Photon interacts with outer orbital electron, imparting some of its energy to the electron, ejecting it from orbit.

The ejected electron (compton electron) leaves the atom with an energy equal to the excess imparted by the photon.

The photon continues on an altered path, scattered, with less energy (longer wavelength) than before the collision.

Figure 2-2 During the Compton effect, the incoming photon loses energy and changes its direction.

b. Atomic electrons are not removed but vibrate because of the deposition of energy from the photon

c. As the electrons vibrate, they emit energy equal to that of the original photon

d. This energy travels in a path slightly different from that of the original photon

e. Ionization has not occurred, although the photon has scattered

4. Pair production
   a. Does not occur in radiography
   b. Produced at photon energies above 1.02 million electron volts
   c. Involves an interaction between the incoming photon and the atomic nucleus

UNITS OF RADIATION MEASUREMENT

A. Traditional units used: roentgen, rad, rem, and curie

B. International System (SI) of Units used: coulomb/kilogram, gray, sievert, and becquerel
   1. Adopted by the International Commission on Radiation Units and Measurements (ICRU) in 1989
   2. Not yet in widespread use in the United States

C. Radiation exposure in air
   1. Measurement of positive and negative particles created when radiation ionizes the atoms in air (x and gamma rays only, up to 3 million electron volts, in-air measurements only)
   2. This is the amount of radiation that may be expected to strike an object placed near the source of radiation
   3. Traditional unit is the roentgen (R); 1 R equals 2.58×10^{-4} coulombs of positive and negative charges produced per kilogram of air
   4. SI unit is the coulomb/kilogram (C/kg)
   5. $1 \text{ R} = 2.58 \times 10^{-4} \text{ C/kg}$
   6. $1 \text{ C/kg} = \frac{1}{2.58} \times 10^{-4} \text{ R}$

D. Unit of absorbed dose
   1. The amount of energy absorbed by the object
   2. Absorption of the energy may result in biologic damage
   3. As the atomic number of the object increases, so does the absorbed dose
   4. Traditional unit is the rad (radiation absorbed dose)—1 rad is 100 ergs of energy deposited per gram of tissue
   5. SI unit is the gray
      a. 1 gray = 1 joule of energy deposited per kilogram of tissue
      b. 1 gray = 100 rads
      c. 1 rad = $\frac{1}{100}$ gray

E. Unit of absorbed dose equivalent
   1. Used to take into account the different biologic effects caused by different types of radiation

2. A quality factor (QF) is used to modify the absorbed dose amount to account for the greater damage inflicted by some forms of ionizing radiation (rad × QF = rem)
   a. QF takes into account linear energy transfer (LET), which is the amount of energy transferred by ionizing radiation per unit length of tissue traveled
   b. LET varies for different types of radiation
   c. High-ionization radiations such as alpha particles and neutrons have high LET (cause more biologic damage)
   d. Lower-ionization radiations such as x and gamma rays have lower LET (cause less biologic damage)
   e. QF for x and gamma rays = 1
   f. Therefore 100 rads of x rays = 100 rem
   g. QF for neutrons = 20
   h. Therefore 100 rads of neutrons = 2000 rem (a higher dose equivalency)
   i. For x and gamma rays with QF = 1: 1 roentgen = 1 rad = 1 rem (approximately)
3. Traditional unit is the rem—1 rem = $\frac{1}{100}$ sievert
4. SI unit is the sievert—1 sievert = 100 rem

F. Radioactivity
   1. Used to measure the quantity of radioactive material (is not used to measure the radiation emitted)
   2. Used primarily in nuclear medicine
   3. Traditional unit is the curie—1 curie = 3.7×10^{10} becquerel
   4. SI unit is the becquerel

ABSORBED DOSE EQUIVALENT LIMITS

A. Agencies involved in dose-response evaluations
   1. National Council on Radiation Protection and Measurements (NCRP)
   2. International Commission on Radiologic Protection (ICRP)
   3. Nuclear Regulatory Commission (NRC)
      a. Enforces standards at the federal level

B. Effective absorbed dose equivalent limit
   1. The upper boundary dose that can be absorbed, either in a single exposure or annually, with a negligible risk of somatic or genetic damage to the individual
   2. As low as reasonably achievable (ALARA)
      a. A concept of radiologic practice that encourages radiation users to adopt measures that keep the dose to the patient and themselves at minimal levels

C. Dose-response relationship
   1. Linear-nonthreshold relationship (Figure 2-3)

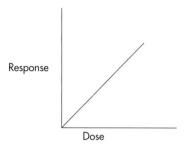

Figure 2-3 Linear-nonthreshold relationship.

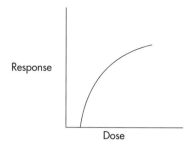

Figure 2-5 Nonlinear-threshold relationship.

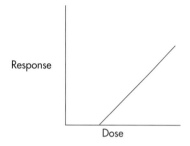

Figure 2-4 Linear-threshold relationship.

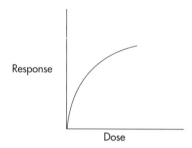

Figure 2-6 Nonlinear-nonthreshold relationship.

    a. States that no level of radiation can be considered completely safe and the degree of response is directly proportional to the amount of radiation received

2. Linear-threshold relationship (Figure 2-4)

    a. States that a dose of radiation exists below which a response does not occur; when that threshold is crossed, the response is directly proportional to the dose received (e.g., cataractogenesis does not occur at low levels of radiation exposure; therefore there is a threshold, or safe, dose)

3. Nonlinear-threshold relationship (Figure 2-5)

    a. States that a safe (threshold) dose of radiation exists that, when exceeded, results in responses that are not directly proportional to the dose received

4. Nonlinear-nonthreshold relationship (Figure 2-6)

    a. States that no level of radiation can be considered completely safe and the degree of the response is not directly proportional to the dose received

5. Stochastic effects: randomly occurring effects of radiation; the probability of such effects is proportional to the dose (increased dose equals increased probability, not severity, of effects)

6. Nonstochastic effects: effects that become more severe at high levels of radiation exposure and do not occur below a certain threshold dose

D. NCRP Report #91

1. Recommends balance between the risk and benefit of using radiation for diagnostic imaging

2. Recommends that somatic and genetic effects be kept to a minimum when using radiation for diagnostic imaging

3. Takes into account all human organs that may be vulnerable to radiation damage

4. Occupational exposure: annual effective absorbed dose equivalent limit for stochastic effects is 5 rem

5. Occupational exposure: annual effective absorbed dose equivalent limits for nonstochastic effects

    a. Lens of the eye: 15 rem

    b. All other organs: 50 rem

6. Occupational cumulative exposure = Age (in years) × 1 rem

7. Students (age 18 and younger): annual effective absorbed dose equivalent limit is 0.1 rem

8. Students (older than age 18): annual effective absorbed dose equivalent limit for skin, extremities, and eye lens is 5 rem

9. General public: annual effective absorbed dose equivalent limit for frequent exposure is 0.1 rem

10. General public: annual effective absorbed dose equivalent limit for infrequent exposure is 0.5 rem

11. General public: annual effective absorbed dose equivalent limit for extremities, skin, and eye lens is 5 rem

12. Embryo-fetus: total dose equivalent for gestation is 0.5 rem

13. Embryo-fetus: dose equivalent limit per month is 0.05 rem

    a. Level of negligible risk is 0.001 rem

REVIEW OF THE CELL

The Cell

A. Contains three main parts
1. Cell membrane
2. Cytoplasm
3. Nucleus

B. Cell membrane
1. Protects cell
2. Holds in water and nucleus
3. Allows water, nutrients, and waste products to pass into and out of the cell (i.e., is semipermeable)

C. Cytoplasm
1. Composed primarily of water
2. Conducts all cellular metabolism
3. Contains organelles
   a. Centrosomes: participate in cell division
   b. Ribosomes: synthesize protein
   c. Lysosomes: contain enzymes for intracellular digestive processes
   d. Mitochondria: produce energy
   e. Golgi apparatus: combines proteins with carbohydrates
   f. Endoplasmic reticulum: acts as a transportation system to move food and molecules within the cell

D. Nucleus
1. Contains deoxyribonucleic acid (DNA—the master molecule) and the nucleolus (with ribonucleic acid [RNA])
2. DNA controls cell division
3. DNA controls all cellular functions

E. Other cell components
1. Proteins: 15% of cell
2. Carbohydrates: 1% of cell
3. Lipids: 2% of cell
4. Nucleic acids: 1% of cell
5. Water: 80% of cell
6. Acids, bases, salts (electrolytes): 1% of cell

F. Cellular life cycle
1. Interphase
   a. Cell growth before mitosis
   b. Consists of three phases: G_1, S, G_2
   c. G_1: pre-DNA synthesis
   d. S: DNA synthesis
   e. G_2: post-DNA synthesis, preparation for mitosis
2. Mitosis: four phases
   a. Prophase
   b. Metaphase
   c. Anaphase
   d. Telophase: division complete—46 chromosomes in each new somatic cell
3. Meiosis
   a. Cell division of sperm or ovum (germ cells) that halves the number of chromosomes in each cell
   b. Sperm and ovum will unite to return the number of chromosomes in each cell of the new individual to 46

Biologic Effects of Ionizing Radiation

A. As LET of radiation increases, so does biologic damage

B. Relative biologic effectiveness (RBE): ability to produce biologic damage; varies with the LET

C. The QF used to calculate rem is a measure of the RBE of the radiation being used

D. Ionizing radiation may change a cell's molecular structure, affecting its ability to function properly

E. Somatic cell exposure may result in a disruption in the ability of the organism to function

F. Reproductive (germ) cell exposure may result in changes called *mutations* being passed on to the next generation

G. Basically, radiation striking a cell will deposit energy in either the DNA (a direct effect) or water in the cytoplasm (an indirect effect) if an interaction occurs

H. Most radiation passes through the body without interacting because matter is composed mainly of empty space

Direct Effect

A. Occurs when radiation transfers its energy directly to the DNA (the master molecule) or RNA

B. As these macromolecules are ionized, disruption in cell processes may occur

C. Some of this damage may be repaired

D. If sufficient damage to the DNA structure occurs, particularly to its nitrogenous bases, a mutation may result

E. Mutation: erroneous information passed to subsequent generations via cell division

F. Results of the direct effect
1. No effect: most common result of LET
2. Disruption of chemical bonds, causing alteration of cell structure and function
3. Cell death
4. Cell line death: death of the tissues or organs that would have been produced from continued cell division had a cell survived; particularly significant if it results in the failure of a major organ or system to develop
5. Faulty information passed on in the next cell division; possible results include mutations, cancer, and abnormal formations

Indirect Effect

A. Because water is the largest constituent of the cell, the probability that it will be struck by radiation is greater

B. Radiolysis of water: occurs as radiation energy is deposited in the water of the cell

C. The result of radiolysis is an ion pair in the cell: a positively charged water molecule (HOH^+) and a free electron

D. Several possibilities exist for chemical reactions at this point; most of them will create further instability in the cell

E. Should the two recombine, no damage occurs

F. Positive and negative water molecules may be formed and then break into smaller molecules such as free radicals

G. Free radicals: highly reactive ions that have an unpaired electron in the outer shell

H. Free radicals may cause biologic damage by transferring their excess energy to surrounding molecules or disrupting chemical reactions

I. Some free radicals may chemically combine to form hydrogen peroxide

J. Hydrogen peroxide is a poison that will cause further damage to the cell

K. The DNA in the cell may be affected by the free radicals or the hydrogen peroxide

L. Such action is called *indirect* because the DNA itself is not struck by the radiation

M. Indirect effect results from ionization or excitation of water molecules

N. Results of the indirect effect
1. No effect: most common response
2. Formation of free radicals
3. Formation of hydrogen peroxide (H_2O_2)

O. Most damage to the body occurs as a result of the indirect effect because most of the body is water and free radicals are readily mobile in water

Target Theory

A. Each cell has a master molecule that directs cell activities

B. Research indicates that DNA is the master molecule

C. If the DNA is the target of radiation damage and is inactivated, the cell will die

D. DNA may be inactivated by either direct or indirect effects

E. All photon-cell interactions occur by chance

F. It cannot be determined whether a given cell death was the result of direct or indirect effects

Radiosensitivity of Cells

A. Law of Bergonié and Tribondeau: cells are most sensitive to radiation when they are immature, undifferentiated, and rapidly dividing

B. If cells are more oxygenated, they are more susceptible to radiation damage (known as the *oxygen enhancement ratio*)

C. As cells mature and become specialized, they are less sensitive to radiation

D. Blood cells: whole body dose of 25 rads depresses blood count
1. Caused by irradiation of bone marrow
2. Lymphocytes are the most radiosensitive blood cells in the body
3. Stem cells in bone marrow are especially radiosensitive

E. Epithelial tissue: is highly radiosensitive, divides rapidly, lines body tissue

F. Muscle: is relatively insensitive because of high specialization and lack of cell division

G. Adult nerve tissue: requires very high doses (beyond medical levels) to cause damage, is very specialized, has no cell division, is relatively insensitive to radiation

H. Reproductive cells
1. Immature sperm cells: are very radiosensitive, divide rapidly, are unspecialized, require 10 rads or more (which is beyond most commonly used diagnostic levels) to increase chances of mutation
2. Ova in female fetus and child are very radiosensitive
3. Ova radiosensitivity decreases until near middle age, then increases again

Somatic Effects of Radiation

A. Somatic effects are evident in the organism being exposed

B. Doses causing these effects are much higher than the levels of radiation used in diagnostic radiography

C. Caused when a large dose of high-LET radiation is received by a large area of the body

D. Examples of early somatic effects of radiation
1. Hematopoietic syndrome: decreases total number of all blood cells; can result in death
2. Gastrointestinal (GI) syndrome: causes total disruption of GI tract structure and function and can result in death
3. Central nervous system syndrome: causes complete failure of nervous system and results in death

E. Examples of late somatic effects
1. Carcinogenesis: causes cancer
2. Cataractogenesis: causes cataracts to form; follows a nonlinear-threshold dose-response curve
3. Embryologic effects: most sensitive during the first trimester of gestation
4. Thyroid is a very radiosensitive organ
5. Shortening of life span: does not occur in modern radiation workers

Genetic Effects of Radiation

A. Caused by damage to DNA molecule, which is passed to the next generation

B. Follows a linear-nonthreshold dose-response curve; no such thing as a safe gonadal dose; any exposure can represent a genetic threat

C. Usually causes recessive mutations, so generally not manifested in the population

D. Doubling dose: amount of radiation that causes the number of mutations in a population to double (is approximately 50 to 250 rads for humans)

E. Genetic mutations will not cause defects that are not already present in the human race from other causes; that is, no defects are unique to radiation exposure

PATIENT EXPOSURE AND PROTECTION

The heart of radiation protection for the patient lies in the concept of ALARA. It is primarily the radiographer's responsibility to see that ALARA is in practice so that patients are properly protected. Taking adequate histories, communicating clearly, using proper immobilization, and conducting radiographic and fluoroscopic examinations calmly and professionally add to the level of safety your patients will encounter while under your care. This section reviews the many technical aspects of the radiographer's practice that contribute to ALARA for the patient.

Beam Limitation

Beam limitation protects the patient by limiting the area of the body and the volume of tissue being irradiated.

A. Collimator
1. Variable aperture device
2. Contains two sets of lead shutters placed at right angles to one another
3. Higher set of lead shutters is placed near the x-ray tube window to absorb off-stem (off-focus) radiation
4. Lower set of lead shutters is placed near the bottom of the collimator box to further restrict the beam as it exits
5. Accuracy of the collimator is subject to strict quality control standards (see Chapter 3)
6. Collimation should be no larger than the size of the image receptor being used
7. Collimators that automatically restrict the beam to the size of the cassette have a feature called *positive beam limitation (PBL)* (also called *automatic collimation*)
8. PBL responds when a cassette is placed in the tray containing sensors that measure its size

B. Cylinder cones
1. Metal cylinders that attach to the bottom of the collimator
2. Used to tightly restrict the beam to a small circle
3. Diameter of the far end of the cone determines field size
4. Cones may be extended an additional 10 to 12 inches by a telescoping action for even tighter restriction of the beam
5. Cones may be used for examination of the os calcis, various skull projections, and cone-down views of vertebral bodies
6. Use of cones results in a restriction of the x-ray beam by cutting out a major portion of the beam
7. mAs must always be increased when using cones to make up for the rays attenuated by the cone
8. Cylinder cones do *not* work by focusing the x-ray beam down the cone; x rays cannot be focused

C. Aperture diaphragm
1. A flat piece of lead with a circle or square opening in the middle
2. Placed as close to the x-ray tube window as possible
3. Has no moving parts

Filtration

A filter is placed in the x-ray beam to remove long wavelength (low-energy) x rays. Low-energy x rays contribute nothing to the diagnostic image but increase patient dose through the photoelectric effect. As low-energy rays are removed, the beam becomes "harder" (predominantly short wavelength, high energy).

A. Two types of filtration: inherent and added

B. Inherent filtration
1. Glass envelope of the x-ray tube
2. Insulating oil around the tube

C. Added filtration
1. Aluminum sheets placed in the path of the beam near the x-ray tube window

D. Total filtration
1. Equals inherent plus added filtration
2. Must equal 2.5-mm aluminum equivalent for x-ray tubes operating above 70 kVp

E. Half-value layer: amount of filtration that reduces the intensity of the x-ray beam to one half of its original value—measured, at least annually, by a qualified radiation physicist

F. Filtration is never adjusted by the radiographer; if it is suspected that the filtration has been altered, the x-ray tube must not be used until checked by a radiation physicist

Gonadal Shields

Gonadal shields are used to protect gonads from unnecessary radiation exposure. They should be used whenever they will not obstruct the area of clinical interest.

A. Gonadal shielding may reduce female gonad dose by up to 50%

B. Gonadal shielding may reduce male gonad dose by up to 95%

C. Proper collimation may also greatly reduce gonadal dose and should be used in conjunction with gonadal shields
D. Most commonly used gonadal shields
1. Flat contact shield: flat piece of lead or a lead apron placed over the gonads
2. Shadow shield: suspended from the x-ray tube housing and placed in the x-ray beam light field; requires no contact with the patient; especially useful during procedures requiring sterile technique

Exposure Factors

Exposure technique determines the quantity and quality of x rays striking the patient.
A. Use optimal kVp for the part being radiographed
B. Use the lowest possible mAs to reduce the amount of radiation striking the patient
C. Part being radiographed should be measured using calipers
D. A reliable technique chart should be consulted to determine the proper exposure factors to use
E. Use of automatic exposure controls (AEC) reduces the number of repeat radiographs

Film-Screen Combinations

Faster film-screen combinations reduce patient dose by allowing for the use of fewer x-ray photons (i.e., lower mAs) to produce a diagnostic image. The efficient conversion of x-ray energy to light energy through the intensifying screens provides the same information with far less radiation exposure to the patient.
A. Use fastest practical film-screen combination for imaging a particular body part
B. Take into account region of the body being irradiated, age of the patient, and requirements for recorded detail

Processing

The automatic processor should be a constant in the production of a visible radiographic image. Elimination of repeat films because of optimal processor performance reduces the dose to the patient and the radiographer.
A. Subject to strict quality control standards to eliminate retakes caused by processor malfunction (see Chapter 4)
B. Exercise care in loading and unloading cassettes
C. Prevent unnecessary exposure of film to safelight

Grids

A. Result in an increase in patient dose because increased mAs are required
B. May result in lower overall patient dose by eliminating retakes caused by poor radiographic contrast
C. Use appropriate type and ratio of grid for part being radiographed and exam being performed

Repeat Radiographs

A. Always result in an increase in radiation dose to the patient
B. Must be kept to a minimum
C. Should be tracked via a departmental discard film analysis
D. Reasons for repeat films should be documented
E. In-service education for areas of frequent repeat films should be conducted by qualified radiographers or radiologists

Technical Standards for Patient Protection

A. Minimum source-to-skin distance for portable radiography: at least 12 inches
B. Fluoroscopy
1. Use of intermittent fluoroscopy (as opposed to a constant beam-on condition)
2. Tight collimation of the beam
3. High kVp
4. Source-to-tabletop distance for fixed fluoroscopes: not less than 15 inches
5. Source-to-tabletop distance for portable fluoroscopes: not less than 12 inches (15 inches preferred)
6. Proper filtration of the beam
7. Fluoro timer that sounds alarm after 5 minutes (300 seconds) of beam-on time
8. Fluoro timer should *not* be reset before alarm goes off; fluoroscopist must be made aware of time that patient and those in the room were exposed
9. Limit dose at the tabletop to no more than 10 R per minute

Other Factors Relating to Patient Dose

A. Measuring patient dose
1. Skin entrance dose
2. Mean marrow dose (MMD): average dose to active bone marrow; indicator of somatic effects on population
B. Genetically significant dose (GSD): radiation dose that, if received by the entire population, would cause the same genetic injury as the total of doses received by the members actually being exposed; the average gonadal dose to the childbearing-age population
C. Pediatrics: children need to be carefully protected from unnecessary exposure; high-speed film-screen combinations should be used along with adequate immobilization
D. Pregnant patients
1. Consideration of the 10-day rule: abdominal radiographic examinations should be performed during the first 10 days following the onset of menstruation
2. The 10-day rule is based on the probability that most females are not pregnant during that time

3. The position of the American College of Radiology is that such exams should be carried out any time they are clinically indicated
4. Radiation doses to the embryo-fetus of less than 15 to 20 rads are considered low risk

RADIATION WORKER EXPOSURE AND PROTECTION

The ALARA concept applies to radiographers as well as to the general public. Many of the steps taken to reduce the dose to the patient will also reduce the dose to the radiographer. However, additional steps may be taken to further protect the radiation worker. Agency standards also apply to the equipment used by radiographers. This section reviews practices and standards used to protect occupationally exposed individuals. As you study the factors involved in protecting the radiation worker, reexamine the annual effective absorbed dose equivalent limits covered previously.

CARDINAL PRINCIPLES OF RADIATION PROTECTION

A. Time: amount of exposure is directly proportional to the duration of exposure
B. Distance: the most effective protection from ionizing radiation
   1. Dose is governed by the inverse square law
   2. The greater the distance from the radiation, the lower the dose
   3. Dose varies inversely according to the square of the distance
   4. Example: if the dose of radiation is 5 R at a distance of 3 feet, stepping back to a distance of 6 feet will cause the dose to decrease to 1.25 R
   5. The inverse square law should always be used during fluoroscopy in which close contact with the patient is not required and during mobile radiography and fluoroscopy
C. Shielding: lead-equivalent shielding will absorb most of the energy of the scatter radiation
   1. A lead apron of at least 0.5-mm lead equivalent should be worn while being exposed to scatter radiation; use of a thyroid shield of at least 0.5-mm lead equivalent should be used for fluoroscopy
   2. The radiographer should *never* be exposed to the primary beam
   3. If radiographer exposure to the primary beam is unavoidable, the exam should not be performed
   4. Family, nonradiology employees, or radiology personnel not routinely exposed should be the first choices to assist with immobilization of the patient for an exam when all other types of immobilization have proven inadequate

5. The radiographer should be the last person chosen to assist with immobilization during an exposure
6. Radiographers and student radiographers should not be viewed as quick and easy-to-use immobilization devices

Radiographer's Source of Radiation Exposure

A. Radiographer's source of radiation exposure is scatter radiation produced by Compton's interactions in the patient
B. Radiographer's greatest exposure occurs during fluoroscopy, portable radiography, and surgical radiography
C. Photons lose considerable energy after scattering
D. Scattered beam intensity is about $\frac{1}{1000}$ the intensity of the primary beam at a 90-degree angle at a distance of 1 meter from the patient
E. Beam collimation helps reduce the incidence of Compton's interactions, resulting in decreased scatter from the patient
F. The use of high-speed image receptors may further reduce the amount of scatter produced

Structural Protective Barriers

A. Primary protective barriers
   1. Consist of $\frac{1}{16}$-inch lead equivalent
   2. Located where the primary beam may strike the wall or floor
   3. If in the wall, extends from the floor to a height of 7 feet
B. Secondary protective barriers
   1. Consist of $\frac{1}{32}$-inch lead equivalent
   2. Extends from where primary protective barrier ends to the ceiling, with a $\frac{1}{2}$-inch overlap
   3. Located wherever leakage or scatter radiation may strike
   4. X-ray control booth is also a secondary protective barrier
      a. Exposure switch must have cord short enough that the radiographer has to be behind the secondary protective barrier to operate the switch
   5. Lead window by control booth is usually 1.5-mm lead equivalent
C. Determinants of barrier thickness
   1. Distance: between the source of radiation and the barrier
   2. Occupancy: who occupies a given area
      a. Uncontrolled area: general public areas such as waiting rooms and stairways; shielded to keep exposure under the annual effective absorbed dose equivalent limit for infrequent exposure of 0.5 rem

b. Controlled area: occupied by persons trained in radiation safety and wearing personnel monitoring devices; shielded to keep exposure under the annual effective absorbed dose equivalent limit of 5 rem
3. Workload: measured in mA minutes per week (mA min/wk); takes into account the volume and types of exams performed in the room
4. Use factor: amount of time the beam is on and directed at a particular barrier

X-Ray Tube Housing

A. X rays may leak through the housing during an exposure
B. The patient and all others present in the room must be protected from excess leakage radiation
C. Leakage radiation may not exceed 100 mR per hour at a distance of 1 meter from the housing

Fluoroscopic Equipment

A. Exposure switch: must be dead-man type
B. Protective curtain: minimum 0.25-mm lead equivalent
C. Bucky slot shield: minimum 0.25-mm lead equivalent
D. Five-minute timer

Portable Radiographic Equipment and Procedure

A. Exposure switch must be on a cord at least 6 feet long
B. Lead aprons should be worn if mobile barriers are unavailable
C. Least scatter is at a 90-degree angle from the patient
D. Apply the inverse square law to reduce dose by using exposure cord at full length
E. Radiographer should *never* hold the cassette in place for a portable exam because of possible exposure to the primary beam
F. Commercial cassette holders, pillows, sponges, and so forth should be used to hold the cassette in place

MONITORING RADIATION EXPOSURE
Monitoring Personnel Exposure

A. Film badges
  1. Consist of plastic case, film, and filters
  2. Plastic case holds film and filters and provides a clip for attaching to clothing
  3. Film used is similar to dental x-ray film and measures doses as low as 10 mrem
  4. Film is sensitive to extremes in temperature and humidity
  5. Filters made of aluminum and copper measure intensity of radiation striking the film badge
  6. Film badges are usually developed monthly, with readings returned to the institution via a film badge report
  7. Film badge report indicates wearer's name, ID number, and radiation dose (expressed in millirem for deep and shallow doses)
  8. Badge reading of *M* indicates exposure below film's sensitivity
B. Thermoluminescent dosimeters (TLDs)
  1. Use lithium fluoride crystals instead of film to record dose
  2. Crystals' electrons are excited by radiation exposure and release this energy on heating
  3. Energy released is visible light, which is measured by a photomultiplier tube
  4. Light is in direct proportion to the amount of radiation received
  5. TLDs are used mainly in ring badges worn by nuclear medicine technologists
  6. Sensitive to exposures as low as 5 mrem
  7. Relatively unaffected by temperature and humidity
  8. Can be worn for longer periods than film badges
  9. TLDs and equipment used to read them are expensive
C. Pocket ionization chambers
  1. Small cylinder, a few inches long, containing gas
  2. Gas is ionized as it is struck by radiation
  3. Small scale that reads from 0 to 200 mR is contained inside
  4. After exposure, chamber is held up to the light and viewed through one end
  5. Exposure scale may be seen, indicating exposure
  6. Limited to 200 mR so that dose above that level cannot be ascertained
  7. Must be reset to zero on a special charging device after each use
  8. Very expensive device that may break if dropped
  9. Not routinely used for personnel monitoring
D. Optically stimulated luminescence (OSL) dosimeters
  1. Use aluminum oxide to record dose
  2. Aluminum oxide layer is stimulated by a laser beam after wear period
  3. Energy released is visible light
  4. Light is in direct proportion to the amount of radiation received
  5. Sensitive to exposures as low as 1 mrem
  6. Relatively unaffected by temperature and humidity
  7. Can be worn up to 3 months at a time
  8. Can be reanalyzed multiple times, if necessary

Monitoring Area Exposure

A. Cutie pie meter (ionization chamber)
  1. Used to measure radiation in an area (e.g., a fluoroscopic room), storage areas for radioisotopes, doses

traveling through barriers, and patients who have radioactive sources within them
2. Not used to monitor short exposure times
3. Measures exposure rates as low as 1 mR per hour
4. Operates on a principle similar to that of the pocket ionization chamber, with internal gas being ionized when struck by radiation

B. Geiger-Mueller detector
1. Used to detect radioactive particles in nuclear medicine facilities
2. Sounds audible alarm when struck by radiation, with sound increasing as radiation becomes more intense
3. Meter reads in counts per minute

REVIEW QUESTIONS

Read the following paragraph. Determine the accuracy of each underlined word or phrase. Then refer to questions **1-8** following the paragraph, and choose the one statement that best corrects and completes the corresponding underlined item.

Background Radiation

Humans' exposure to ionizing radiation comes from two sources: natural background and artificial radiation. Natural background radiation represents (1) <u>18% to 20%</u> of this exposure. It includes cosmic radiation from space, exposure from radioactive minerals, and the human body itself. Of these, the greatest source is (2) <u>cosmic radiation.</u> (3) <u>Cosmic radiation tends to concentrate over land masses and in low-lying areas.</u> Of recent discovery, but (4) <u>in extremely low doses,</u> is exposure to radon gas. (5) <u>Also included in this category are gamma rays, which are naturally occurring in radioisotopes that are used in nuclear medicine procedures.</u> Artificial sources of radiation include (6) <u>fallout from nuclear weapons testing, consumer products, and medical and dental procedures not included in natural background radiation.</u> Exposure to artificial background radiation constitutes the other (7) <u>80% to 82%</u> of humans' exposure. Most exposure to artificial radiation comes from (8) <u>fallout from the nuclear bombings in World War II, which remains in the upper atmosphere.</u>

1. a. The underlined word or phrase is accurate as written
   b. 20% to 25%
   c. 82%
   d. 92%

2. a. The underlined word or phrase is accurate as written
   b. Radon gas
   c. Radioactive materials
   d. The body itself

3. a. The underlined word or phrase is accurate as written
   b. Cosmic radiation is present only in space
   c. Cosmic radiation is a source of exposure only to those who lie in the sun
   d. Cosmic radiation is greater at higher altitudes because of a thinner atmospheric shield

4. a. The underlined word or phrase is accurate as written
   b. In extremely high doses
   c. In doses proportional to other sources
   d. Exposure to radon gas is the greatest source of natural background radiation: 55% of annual background dose

5. a. The underlined word or phrase is accurate as written
   b. False; gamma rays are not used in nuclear medicine procedures
   c. False; gamma rays used in nuclear medicine procedures are part of artificial background radiation
   d. Statement should also include natural x rays

6. a. The underlined word or phrase is accurate as written
   b. Should also include radon
   c. Should also include microwave ovens
   d. There are no medical or dental procedures included in natural background radiation

7. a. The underlined word or phrase is accurate as written
   b. 18%
   c. 8%
   d. 75%

8. a. The underlined word or phrase is accurate as written
   b. Microwave ovens
   c. Smoke alarms
   d. Medical and dental procedures using ionizing radiation

Use the list that follows to answer questions **9-22.** Items may be used more than once. Choose the one best answer for each question.

- **A.** Photoelectric interaction
- **B.** Compton's interaction
- **C.** Coherent scatter
- **D.** Pair production
- **E.** Primary radiation; exit radiation

9. Occurs above 1.02 million electron volts D

10. Also called *incoherent scattering*

11. Radiation coming from the anode; radiation exiting the patient E

12. Photon-tissue interaction that never occurs in diagnostic radiography C

13. Responsible for producing contrast on the radiograph A

14. Produces scatter radiation that exits the patient and may fog the radiograph B

15. Produces scatter energy as a result of vibration of orbital electrons C

16. Radiation striking the patient; image-forming radiation E

17. Results in total absorption of incident photon A

18. Only photon-tissue interaction that does not result in ionization C

19. Only photon-tissue interaction that involves an incident photon and atomic nucleus

20. Photon-tissue interaction that primarily involves *K*-shell electrons

21. Photon-tissue interaction that primarily involves loosely bound outer-shell electrons

22. Results in the production of a photoelectron that is ejected from the atom

For questions **23-25,** determine whether the statement is correct or complete. If it is incorrect, choose the answer that best corrects it. If it is incomplete, choose the answer that is more complete and accurate. If the answer is accurate as written, choose *a.*

23. The unit of absorbed dose is the rad
- a. This statement is correct, complete, and accurate as written; no choices below correct or complete it
- b. The unit of absorbed dose is the rad, which equals rem times a quality factor
- c. The unit of absorbed dose is the rad, which is the amount of energy absorbed by an object
- d. The unit of absorbed dose is the rad, which equals 100 ergs of energy deposited per gram of tissue; the SI unit of absorbed dose is the gray

24. The unit of radiation exposure in air is the roentgen; this unit in the SI system is the coulomb/kilogram
- a. This statement is correct, complete, and accurate as written; no choices below correct or complete it
- b. The unit of radiation exposure in air is the roentgen; this unit in the SI system is the coulombs/kilogram; the roentgen is equal to 2.58×10^{-4} coulombs/kilogram
- c. The unit of radiation exposure in air is the roentgen; this unit in the SI system is the coulombs/kilogram; the roentgen is equal to 2.58×10^{-4} coulombs/kilogram; it measures positive and negative charges produced in air
- d. The unit of radiation exposure in air is the roentgen; this unit in the SI system is the coulombs/kilogram; the roentgen is equal to 2.58×10^{-4} coulombs/kilogram; it measures positive and negative charges produced in air; the roentgen measures the amount of radiation received by the patient during fluoroscopy and is reported on film badge reports

25. The unit of dose equivalency is the rem; it is calculated using the following equation: rads × quality factor; the SI unit of absorbed dose equivalent is the sievert
   a. This statement is correct, complete, and accurate as written; no choices below correct or complete it
   b. The unit of dose equivalency is the rem; it is calculated using the following equation: rads × quality factor; the SI unit of absorbed dose equivalent is the sievert; the rem takes into account different biologic effects caused by various sources of radiation; the rem is the unit reported on film badge reports
   c. The unit of dose equivalency is the rem; it is calculated using the following equation: rads × quality factor; the SI unit of absorbed dose equivalent is the sievert; the rem takes into account different biologic effects caused by various sources of radiation
   d. The unit of dose equivalency is the rem; it is calculated using the following equation: rads × quality factor; the SI unit of absorbed dose equivalent is the sievert; the rem is the unit reported on film badge reports

For each of the following questions, choose the single best answer.

26. The amount of energy deposited by radiation per unit length of tissue being traversed is:
   a. LET, which determines the use of a QF when calculating the absorbed dose equivalent
   b. Linear energy transfer
   c. Higher for wave radiations than for particulate radiations
   d. LET, which is expressed as a QF when calculating absorbed dose

27. The agency that publishes radiation protection standards based on scientific research is the:
   a. Nuclear Regulatory Commission (NRC)
   b. International Commission on Radiation Protection (ICRP)
   c. National Council on Radiation Protection and Measurements (NCRP)
   d. Bureau of Radiological Health (BRH)

28. The agency that enforces radiation protection standards at the federal level is the:
   a. Nuclear Regulatory Commission (NRC)
   b. International Commission on Radiation Protection (ICRP)
   c. National Council on Radiation Protection and Measurements (NCRP)
   d. Bureau of Radiological Health (BRH)

29. Effective absorbed dose equivalent limit is defined as the upper boundary dose that:
   a. Can be absorbed annually with a negligible risk of somatic or genetic damage to the individual
   b. Can be absorbed, either in a single exposure or annually, with no risk of damage to the individual
   c. Can be absorbed, either in a single exposure or annually, with no risk of somatic or genetic damage to the individual
   d. Can be absorbed, either in a single exposure or annually, with a negligible risk of somatic or genetic damage to the individual

30. *ALARA* is an acronym for:
   a. As long as reasonably achievable
   b. As little as reasonably achievable
   c. As long as radiologist allows
   d. A radiation protection concept that encourages radiation users to keep the dose to the patient as low as reasonably achievable

Use the list that follows to answer questions **31-36.** Items may be used more than once.

   A. Nonlinear-nonthreshold effect
   B. Linear-nonthreshold effect
   C. Linear-threshold effect
   D. Nonlinear-threshold effect
   E. Dose-response curves

31. Graphs that show the relationship between dose of radiation received and incidence of effects

32. Basis for all radiation protection standards

33. There is no safe level of radiation, and the response to the radiation is not directly proportional to the dose received

34. There is no safe level of radiation, and the response to the radiation is directly proportional to the dose received

35. There is a safe level of radiation for certain effects, and those effects are directly proportional to the dose received when the safe level is exceeded

36. There is a safe level of radiation for certain effects, and those effects are not directly proportional to the dose received when the safe level is exceeded

For each of the following questions, choose the single best answer.

37. Effects of radiation that occur randomly, with the probability of such effects being proportional to the dose received, are called:
   a. Dose-response curves
   b. Stochastic effects
   c. Genetic effects
   d. Somatic effects

38. Effects of radiation that, once the threshold dose is exceeded, become more severe at higher levels of exposure are called:
   a. Dose-response curves
   b. Nonstochastic effects
   c. Genetic effects
   d. Somatic effects

Use the list that follows to answer questions **39-46.** Items may be used more than once.

   A. 5 rem
   B. 0.1 rem
   C. 0.5 rem
   D. 0.05 rem
   E. 1 rem

39. Embryo-fetus dose equivalent limit per month

40. Occupational cumulative exposure = age in years multiplied by this dose

41. Annual occupational effective absorbed dose equivalent limit for stochastic effects

42. Annual effective absorbed dose equivalent limit for students age 18 or younger

43. Annual effective absorbed dose equivalent limit for general public—infrequent exposure

44. Embryo-fetus dose equivalent limit for gestation

45. Annual effective absorbed dose equivalent limit for general public—frequent exposure

46. Annual effective absorbed dose equivalent limit for general public for extremities, skin, and lens of eye

For each of the following questions, choose the single best answer.

47. The QF used in calculating rem takes into account:
   a. Duration of exposure
   b. Source of exposure
   c. LET
   d. b and c

48. LET and biologic damage are:
   a. Directly proportional
   b. Indirectly proportional
   c. Inversely proportional
   d. Unrelated

49. The ability of different types of radiation to produce the same biologic response in an organism is called:
   a. LET
   b. QF
   c. RBE
   d. Doubling dose

50. The phases of the cellular life cycle, in order, are:
   a. Prophase, metaphase, anaphase, telophase
   b. Interphase, prophase, metaphase, anaphase, telophase
   c. G_1, S, G_2, telophase
   d. Interphase (G_1, S, G_2), prophase, metaphase, anaphase, telophase

51. The process of cell division for germ cells is called:
   a. Mitosis
   b. Spermatogenesis
   c. Organogenesis
   d. Meiosis

Use the list that follows to answer questions **52-60.** Items may be used more than once.

   A. Indirect effect
   B. Target theory
   C. Direct effect
   D. Doubling dose
   E. Mutations

52. Occurs when radiation transfers its energy to DNA

53. States each cell has a master molecule that directs all cellular activities and that, if inactivated, will result in cellular death

54. Amount of radiation required to increase the number of mutations in a population by a factor of 2

55. Occurs when radiation transfers its energy to the cellular cytoplasm

56. Induces radiolysis

57. Changes in genetic code passed on to next generation

58. Responsible for producing free radicals

59. Occurs when master molecule is struck by radiation

60. Poisons the cell with H_2O_2

For the following question, choose the single best answer.

61. Most of the damage to a cell occurs as a result of:
   a. Direct effect
   b. Mutations
   c. Law of Bergonié and Tribondeau
   d. Indirect effect

Read the following paragraph. Determine the accuracy of each underlined word or phrase. Then refer to questions **62-68** following the paragraph, and choose the one statement that best corrects and completes the corresponding underlined item.

Cell Radiosensitivity

Cell radiosensitivity is described by the (62) Law of Bergonié and Tribondeau, (63) which states that cells are most sensitive to radiation when they are specialized and rapidly dividing. Furthermore, it is believed that (64) cells are more radiosensitive when fully oxygenated. (65) Blood count can be depressed with a whole body dose of 25 rem, which is a result of irradiation of the bone marrow. However, (66) the most radiosensitive cells in the body are lymphocytes. Other highly radiosensitive cells are (67) epithelial cells, nerve cells, sperm, and muscle cells. Less radiosensitive are (68) ova in women of reproductive age.

62. a. The underlined word or phrase is accurate as written
   b. There is no law used by these scientists
   c. Bergonié and Tribondeau described dose-response relationships
   d. This law is really just a hypothesis

63. a. The underlined word or phrase is accurate as written
   b. False; cells are equally radiosensitive at all times
   c. False; cells are most sensitive to radiation when they are nonspecialized, immature, and dividing rapidly
   d. False; cells are most radiosensitive when they are specialized, mature, and rapidly dividing

64. a. The underlined word or phrase is accurate as written
   b. False; cells are most radiosensitive when least oxygenated, such as when they are cells in a patient who has cancer
   c. False; cells are equally radiosensitive regardless of their state of oxygenation
   d. False; cells are most radiosensitive when in a state of high concentration of CO_2

65. a. The underlined word or phrase is accurate as written
   b. False; the whole body dose required is at least 125 rem
   c. False; the dose does not need to be whole body
   d. False; the absorbed dose is expressed in rads

66. a. The underlined word or phrase is accurate as written
   b. False; the most radiosensitive cells are sperm
   c. False; the most radiosensitive cells are ova
   d. False; the most radiosensitive cells are epithelial cells

67. a. The underlined word or phrase is accurate as written
   b. False; nerve cells and muscle cells are relatively insensitive
   c. False; epithelial cells and sperm are relatively insensitive, especially in adults
   d. False; all cells listed are relatively insensitive to radiation effects

68. a. The underlined word or phrase is accurate as written
   b. False; this is why gonadal shielding must be used whenever possible
   c. False; this is why the 10-day rule must be followed, as recommended by the ACR
   d. False; this is a common misconception

Read the following paragraph. Determine the accuracy of each underlined word or phrase. Then refer to questions **69-71** following the paragraph, and choose the one statement that best corrects and completes the corresponding underlined item.

Somatic and Genetic Effects of Radiation

Most somatic effects occur at (69) <u>doses delivered during diagnostic radiography.</u> Somatic effects manifest themselves (70) <u>in the person who has been irradiated.</u> Examples of early somatic effects are GI syndrome, central nervous system syndrome, and hematopoietic syndrome. Examples of late somatic effects are (71) <u>carcinogenesis, genetic effects, embryologic effects, and shortening of the life span.</u>

69. a. The underlined word or phrase is accurate as written
   b. True; this is the basis for radiation protection standards; this is a more complete answer than choice *a*
   c. False; most somatic effects occur at doses far beyond diagnostic levels
   d. False; all somatic effects occur during radiation therapy, which is what makes it so effective

70. a. The underlined word or phrase is accurate as written
   b. False; because the gonads are also irradiated, these effects are also manifested in the next generation
   c. False; genetic effects are manifested in the person irradiated if it is a child
   d. False; both somatic and genetic effects are manifested in the person being irradiated; this is the basis for the formation of mutations

71. a. The underlined word or phrase is accurate as written
   b. False; genetic effects are considered early somatic effects
   c. False; these are all the result of genetic effects because the genes in the cells have been irradiated, causing the effect
   d. False; genetic effects are not considered somatic effects

For each of the following questions, choose the single best answer.

72. Methods of limiting the area of the patient being irradiated include the use of:
   a. Cylinder cones
   b. Aperture diaphragms
   c. Collimators
   d. All of the above

73. Which of the following statements concerning gonadal shields is (are) accurate?
   a. Gonadal shields should be used on all patients
   b. Gonadal shields may reduce male gonad dose by up to 50%
   c. Gonadal shields may reduce female gonad dose by up to 95%
   d. All of the above

74. Which of the following sets of exposure factors would result in the lowest dose to the patient?
   a. High mAs, low kVp, 400-speed film-screen combination
   b. Low mAs, high kVp, 400-speed film-screen combination
   c. Low mAs, high kVp, small focal spot, 100-speed film-screen combination
   d. Low mAs, high kVp, large focal spot, 100-speed film-screen combination

75. Which of the following is used as part of an effort to observe the ALARA concept?
   a. More than one but not all of the following
   b. Collimation
   c. High-speed film-screen combinations
   d. Grids

76. The cardinal rules of radiation protection include:
   a. Collimation, gonadal shielding, no repeats
   b. Collimation, short exposure time, no repeats
   c. Shielding, distance, time
   d. Time, distance, collimation

Use the list that follows to answer questions **77-85**. Items may be used more than once.

    A. TLD
    B. Film badge
    C. Pocket ionization chamber
    D. Cutie pie monitor
    E. Geiger-Mueller detector

77. Used to survey an area for radiation detection and measurement

78. Accurate as low as 10 mrem

79. Includes filters for measurement of radiation energy

80. Measures in-air exposures from 0 to 200 mR

81. Detection device that sounds an alarm to indicate the presence of radioactivity

82. Accurate as low as 5 mrem

83. Must be reset for each use

84. May be used up to 3 months at a time

85. Sensitive to extremes in environment

For each of the following questions, choose the single best answer.

86. An indicator of somatic effects on the population as a whole (which is the average dose to active bone marrow) is called:
    a. GSD
    b. ALARA
    c. MMD
    d. MPD

87. The radiation dose that would cause the same genetic injury to the population as the sum of doses received by individuals actually being exposed is called:
    a. GSD
    b. ALARA
    c. MMD
    d. MPD

88. The timer used in fluoroscopy:
    a. Must be 3 minutes
    b. Should always be reset before the alarm sounds so that it will not annoy the radiologist
    c. Sounds an alarm after 3 minutes
    d. Is used to alert the fluoroscopist after 5 minutes of fluoroscopy have elapsed

89. The most effective protection against radiation exposure for the radiographer is:
    a. Lead aprons
    b. Lead gloves
    c. Lead glasses
    d. Distance

90. If the dose of scatter radiation in fluoroscopy to the radiographer is 10 mR at a distance of 2 feet from the table, where should the radiographer stand to reduce the dose to 2.5 mR?
    a. 8 feet from the table
    b. 4 feet from the table
    c. At the foot of the table
    d. Directly behind the fluoroscopist

91. Lead aprons used in fluoroscopy must be at least:
    a. 0.5-mm lead
    b. 0.25-mm lead
    c. 0.1-mm lead
    d. 0.25-mm lead equivalent

92. Which of the following statements is true concerning the holding of patients for radiographic examinations?
    a. May be performed routinely to obtain a diagnostic examination
    b. Should be done only when absolutely necessary and then the holding should be done by a competent radiographer so that a repeat will not be needed
    c. Should be done only when absolutely necessary and then the holding should be done by a non-pregnant member of the patient's family
    d. May be performed using a student radiographer to hold because students are not exposed as often as staff radiographers

93. The factor(s) that must be considered when designing structural shielding for a radiology room or department include:
    a. Use factor
    b. Occupancy
    c. Workload
    d. All of the above

94. The lowest intensity of scatter radiation from the patient is located:
    a. At the head of the table
    b. At a 90-degree angle from the patient
    c. At a 180-degree angle from the patient
    d. At the foot of the table

95. A film badge reading of *M* means:
   a. A dose below 10 mrem has been received
   b. A maximum dose has been received
   c. A mean (average) dose has been received
   d. Much radiation has been received

96. A reading of 200 mR with a pocket ionization chamber means:
   a. 200 roentgens have been received
   b. At least 200 milliroentgens have been received
   c. 200 millirads have been received
   d. 2 roentgens have been received

97. Which of the following doses are considered low risk to the embryo-fetus?
   a. <100 rads
   b. <50 rads
   c. <15 to 20 rads
   d. <30 rads

98. Minimum source-to-skin distance for mobile radiography must be at least:
   a. 15 inches
   b. 12 inches
   c. 36 inches
   d. 55 inches

99. Positive beam limitation is also known as:
   a. Use of collimators
   b. Beam limitation used for all exams
   c. Use of beam restrictors
   d. Automatic collimation

100. Filtration should be adjusted by the radiographer:
   a. To "harden" the x-ray beam
   b. To remove the soft rays from the x-ray beam
   c. To exercise radiation protection
   d. Never

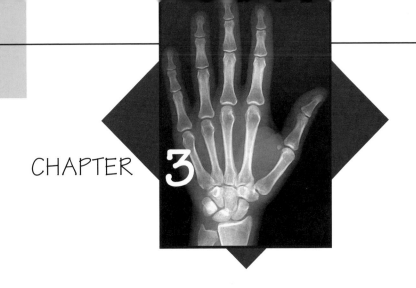

CHAPTER **3**

Review of Equipment Operation and Maintenance

BASIC PHYSICS TERMINOLOGY

Matter   has form or shape and occupies space

Mass   the amount of matter in an object; generally considered the same as weight

Energy   the ability to do work

Potential energy   the energy of position

Kinetic energy   the energy of motion

Chemical energy   energy from a chemical reaction

Electrical energy   a result of the movement of electrons

Thermal energy   heat energy resulting from the movement of atoms or molecules

Nuclear energy   energy from the nucleus of an atom

Electromagnetic energy   energy that is emitted and transferred through matter

Ionizing radiation   electromagnetic radiation that is able to remove an electron from an atom

Ionization   the removal of an electron from an atom

MEASUREMENT STANDARDS

Length   meter

Mass   kilogram

Time   second

SI system   meter, kilogram, second

MKS system   meter, kilogram, second

CGS system   centimeter, gram, second

British system   foot, pound, second

Velocity (speed)   how fast an object is moving

Acceleration   the rate of change of speed per unit of time

Work   force applied on an object over a distance

Power   the rate of doing work (measured in watts)

ATOMIC STRUCTURE

Atomic nucleus   contains protons (positive charges) and neutrons (no charge); contains most of the mass of an atom

Atomic mass   number of protons plus number of neutrons; represented by the letter A

Electron shells   contain orbital electrons (negative charges); electron shells represented by the letters K, L, M, N, O, P, and Q; in a stable atom the number of electrons and protons is equal

Atomic number of an atom   equals the number of protons in the nucleus; represented by the letter Z; the atomic number determines the chemical element; all chemical elements are represented in the periodic table of the elements

Isotopes   atoms with the same number of protons but with a different number of neutrons

Electron-binding energy   force that holds electrons in orbit around the nucleus

Octet rule   the outer shell of an atom may not contain more than eight electrons

Particulate radiation   alpha particles (helium nucleus: two protons and two neutrons); beta particles (electron-like particles emitted from the nucleus of a radioactive atom)

CHARACTERISTICS OF ELECTROMAGNETIC RADIATION

Photon the smallest amount of any type of electromagnetic radiation; also considered a bundle of energy called a *quantum*; travels at the speed of light; travels in waves in a straight path

Sine waves waves of electromagnetic radiation; wave height is called *amplitude*; distance between the peaks of the waves is called *wavelength*; as photon wavelength decreases, photon energy increases

Frequency number of wavelengths passing a given point per unit time; measured in hertz (Hz)

Speed of travel electromagnetic radiation travels at the speed of light (186,000 miles per second); travel at the speed of light is constant regardless of wavelength or frequency; wavelength and frequency of electromagnetic radiation are inversely proportional

Gamma rays electromagnetic rays produced in the nucleus of radioactive atoms; x rays and gamma rays differ only in their origin

Wave-particle duality the concept that although x-ray photons exist as waves, they exhibit properties of particles

Attenuation partial absorption of the energy of an x-ray beam as it traverses an object

Inverse square law law that governs the intensity of x radiation; states that the intensity of the x-ray beam is inversely proportional to the square of the distance between the source of the x rays and the object

Law of conservation of matter matter cannot be created or destroyed

Law of conservation of energy energy cannot be created or destroyed

PRINCIPLES OF ELECTRICITY AND MAGNETISM

Electrostatics stationary electric charges (static electricity)

Electrification movement of electrons between objects

Laws of electrostatics unlike charges attract, and like charges repel; electrostatic charges reside on the outer surface of a conductor and are concentrated at the area of greatest curvature; only negative charges move; inverse square law

Methods of electrification friction, contact, and induction

Conductor material that allows the free flow of electrons

Insulator object that prohibits the flow of electrons

Electric current the movement of electrons along a conductor or pathway (electric circuit); measured in amperes

Electromotive force (EMF) measured in volts; the force with which electrons move in an electric circuit

Electrodynamics electric charges in motion

Semiconductor material that may act as an insulator or conductor under different conditions

Electric resistance measured in ohms

Ohm's law voltage in the circuit is equal to the current times resistance

Electric circuits path along which electrons flow; may be wired as series circuits or parallel circuits

Alternating current (AC) electric circuit in which the current of electrons oscillates back and forth

Direct current (DC) unidirectional flow of electrons in an electric conductor

Sine wave representation of electron flow as alternating current

Magnetic field energy field surrounding an electric charge in motion; can magnetize a ferromagnetic material, such as iron, if the material is placed in the magnetic field

Magnetic poles every magnet has a north pole and a south pole

Laws of magnetics like poles repel, and unlike poles attract; the force of attraction between poles is governed by the inverse square law

Electromagnetism movement of electrons in a conductor produces a magnetic field around the conductor; a coiled conductor (i.e., a wire), through which an electric current is flowing, will have overlapping magnetic fields

Solenoid stacks of wire coil through which electric current flows, creating overlapping force field lines; a magnetic field is concentrated through the center of the coil

Electromagnet a solenoid with an iron core that concentrates the magnetic field

Electromagnetic induction the process of causing an electric current to flow in a conductor when it is placed within the force field of another conductor; two types of electromagnetic induction are self-induction and mutual induction

Self-induction opposing voltage created in a conductor by passing alternating current through it

Mutual induction inducing current flow in a secondary coil by varying the current flow through a primary coil

Electric generator device that converts mechanical energy to electrical energy; usual output of an electric generator is alternating current

Single-phase, two-pulse alternating current the simplest type of current; voltage (and accompanying current) flows as a sine wave (~); voltage begins at zero, peaks at full value at the crest of the wave, returns to zero, reverses, and again peaks on the inverse portion of the cycle at the trough

Three-phase alternating current special wiring patterns (wye, star, delta) used to create voltage waveforms that are placed 120 degrees out of phase with one another; these voltage waveforms are called *three-phase*; three-phase waveforms may have 6 pulses per cycle or 12 pulses per cycle; three-phase, six-pulse waveforms contain 360 pulses per second; three-phase, twelve-pulse contain 720 pulses per second; high-frequency generators produce high-frequency electricity (thousands of hertz)

Electric motor   device that converts electric to mechanical energy

Transformer   changes electric voltage and current into higher or lower values; transformer operates on the principle of mutual induction, so it requires alternating current

Step-up transformer   transformer that increases voltage from the primary to the secondary coil and decreases current in the same proportion; a step-up transformer has more turns in the secondary than in the primary coil; a step-up transformer is used in the x-ray circuit to increase voltage to the kilovoltage level for x-ray production

Step-down transformer   transformer that decreases voltage from the primary to the secondary coil and increases current in the same proportion; a step-down transformer has more turns in the primary than in the secondary coil; a step-down transformer is used in the filament portion of the x-ray circuit to increase current flow to the cathode

Autotransformer   a transformer that contains an iron core and a single winding of wire; an autotransformer is used in the x-ray circuit to provide a small increase in voltage before the step-up transformer; it is at the autotransformer that the kVp settings are made

Rectification   the process of changing alternating current to direct current

Line voltage compensation   x-ray circuit depends on a constant source of power; power coming into radiology department may vary; line voltage compensator keeps incoming voltage adjusted to proper value; usually operates automatically, but may be manually adjusted on older equipment

CONDITIONS NECESSARY FOR THE PRODUCTION OF X RAYS

A. Source of electrons
B. Acceleration of electrons
C. Sudden stoppage of electrons against target material

Equipment Used in the Production of X Rays

A. Autotransformer (Figure 3-1)
  1. Also known as a *variable transformer*
  2. Provides for the variation of voltage flowing in the x-ray circuit
  3. Single coil of wire with an iron core
  4. Source for selecting kVp
  5. Operates on the principle of self-induction
     a. Single winding of wire incorporates both the primary and secondary coils of the transformer
  6. Primary turns (primary taps) are fed 220 V from the radiology department's incoming line
  7. Secondary turns (secondary taps) are selected by the radiographer using the kVp select control
  8. Voltage is then stepped up or stepped down by only a small amount and sent to the primary side of the high-voltage step-up transformer
  9. The high-voltage step-up transformer then boosts the voltage to the kVp that was selected

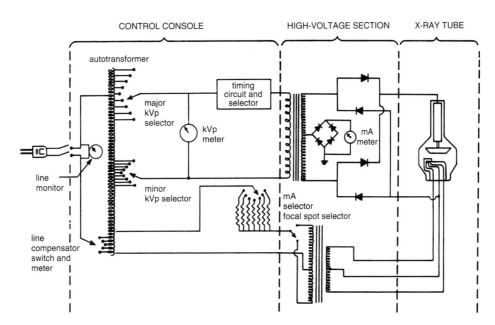

Figure 3-1   Simplified electric circuit diagram for x-ray machine.

B. Prereading voltmeter
1. The voltmeter in the x-ray circuit indicates the voltage that is selected
2. Called *prereading* because it indicates the kilovoltage that will be flowing through the tube once the exposure is made
3. Placed in the circuit between the autotransformer and the high-voltage transformer

C. Timer
1. Used to regulate the duration of the x-ray exposure
2. Wired in the circuit between the autotransformer and the high-voltage transformer
3. Synchronous timer
    a. Operates from a motor with a frequency of 60 Hz turning at 60 rotations per second
    b. Timer increments are in multiples of $\frac{1}{60}$ (i.e., $\frac{1}{30}$, $\frac{1}{15}$, etc.)
    c. Shortest time possible is $\frac{1}{60}$ second
4. Impulse timer
    a. Counts voltage pulses
    b. In a 60-Hz, full-wave rectified current, there are 120 pulses per second; therefore a setting of one pulse would yield an exposure of $\frac{1}{120}$ second
5. mAs timer
    a. Provides the safest tube current in the shortest time possible
    b. Measures total tube current
    c. Located after the secondary coil of the high-voltage transformer
6. Electronic timer
    a. Microprocessor controlled
    b. Contained in most radiographic equipment
    c. Allows exposure times as low as 1 ms (0.001 s)
7. Automatic exposure control (AEC)
    a. Is used to provide consistency of radiographic quality
    b. Relies on excellent positioning skills and extensive knowledge of surface and internal anatomy because the part being radiographed must be accurately positioned over ionization sensors
    c. Consists of a flat ionization chamber that is located between the patient and the image receptor; some units use a photomultiplier tube placed behind the film that senses the brightness produced by a fluorescent screen
    d. As radiation passes through the ionization chamber, it ionizes the gas contained inside
    e. The level of ionization is directly proportional to the density that will appear on the film
    f. When a predetermined level of ionization is reached (allowing time for a sufficient amount of radiation to pass through to strike the film), an electronic switch terminates the exposure

    g. Backup timer must be set to terminate the exposure in the event of a malfunction
    h. Backup timer protects the patient from overexposure and the x-ray tube from overheating
    i. Minimum response time: shortest time possible with an AEC because of the time it takes to operate
    j. Shortest time with an AEC is 1 ms (0.001 s)
8. Falling load generator
    a. Modern generator that takes advantage of extremely short time capabilities and tube heat loading potential
    b. Radiographer sets mAs and kVp
    c. Falling load generator calculates the most efficient method of obtaining the required mAs
    d. X-ray tube current starts at highest level possible for first portion of the exposure
    e. When the tube's maximum heat load has been reached for that mA, the generator drops the mA to the next lower level that the tube can handle
    f. The exposure continues at progressively lower levels of mA for the shortest times possible until the desired mAs has been reached
    g. Falling load generator always uses the shortest times possible to obtain a given mAs
    h. Disadvantages: exams in which long exposure times are used (e.g., breathing techniques for lateral thoracic spine); rapid sequence exposures in which heat buildup in the tube may cause exposure times to increase

D. Step-up transformer (high-voltage transformer)
1. Consists of primary coils and secondary coils
2. Requires alternating current to operate
3. Primary coil receives voltage from the autotransformer
4. Operates on principle of mutual induction
    a. Force field surrounding a wire with electricity flowing through it will induce (cause) electricity to flow in a second wire placed within the force field
5. Voltage in the primary coil is boosted to the kilovoltage level (thousands of volts) in the secondary coil
    a. Number of turns of wire in the primary coil compared with the number of wire turns in the secondary coil is called the *turns ratio*
    b. Turns ratio determines how much the voltage is stepped up
    c. The greater the turns ratio, the higher the resulting kilovoltage
    d. Voltage is being induced in the secondary coil, which has many more wire turns than the primary coil
6. The turns ratio may be 500 to 1000, depending on the machine
7. Voltage is varied at the autotransformer
8. Turns ratio in the step-up transformer is not varied

E. Rectifier
1. X-ray tube requires direct current to operate properly
2. Rectifier changes alternating current coming from the step-up transformer to direct current
3. Rectifiers are solid-state semiconductor diodes
   a. Consist of silicon-based n-type and p-type semiconductors
4. Located between the step-up transformer and the x-ray tube
5. Unit with four diodes provides full-wave rectification for single-phase generator
   a. Full-wave rectification produces pulsating direct current
   b. Resultant waveform contains two pulses per cycle (120 pulses per second)
   c. Uses both portions of rectified alternating current
   d. Results in 100% ripple, with voltage dropping to zero 120 times per second
   e. X-ray production ceases 120 times per second
6. Unit with 6 or 12 diodes provides full-wave rectification for three-phase equipment
   a. Because three-phase current is used, voltage never drops to zero during the exposure
   b. Voltage ripple for three-phase, six-pulse is approximately 13%; therefore the voltage actually used is about 87% of the kVp set
   c. Voltage ripple for three-phase, twelve-pulse is approximately 4%; therefore the voltage actually used is about 96% of the kVp set
   d. Voltage ripple for high-frequency generators is approximately 1%; therefore the voltage actually used is about 99% of the kVp set
   e. High-frequency units result in lower patient dose
   f. Three-phase, full-wave rectified waveforms produce higher average photon energy (35% higher for three-phase, six-pulse; 41% higher for three-phase, twelve-pulse)
   g. Three-phase and high-frequency units produce 12% to 16% more x rays than single-phase units
   h. kVp values used with single-phase equipment may be decreased 12% to 16% when performing the same exam on three-phase or high-frequency equipment
F. Milliammeter (mA meter)
1. Measures tube current in milliamperes
2. Wired between the rectifier and x-ray tube
G. mA control (filament circuit)
1. Regulates the number of electrons available at the filament to produce x rays
2. Voltage is provided by tapping windings of the autotransformer and varying the voltage being sent to the step-down transformer
   a. Step-down transformer reduces voltage and increases current in response to the use of variable

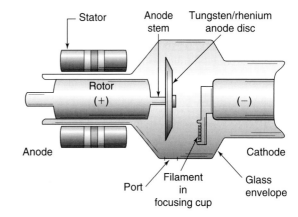

Figure 3-2 Structure of a typical x-ray tube, including the major operational parts.

resistors (rheostats) manipulated by the radiographer via the mA stations on the control panel
   b. Resultant high current is sent on to heat the filament
   c. A filament ammeter may also be connected
H. X-ray tube (Figure 3-2)
1. Cathode assembly: negative electrode in the x-ray tube
   a. Contains two filaments: a small and a large
   b. Filaments are made of tungsten (because of its high melting point); a small amount of thorium is added to reduce vaporization and to prolong tube life
   c. Filaments are heated slightly when the x-ray machine is turned on; no electrons are ejected at this low level of heating
   d. During x-ray exposure, one filament will be heated to a level that causes electrons to be "boiled off" in preparation for x-ray production (which is known as *thermionic emission*)
   e. Over time, filaments will vaporize and coat the inner surface of the x-ray tube with tungsten, leading to tube failure
   f. Cathode assembly also includes the focusing cup
   g. Focusing cup surrounds the filaments on three sides
   h. Focusing cup has negative charge applied, which tends to concentrate electrons boiling off the filaments into a narrower stream and repels them toward the anode
   i. Electron concentration keeps the electrons aimed at a smaller area of the anode
   j. Some x-ray tubes use the focusing cup as an electronic grid that can turn the current on and off rapidly, allowing for very short and precise exposure times, such as those needed for rapid serial exposures (referred to as a *grid-controlled tube*)

2. Anode: positive electrode in the x-ray tube
   a. Consists of a metal target made of a tungsten-rhenium alloy (because of its high melting point and high atomic number) embedded in a disk (or base) of molybdenum with a motor to rotate the target
   b. Must be able to tolerate extremely high levels of heat produced during x-ray production
   c. Anode rotates from 3,300 to 10,000 rpm, depending on tube design
   d. Rotation is achieved by the use of an induction motor located outside of the x-ray tube, which turns a rotor located inside the x-ray tube; the target is attached at the end of the rotor
   e. Rotation of the target allows greater heat dissipation
   f. Rotation of the target is stopped by a braking action provided by the induction motor
   g. The x-ray machine should never be shut off immediately after an exposure until the target has stopped rotating
   h. Without the braking action the target may spin for up to 30 minutes, causing great strain on the bearings
   i. Electrons strike the target on the focal track (sometimes called the *focal spot*)
   j. Focal track is beveled, producing the target angle
   k. The target angle allows for a larger actual focal spot (area bombarded by electrons) while producing a smaller effective focal spot (the area seen by the image receptor)
   l. The larger the actual focal spot, the greater the heat capacity; the smaller the effective focal spot, the greater the radiographic image sharpness
   m. This effect is called the *line-focus principle*
   n. Target angle may be from 7 to 20 degrees, depending on tube design
   o. The exposure switch should be activated in one continuous motion, activating the rotor and then the exposure button
   p. The equipment allows the rotor to come up to speed before making the exposure
   q. The radiographer does not control this by activating the rotor and waiting to press the exposure button
   r. Activating the rotor and allowing it to operate by itself results only in unnecessary heating of the filament and wear on the induction motor, shortening tube life
3. Glass envelope with window
   a. Cathode and target are inside the glass envelope; some models use a partial metal envelope
   b. Glass envelope also contains a vacuum so that electrons from the filament do not collide with atoms of gas
   c. Tube window: thinner section of glass envelope that allows x rays to escape
4. Tube housing: encases x-ray tube
   a. Made of aluminum with lead lining
   b. Supports and protects the tube, restricts leakage radiation during exposure, and provides electrical insulation
   c. Also contains oil in which the x-ray tube is immersed to assist with cooling and additional electrical insulation

X-Ray Production

A. Overview of the x-ray production circuit
   1. The x-ray machine is turned on, and a small amount of current is sent to the filament to warm it and ready it for much higher current
   2. Radiographer takes equipment through warm-up exposures to further warm the filament and the anode
   3. Radiographer chooses exposure factors on control console for the examination to be performed
   4. Electricity coming into the radiology department is adjusted by the line voltage compensator in the x-ray equipment to maintain it at a constant level
   5. When making the exposure, the radiographer presses the rotor switch and exposure switch in one continuous motion
   6. The induction motor begins spinning the anode as the filament gets hotter
   7. When the exposure switch is closed, the voltage selected by the mA control flows from the autotransformer, through the variable resistors, and into the step-down transformer in the filament circuit
   8. The filament heats considerably, boils off electrons (thermionic emission), and creates a space charge or electron cloud around the filament
   9. At the same time, the alternating current and voltage selected by choosing taps off the autotransformer are sent to the primary coils of the high-voltage step-up transformer, where they are boosted to kilovoltage levels
   10. After leaving the secondary coils of the step-up transformer, the voltage and alternating current are sent through the rectifier, which changes the alternating current to pulsating direct current
   11. The kilovoltage creates a high potential difference in the x-ray circuit, making the anode less negative (relatively positive) and the cathode highly negative
   12. This high potential difference causes the electrons to move at very high speed (approximately half the speed of light) from the cathode to the anode

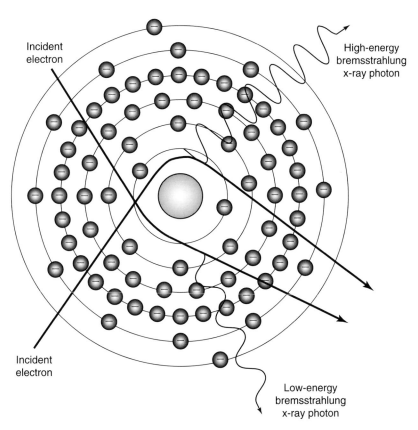

Incident electron

Incident electron

High-energy bremsstrahlung x-ray photon

Low-energy bremsstrahlung x-ray photon

Figure 3-3 A bremsstrahlung interaction.

13. The collision of these projectile electrons with the atoms of the target material causes a conversion of the electrons' kinetic energy (100%) to heat (99.8%) and x rays (0.2%)

14. Heat is produced by the projectile electrons striking the outer-shell electrons of the target material and placing them in an excited state, which causes them to emit infrared radiation

15. The production of x rays comes from two interactions with the anode

B. Brems radiation (Figure 3-3)

1. A projectile electron misses outer-shell electrons in the target and moves in close to the nucleus

2. Because the nucleus is positive and the electron is negative, it is slowed or braked

3. The reduction in kinetic energy causes the electron to slow and release energy as an x-ray photon

4. The resultant x rays are called *bremsstrahlung (braking) x rays* because they are produced by the slowing (braking) of projectile electrons

5. At diagnostic levels, most x rays produced are from brems interaction

C. Characteristic radiation (Figure 3-4)

1. A projectile electron collides with an inner-shell electron of a target atom

2. It removes that electron from orbit and ionizes the atom

3. A hole exists in the inner shell from the vacated electron

4. An electron from the next outer shell falls in to fill the hole

5. As the electron falls in, energy is given off in the form of an x-ray photon

6. This creates a hole in its shell of origin, and an electron from the next outer shell falls in to fill this vacancy; this continues until the atom is once again stable

7. Each time an electron falls in to fill a hole, an x-ray photon is given off

8. Each x-ray photon has a specific energy, equal to the difference in the binding energies of the two shells involved

9. Only x rays produced at the *K* shell are of sufficient energy to be used in diagnostic radiography

10. Because the x rays possess energy characteristic of the specific binding energies of the atom involved, they are called *characteristic x rays*

11. Characteristic x rays are produced at kVp levels above 70 but only in small numbers

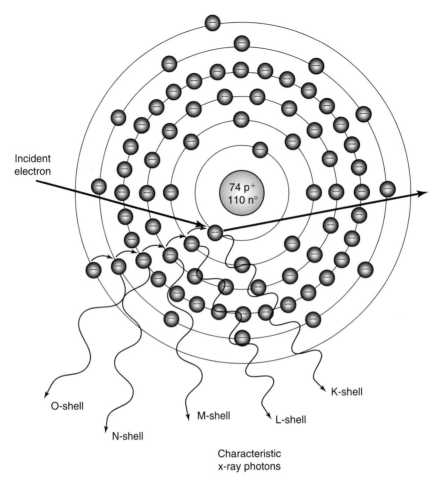

Incident electron

74 p+
110 n°

O-shell

N-shell

M-shell

L-shell

K-shell

Characteristic
x-ray photons

Figure 3-4 A characteristic interaction.

D. X-ray properties
1. Part of the electromagnetic radiation spectrum
2. Highly penetrating
3. Invisible
4. Travel at the speed of light (186,000 miles per second)
5. Travel in straight lines as waves
   a. Wavelength of diagnostic x rays: 0.1 to 0.5 angstroms (1 angstrom = 10^{-10} m, which is one ten-billionth of a meter)
   b. Wavelength is the distance from crest to crest or trough to trough, or the distance covered by one complete sine wave
   c. Frequency: the number of waves passing a given point per unit time
   d. Wavelength and frequency are inversely proportional to one another: as wavelength increases, frequency decreases; as wavelength decreases, frequency increases
   e. Short-wavelength rays are more penetrating; long-wavelength rays are less penetrating

6. Invisible to the human eye
7. Have characteristics of waves and particles; travel in bundles or packets of energy called *photons*
8. Exist in a wide range of wavelengths and energies
9. Can ionize matter and gases
10. Cause fluorescence of phosphors
11. Unable to be focused by a lens
12. Liberate a small amount of heat when passing through matter
13. Electrically neutral
14. Affect photographic film
15. Cause biologic and chemical changes through excitation and ionization
16. Scatter and produce secondary radiation

E. X-ray beam characteristics
1. Because x rays are produced by brems and characteristic interactions at the anode, the resultant x-ray beam contains many different energies
2. An x-ray beam containing many different energies is called *heterogeneous*
3. The collection of all different energies (wavelengths) of x rays is called the *x-ray emission spectrum*

4. Discrete x-ray spectrum: produced by characteristic x rays because energies involved are specific to the target atom and are predictable
5. Continuous x-ray spectrum: produced by brems radiation because these energies are all different (from the peak electron energy down to zero energy)
6. The maximum energy an x-ray photon can have corresponds to the kVp that was used
7. Beam characteristics may be altered by using filtration
   a. A filter is usually a sheet of aluminum placed in the primary beam just as it exits the x-ray tube and before it reaches the collimator
   b. The tube housing and glass envelope of the x-ray tube offer inherent filtration
   c. Total beam filtration equals inherent filtration plus added filtration
   d. Total filtration must be at least 2.5-mm aluminum equivalent
   e. Filtration removes the low-energy (long-wavelength, "soft") rays from the beam
   f. The result of removing soft rays from the beam is lower patient skin dose
   g. Other types of filters that directly affect the radiographic image may be used: trough filter, wedge filter
   h. Half-value layer: amount of filtration that reduces the beam intensity by half

F. Heat units and their management
1. Heat units are a calculation of the total heat produced during an x-ray exposure
2. Heat units are calculated using the following equations:
   a. Single-phase, full-wave rectified equipment: kVp × mAs
   b. Three-phase, six-pulse, full-wave rectified equipment: kVp × mAs × 1.35 (Remember: this equipment produces x-ray photons with 35% higher average photon energy)
   c. Three-phase, twelve-pulse, full-wave rectified equipment: kVp × mAs × 1.41 (Remember: this equipment produces x-ray photons with 41% higher average photon energy)
3. X-ray tubes and tube housing are constructed to absorb certain levels of heat units
4. Most modern x-ray equipment will automatically prevent the user from making an exposure capable of producing too much heat in the tube; this is indicated on some control panels by the warning "technique overload," a red light, or a failure to get a green light indicating that the anode is ready
5. Most modern x-ray equipment will prevent overloading the tube during a series of exposures and will not allow additional exposures until the tube has cooled sufficiently

OTHER IMAGING EQUIPMENT

A. Fluoroscopy
1. Provides dynamic visualization of internal structures
2. Consists of x-ray table to hold patient, with x-ray tube inside the table, the spot film device and image intensifier (image receptors) over the table, and a television monitor nearby
3. Spot film device allows the fluoroscopist to take radiographs of an area of interest as it is seen "live" on the television monitor
4. X-ray tube and image receptor(s) are connected with a C arm to keep them the appropriate distance apart, regardless of the movement of the equipment
5. X-ray tube for fluoroscopy is operated at 3 to 5 mA
6. Regulation of kVp and mA for fluoroscopy depends on the part being examined
7. kVp and mA determine the brightness level of the fluoroscopic image
   a. kVp and mA are automatically adjusted during fluoroscopy by a process known as *automatic brightness control* (also called *automatic brightness stabilization* and *automatic gain control*)
8. Visible image on the television monitor is a result of image intensification
9. Image-intensifier tube converts x-ray energy into visible light and then into an electronic signal that is displayed as an image on the monitor
10. Image-intensifier tube consists of the following parts (Figure 3-5):
    a. Input phosphor: made of cesium iodide; receives exit rays from the patient and converts them into visible light
    b. Visible light from input phosphor strikes the photocathode, a thin layer next to the input phosphor; it releases electrons in amounts directly proportional to the visible light striking it
    c. The electrons are concentrated and directed toward the other end of the image-intensifier tube (anode) by a series of electrostatic lenses and by 25 kVp applied through the tube
    d. The electrons strike the output phosphor, which is made of zinc cadmium sulfide
    e. The energy of the electrons is converted by the phosphors to visible light in amounts 50 to 75 times greater than at the photocathode
    f. This increase in brightness caused by acceleration of the electrons is called *flux gain*
    g. The output phosphor is smaller than the input phosphor, resulting in an increase in brightness called *minification gain*
    h. Total brightness gain is a product of minification gain and flux gain

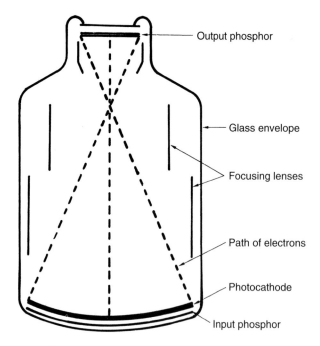

— Output phosphor

— Glass envelope

— Focusing lenses

— Path of electrons

— Photocathode

— Input phosphor

Figure 3-5 Diagram of the image intensifier.

    i. Total brightness gain ranges from 5,000 to 20,000 and decreases as the tube ages

    j. Varying the voltage flowing through the image-intensifier tube taps different areas of the input phosphor/photocathode assembly for electrons; this results in the ability to perform magnification during fluoroscopy

    k. Magnification is possible only with dual-focus or trifocus tubes, which result in increased patient dose

  11. Viewing and recording of fluoroscopic image

    a. Image may be sent to various viewing and recording devices using an image distributor located near the output phosphor

    b. The signal may be sent to a television monitor for viewing by using vidicon or Plumbicon video tubes or a charge-coupled device (CCD)

    c. The signal may be sent to a spot film camera (using 70-, 90-, or 105-mm cut film) or a cine camera (using 16- or 35-mm movie film)

    d. The fluoroscopic image may be recorded on videotape or magnetic disk

    e. Digital fluoroscopy provides computerized images from the output phosphor

B. Mobile radiographic and fluoroscopic units

  1. Mobile fluoroscopic units are usually called *C arms*

    a. X-ray tube and image intensifier are located on opposite cusps of the C, just as in stationary fluoroscopy

    b. Mobile units are capable of providing stationary images (using a last-image-hold feature) and dynamic images

    c. They are used primarily in surgery

  2. Mobile radiographic units allow radiography to be performed under almost any conditions

    a. Most common mobile radiographic units operate on nickel-cadmium batteries

    b. These batteries are recharged by plugging the machine into an outlet

    c. The batteries provide power to propel the unit and operate the x-ray tube

    d. Capacitor-discharge mobile radiographic units must be plugged into a wall outlet for power, and the capacitor must be charged before each exposure

    e. High-frequency mobile radiographic units are smaller and provide ripple-free output

C. Other dedicated x-ray equipment

  1. Mammographic equipment

  2. Head (skull) units

  3. Tomographic equipment

D. Maintenance of x-ray–producing equipment

  1. Quality assurance: a complete program in a radiology department that addresses all aspects of quality, including customer service, image interpretation, accuracy of diagnosis, and distribution of radiologist's reports

  2. Quality control: a program that specifically addresses the safe and reliable operation of equipment

  3. Quality control program is required by the Joint Commission on Accreditation of Healthcare Organizations (JCAHO)

  4. Responsibility for quality control program: radiologist, radiology manager, radiation physicist, quality control technologist (sometimes a separate position; sometimes a staff radiographer's duties; depends on the size of the radiology department)

  5. Many different tests may be performed as part of a quality control program

  6. Filtration-beam quality: tested using a digital dosimeter; half-value layer measurement is required

  7. Collimator: must be accurate to within 2% of the source-to-image distance (SID)

  8. Effective focal spot size: measured using the slit camera, pinhole camera, or star test pattern; should be within 50% of size stated in equipment specifications

  9. kVp: tested using the Wisconsin kVp test cassette or similar devices or using a digital kVp meter; kVp must be accurate to within 4 kVp of that chosen

  10. Timer

    a. Timer on single-phase equipment may be tested using a spinning top test; one dot appears on radiograph for each $\frac{1}{120}$-second exposure (assuming full-wave rectification)

    b. Timer on three-phase equipment may be tested using a motorized spinning top, which indicates an arc on the finished radiograph; amount of arc in degrees (fractions of 360 degrees) indicates exposure time

  c. Timer on three-phase equipment may also be tested using a digital testing device

11. Exposure linearity: tested using a digital dosimeter; various mA-time combinations for a given mAs are checked; adjacent mA stations should be within 10% of one another

12. Exposure reproducibility: tested using digital dosimeter; tests kVp, mA, and time in successive exposures; variation in measured radiation intensity should not be more than 5%

13. Automatic exposure controls: tested to verify reproducibility of exposure using phantoms to simulate variations in patient thickness

14. Fluoroscopy exposure rate: tested using digital dosimeter; entrance skin dose should not be more than 5 rads per minute

15. Patient dose is measured using cassette spot films and spot film cameras

16. Automatic brightness control on image intensifier: checked to ensure that radiation dose hitting the input phosphor is constant

17. Resolution of television system: tested using resolution test patterns

18. Other equipment used affecting the recorded image must also be part of a quality control program (see Chapter 4)

REVIEW QUESTIONS

For the following question, choose the single best answer.

1. Which of the following definitions are accurate?
1. Ionization is the removal of an electron from an atomic nucleus
2. Matter has form and occupies space
3. Kinetic energy is the energy of position
4. Mass is the amount of matter in an object
5. Electrical energy results from the heat produced when electrons are in motion
6. The radiations in the electromagnetic spectrum are all ionizing
   a. All are accurate
   b. 1, 3, 5, 6
   c. 2, 4
   d. 1, 2, 4

Read the following paragraph. Determine the accuracy of each underlined word or phrase. Then refer to questions **2-10** following the paragraph, and choose the one statement that best corrects and completes the underlined items.

Atomic Structure

The atom consists of a (2) <u>positively charged</u> nucleus and electrons in orbital shells. The orbital shells are designated by the letters (3) <u>*A, B, C, D,* etc.</u> Most of the mass of the atom is contained in the (4) <u>electrons.</u> The atomic number of an atom is the (5) <u>number of protons in the nucleus and is represented by the letter *Z*.</u> Atomic mass is (6) <u>the number of electrons in the atom and is represented by the letter *A*.</u> In a stable atom (7) <u>the number of electrons and protons is equal.</u> Atoms with the same number of protons but with a different number of neutrons are called (8) <u>ionized.</u> Electrons are held in orbit around the nucleus by a force called (9) <u>electromagnetic induction.</u> The law stating that the outer shell of an electron must always contain eight electrons is called the (10) <u>octet rule.</u>

2. a. The underlined word or phrase is accurate as written
   b. Negatively charged
   c. Neutral

3. a. The underlined word or phrase is accurate as written
   b. *Z, Y, X,* etc.
   c. *K, L, M,* etc.
   d. 1, 2, 3, 4, etc.

4. a. The underlined word or phrase is accurate as written
   b. Protons
   c. Neutrons
   d. Nucleus

5. a. The underlined word or phrase is accurate as written
   b. Number of electrons in the orbital shells and is represented by the letter *A*
   c. Number of electrons in the orbital shells and is represented by the letter *Z*
   d. Number of protons in the nucleus and is represented by the letter *A*

6. a. The underlined word or phrase is accurate as written
   b. Number of protons and neutrons in the nucleus and is represented by the letter *A*
   c. Number of protons in the nucleus and is represented by the letter *Z*
   d. Number of electrons in the nucleus and is represented by the letter *Z*

7. a. The underlined word or phrase is accurate as written
   b. The number of electrons is greater than the number of protons
   c. The number of protons is greater than the number of electrons
   d. The number of protons and electrons is equal, but there is a different number of neutrons

8. a. The underlined word or phrase is accurate as written
   b. Electrified
   c. Antimatter
   d. Isotopes

9. a. The underlined word or phrase is accurate as written
   b. Mutual induction
   c. Electron-binding energy
   d. Gravity

10. a. The underlined word or phrase is accurate as written
   b. Outer-shell rule
   c. Eight-electron rule
   d. There is no such rule

For the following question, choose the single best answer.

11. Examples of particulate radiation are:
   a. X rays, gamma rays, and cosmic rays
   b. Helium nuclei and beta particles
   c. Electrons, protons, and meteorites
   d. X rays and quarks

Read the following paragraph. Determine the accuracy of each underlined word or phrase. Then refer to questions **12-22** following the paragraph, and choose the one statement that best corrects and completes the corresponding underlined item.

Electromagnetic Radiation

Electromagnetic radiation travels (12) <u>in waves along a straight path.</u> (13) <u>It travels as bundles of energy called *protons.*</u> The speed of electromagnetic radiation is equal to the speed of (14) <u>light.</u> (15) <u>The waves of radiation are called *sign waves,*</u> each of which has wavelength and frequency. Wavelength is the distance from the (16) <u>source of radiation to the object it strikes.</u> (17) Frequency is the number of <u>times the radiation strikes an object.</u> As wavelength increases and frequency decreases, (18) <u>the speed of the radiation also decreases.</u> Generally speaking, wavelength and frequency (19) <u>are proportional to one another.</u> (20) <u>As radiation strikes and travels through matter, a process called *attenuation* occurs, which results in partial or full transfer of the</u>

radiation's energy to the atoms. Radiation is governed by the inverse square law, which states that (21) <u>the intensity of radiation is directly proportional to the square of the distance between the source of radiation and the point at which it is measured.</u> Finally, (22) <u>as the radiation strikes matter, the energy of the rays is destroyed, as are the atoms with which it interacts.</u>

12. a. The underlined word or phrase is accurate as written
b. In straight lines along a straight path
c. As electrons in waves along a straight path
d. Radiation travels only through a vacuum

13. a. The underlined word or phrase is accurate as written
b. It travels as bundles of energy called *electrons*
c. It travels as bundles of energy called *photons*
d. It travels as bundles of energy called *phasers*

14. a. The underlined word or phrase is accurate as written
b. Sound
c. Half the speed of light
d. Half the speed of sound

15. a. The underlined word or phrase is accurate as written
b. The waves of radiation are called *current*
c. The waves of radiation are called *signal waves*
d. The waves of radiation are called *sine waves*

16. a. The underlined word or phrase is accurate as written
b. Crest of a wave to the crest of the next wave
c. Trough of a wave to the trough of the next wave
d. b and c

17. a. The underlined word or phrase is accurate as written
b. Electrons that are transferred by radiation to the object
c. Waves that pass a given point per unit time
d. Seconds it takes for waves to pass a given point per unit time

18. a. The underlined word or phrase is accurate as written
b. The speed of radiation increases
c. The speed of radiation remains constant
d. The speed of radiation depends on the presence or absence of a vacuum

19. a. The underlined word or phrase is accurate as written
b. Are inversely proportional to one another
c. Are directly proportional to one another
d. Are inversely proportional to the square of their values

20. a. The underlined word or phrase is accurate as written
b. As radiation strikes and travels through matter, a process called *electrification* occurs, which results in partial or full transfer of energy
c. As radiation strikes matter, all energy is surrendered by a process known as *attenuation*
d. As radiation strikes matter, its energy is destroyed and the photons cease to exist

21. a. The underlined word or phrase is accurate as written
b. The intensity of radiation is inversely proportional to the distance between the source of radiation and the point at which it is measured
c. The intensity of radiation is inversely proportional to the square of the distance between the source of radiation and the point at which it is measured
d. The intensity of radiation is inversely proportional to the square of the distance between the source of radiation and the point at which it is measured and is calculated using the following equation

$$\text{Old R/New R} = \text{Old D}^2/\text{New D}^2$$

22. a. The underlined word or phrase is accurate as written
b. As the radiation strikes matter, the energy of the rays is increased from acquiring the energy of the atoms
c. As the radiation strikes matter, the energy of the rays is not destroyed but converted to matter
d. As the radiation strikes matter, the energy of the rays is transferred to the atoms according to the law of conservation of energy

For the following questions, choose the single best answer.

23. Which of the following statements are true regarding electrostatic charges?

✓ 1. Electrostatics is the study of electric charges at rest

2. The movement of electrons from one object to another is called *ionization*

3. Like charges attract, and unlike charges repel

✓ 4. Electrostatic charges concentrate on a conductor in the area of greatest curvature

5. Friction, contact, and induction are methods of ionization

   a. 2, 3, 5
   b. 1, 4
   c. All are accurate
   d. None are accurate

24. Which of the following statements are false?

1. A magnetic field always surrounds an electrical charge in motion

2. Current flows back and forth in AC

3. Current flows in one direction in DC

4. The volt is the unit of electric current

5. A conductor allows the free flow of electrons

6. The ampere is the unit of electromotive force

7. The volt is the unit of potential difference

8. The path of electric current is called the *circuit*

9. Ohm's law is calculated using the equation VI = R

10. A semiconductor is a material that may act as a conductor under some conditions and as an insulator under other conditions

   a. 4, 6, 9
   b. 1, 2, 3, 5, 7, 8, 10
   c. 1, 7, 10
   d. 4, 6, 9, 10

Read the following paragraph. Determine the accuracy of each underlined word or phrase. Then refer to questions **25-33** following the paragraph, and choose the one statement that best corrects and completes the corresponding underlined item.

Electromagnetic Induction

Electromagnetic induction is the process of causing an electric current to flow in a conductor (25) <u>when it is placed in contact with another conductor.</u> The two types of electromagnetic induction are (26) <u>autoinduction and mutual induction.</u> (27) <u>Autoinduction is used in the operation of the autotransformer.</u> Mutual induction is used in the operation of the step-up and step-down transformers. Because the wires in the transformers are coiled, (28) <u>their magnetic fields lie next to one another, thereby increasing the strength of the fields.</u> Electricity is provided by a device known as a (29) <u>*motor.*</u> The electricity provided to the radiology depart-

ment is (30) <u>120-Hz AC.</u> This current is single-phase, two-pulse current, providing (31) <u>120</u> pulses per second. Using special wiring patterns called *wye, star,* or *delta* converts the current to three-phase current. Three-phase power uses three waveforms placed 120 degrees out of phase with one another. (32) <u>Three-phase, six-pulse power has 240 pulses per second, whereas three-phase, twelve-pulse power has 360 pulses per second.</u> The primary advantage of three-phase power is that (33) <u>voltage drops to zero only three times per second.</u>

25. a. The underlined word or phrase is accurate as written

b. When it is placed near a generator

c. When it is placed in the electromagnetic field of another conductor

d. When it is placed in the electromagnetic field created by the x-ray beam

26. a. The underlined word or phrase is accurate as written

b. Solenoid induction and mutual induction

c. Generated induction and self-induction

d. Self-induction and mutual induction

27. a. The underlined word or phrase is accurate as written

b. Self-induction is used in the operation of the autotransformer

c. Mutual induction is used in the operation of the autotransformer

d. Direct current is used in the operation of the autotransformer

28. a. The underlined word or phrase is accurate as written

b. Their magnetic fields overlap, thereby decreasing the strength of the fields and making them less effective

c. Their magnetic fields overlap, thereby increasing the strength of the fields

d. Their magnetic fields remain separate around each turn of the wire

29. a. The underlined word or phrase is accurate as written

b. Solenoid

c. An induction motor

d. Generator

30. a. The underlined word or phrase is accurate as written

b. 60-Hz AC

c. 60-Hz DC

d. 120-Hz DC

31. a. The underlined word or phrase is accurate as written
   b. 60
   c. 30
   d. 2

32. a. The underlined word or phrase is accurate as written
   b. Three-phase, six-pulse power has 120 pulses per second, whereas three-phase, twelve-pulse power has 360 pulses per second
   c. Three-phase, six-pulse power has 360 pulses per second, whereas three-phase, twelve-pulse power has 720 pulses per second
   d. Three-phase, six-pulse power has 6 pulses per second whereas three-phase, twelve-pulse power has 12 pulses per second

33. a. The underlined word or phrase is accurate as written
   b. Voltage drops to zero only six times per second
   c. Voltage drops to zero only 12 times per second
   d. Voltage never drops to zero

For questions **34-38,** choose the single best answer.

34. A variable transformer that is used to select kVp for the x-ray circuit is the:
   a. Step-up transformer
   b. Autotransformer
   c. Step-down transformer
   d. Rectifier

35. A transformer that has more turns in the secondary than in the primary coil is called a:
   a. Step-up transformer
   b. Solenoid
   c. Step-down transformer
   d. Filament transformer

36. The transformer used to boost voltage to kilovoltage levels is called a(n):
   a. Autotransformer
   b. Step-down transformer
   c. Step-up transformer
   d. Low-voltage transformer

37. Voltage coming to the x-ray machine is kept constant through the use of a(n):
   a. Autotransformer
   b. Step-down transformer
   c. Rectifier
   d. Line voltage compensator

38. A step-down transformer:
   a. Steps down voltage
   b. Steps down current
   c. Steps up voltage
   d. Steps up resistance

Use the list that follows to answer questions **39-47.** Items may be used more than once. Choose the one best answer for each question.

   A. Step-down transformer
   B. Rectifier
   C. Cathode
   D. Timer
   E. kVp meter

39. The site of the process of thermionic emission *C*

40. Prereading device *E*

41. Reduces voltage and provides current to produce electron cloud or space charge *A*

42. Usually electronic, with increments as low as 0.001 s *D*

43. Changes AC to DC *B*

44. Surrounded by negatively charged focusing cup *C*

45. Composed of solid-state, silicon-based diodes *B*

46. Regulates the duration of x-ray production *D*

47. Located in x-ray circuit between high-voltage transformer and x-ray tube *AB*

Use the list that follows to answer questions **48-56.** Items may be used more than once. Choose the one best answer for each question.

    A. Anode
    B. mA meter
    C. Ionization chamber
    D. Falling load generator
    E. Step-up transformer

48. Measures tube current *B*

49. Spins at 3,300 to 10,000 rpm *A*

50. Uses maximum heat storage ability of tube to deliver mAs *D*

51. Source of bremsstrahlung and characteristic rays *A*

52. Increases voltage approximately 500 times *E*

53. Most commonly used AEC *C*

54. Always delivers shortest exposure time possible *D*

55. Turned by a rotor *A*

56. Located between the patient and the image receptor *C*

Read the following paragraph. Determine the accuracy of each underlined word or phrase. Then refer to questions **57-66** following the paragraph, and choose the one statement that best corrects and completes the corresponding underlined item.

The Production of X Radiation

(57) <u>The filament is kept warmed with a standby current from the time the x-ray machine is turned on.</u> (58) <u>The machine is immediately ready for use.</u> The proper exposure factors are selected, and the patient is accurately positioned. If a student radiographer is performing the positioning, (59) <u>activating the rotor will accelerate the process.</u> (60) <u>When ready to make the exposure, the radiograph activates the rotor switch for several seconds to bring the rotor up to speed and heat the filament. At this time the exposure switch is depressed.</u> Electrons are boiled off the filament, and the electron stream is aimed at the target with the assistance of a (61) <u>positively charged focusing cup.</u> The electron stream moves toward the anode because of the kilovoltage being passed through the tube, which creates a high potential difference between the two electrodes. (62) <u>As the electrons strike the anode, they break apart and a great amount of heat is liberated.</u> However, (63) <u>most of the energy is converted to x rays.</u> (64) <u>Some electrons strike and remove K-shell (outer-shell) electrons from the target mate-</u>

rial. (65) <u>As these vacancies are filled by L-shell electrons, energy is given off in the form of x rays.</u> (66) <u>Other incident electrons miss hitting orbital electrons and instead are slowed as they get closer to the nucleus of the target material. This braking action produces heat and x rays.</u>

57. a. False; turning on the machine activates the control panel only
    b. This statement is true
    c. This statement is true only if the machine has a three-phase generator
    d. False; because the exposure switch has not been activated, the filament cannot be heated

58. a. True; modern x-ray equipment is all electronic, so it needs no preparation for use
    b. False; a high-kVp, high-mAs technique must first be used to warm up the generator
    c. False; modern x-ray equipment requires time to warm up before making the first exposure of the day
    d. False; x-ray equipment must first be put through a series of low-heat unit warm-up exposures designed to heat the filament and anode before making diagnostic exposures

59. a. This always works and should be used to build confidence in students
    b. Activating the rotor begins a series of events that results in unnecessary exposure to the student and patient
    c. Because thermionic emission begins each time the rotor switch is activated, all this does is reduce the life of the x-ray tube by burning up the filament
    d. This action prolongs the life of the x-ray tube by keeping current flowing as often as possible

60. a. False; the rotor and exposure switch should be activated in one fluid motion as prescribed by most equipment manufacturers
    b. True; the equipment must be ready to make the exposure, and the radiographer has full control of the process
    c. False; the filament is already heated to incandescence when the mA station is selected
    d. True; because x rays are produced along the focal track, the anode does not need to be at full speed before the exposure begins as long as it is spinning at full speed by the termination of the exposure

61. a. False; focusing cup has a neutral charge
    b. False; focusing cup has a negative charge
    c. False; focusing cup has a positive charge, but it becomes negative from the thermionic emission
    d. False; focusing cup is negative so that it can repel the electron cloud

62. a. True; most of the energy is converted to heat rather than x rays
   b. False; the electrons do not break apart; however, the process of x-ray production yields a great amount of heat
   c. True; it is the breaking of electron bonds that produces the heat
   d. False; the electrons do not break apart

63. a. True; of all the energy involved, 99.8% is converted to x rays and 0.2% is converted to heat
   b. True; this is how a sufficient number of x rays are produced for diagnostic imaging
   c. False; of all the energy involved, 99.8% is converted to heat and 0.2% is converted to x rays
   d. False; more than 99% of the energy is converted to heat, which in turn converts to x rays at the anode

64. a. Statement is false
   b. False; *K*-shell electrons are not removed, just caused to vibrate
   c. False; electrons cannot be removed from the *K* shell because of its extremely high binding energy
   d. False; the *K* shell is the inner shell

65. a. True
   b. True; such x rays are called *brems rays*
   c. True; such x rays are called *characteristic x rays*
   d. True; but such x rays have a long wavelength and are not considered diagnostic

66. a. True; these rays are called *brems rays*
   b. True; these rays are called *characteristic rays*
   c. False; all incident electrons strike orbital electrons; the target atoms are so large they cannot be missed
   d. False; only characteristic x-ray production produces heat

For the following questions, choose the single best answer.

67. Which of the following are properties of x rays?
   1. Electrically negative
   2. Affect film emulsion
   3. Scatter and produce secondary radiation
   4. Invisible to the human eye
   5. Travel at the speed of light (186,000 miles per hour)
   6. Possess wavelengths between 1 and 5 angstroms
   7. Travel in bundles of energy called *photons*
   8. Can ionize matter and gases
   9. Can be focused by collimators
   10. Cause phosphors to fluoresce
   a. All are accurate
   b. 2, 3, 4, 7, 8, 10
   c. 1, 5, 6, 9
   d. 2, 3, 4, 6, 8, 9, 10

68. The x-ray beam is:
   a. Heterogeneous; all rays possess the same energy
   b. Homogeneous; all rays possess the same energy
   c. Monoenergetic; all energies correspond to the kVp
   d. Heterogeneous or polyenergetic, consisting of many different energies (wavelengths)

69. The x-ray emission spectrum consists of:
   a. Brems and characteristic rays
   b. Discrete spectrum (produced by brems rays) and continuous spectrum (produced by characteristic rays)
   c. Discrete spectrum (produced by characteristic rays) and continuous spectrum (produced by brems rays)
   d. X rays and electrons, both part of the electromagnetic spectrum

70. The primary purpose of filtration is:
   a. Radiation protection
   b. Removal of short-wavelength (soft) rays
   c. To harden the beam for imaging
   d. Removal of long-wavelength (hard) rays

71. The amount of material needed to reduce the intensity of the beam by ¹⁄₁₀ is called:
   a. Half-value layer
   b. Tenth-value layer
   c. Total filtration
   d. Inherent filtration

72. Which of the following statements regarding filtration is true?
   a. Total filtration must not be less than 2-mm aluminum equivalent
   b. Total filtration must remove all soft rays from the beam
   c. Total filtration (added + compensating) must not be less than 2.5-mm aluminum equivalent
   d. Total filtration (not less than 2.5-mm aluminum equivalent) = inherent filtration (glass envelope, tube housing, oil) + added filtration (aluminum)

73. Calculating heat units for three-phase, twelve-pulse equipment requires the use of _____ as a constant; calculating heat units for single-phase equipment requires the use of _____ as a constant; calculating heat units for three-phase, six-pulse equipment requires the use of _____ as a constant.
   a. 1, 1.35, 1.41
   b. 1.35, 1, 1.41
   c. Calculating heat units does not require the use of a constant because all x rays possess the same ionizing potential
   d. 1.41, 1, 1.35 because average photon energy is different with each type of equipment

74. Which of the following charts may be consulted to determine the safety of a single x-ray exposure?
a. Anode cooling curve
b. H & D curve
c. Characteristic tube chart
d. Tube rating chart

75. Which of the following charts may be consulted to determine the safety of a series of x-ray exposures?
a. Anode cooling curve
b. H & D curve
c. Characteristic tube chart
d. Tube rating chart

76. The portion of the image-intensifier tube that converts electron energy to visible light is the:
a. Output phosphor
b. Photocathode
c. Input phosphor
d. Brightness gain

77. The portion of the image-intensifier tube that converts visible light to an electronic image is the:
a. Output phosphor
b. Photocathode
c. Input phosphor
d. Brightness gain

78. The input phosphor of the image-intensifier tube converts:
a. Electron energy to x-ray energy
b. X rays and heat to visible light
c. X-ray energy to visible light
d. X-ray energy to an electronic image

79. Total brightness gain achieved using an image intensifier equals:
a. Flux gain times minification gain
b. Diameter of input phosphor times diameter of output phosphor
c. Intensification factor: brightness without an image intensifier divided by brightness with an image intensifier
d. Total light emitted at photocathode

80. Single-phase, full-wave rectification produces:
a. Direct current
b. Pulsating direct current
c. Pulsating direct current with 120 pulses per second
d. Pulsating direct current with 120 pulses per second and 100% ripple

81. Three-phase, six-pulse full-wave rectification produces:
a. Direct current with 13% ripple
b. Direct current with 4% ripple
c. Direct current with 100% ripple
d. Alternating current with 13% ripple

82. Three-phase, twelve-pulse full-wave rectification produces:
a. Direct current with 13% ripple
b. Direct current with 4% ripple
c. Direct current with 100% ripple
d. Alternating current with 13% ripple

83. The increase in average photon energy when using three-phase, six-pulse equipment compared with single-phase equipment is:
a. 1.35%
b. 41%
c. 1.41%
d. 35%

84. The increase in average photon energy when using three-phase, twelve-pulse equipment compared with single-phase equipment is:
a. 1.35%
b. 41%
c. 1.41%
d. 35%

85. Average photon energy is the same as three-phase, six-pulse. Programs that deal with the safe and reliable operation of equipment and those that address all aspects of the delivery of radiology services are called, respectively:
a. Quality assurance and quality control
b. Total quality improvement
c. Quality control and quality assurance
d. Total quality management

86. Examples of dedicated x-ray equipment include:
a. Mammography units
b. Tomography units
c. Mobile x-ray machines
d. All of the above

For each of the quality checks in items **87-90**, choose the parameters that must be met from the list that follows:

    A. 4
    B. 5%
    C. 2% of SID
    D. 10%
    E. 4%

87. Collimator

88. kVp D (A)

89. Exposure linearity D

90. Exposure reproducibility B

For the following questions, choose the single best answer.

91. When a spinning top test is performed on single-phase equipment, a radiograph exhibiting four dots would indicate:
    a. An accurate timer, if set on ¹⁄₂₀ second
    b. A malfunctioning timer, if set on ¹⁄₃ second
    c. An accurate timer, if set on ¹⁄₃₀ second
    d. b and c

92. When a spinning top test is performed on three-phase equipment, a timer setting of ¹⁄₆₀ second should indicate the following on the resultant radiograph:
    a. 2 dots
    b. 60 dots
    c. A 6-degree arc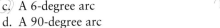
    d. A 90-degree arc

93. The test that measures the accuracy of adjacent mA stations is:
    a. Exposure reproducibility
    b. Spinning top test
    c. Pinhole camera
    d. Exposure linearity

94. The test that measures the accuracy of successive exposures is:
    a. Exposure reproducibility
    b. Spinning top test
    c. Pinhole camera
    d. Exposure linearity

95. Effective focal spot size may be measured using the following tool(s):
    a. Slit camera
    b. Star test pattern
    c. Pinhole camera
    d. All of the above

96. Resolution of the television system may be measured using the following tool(s):
    a. Wire mesh test
    b. Line pairs–per–millimeter resolution tool
    c. Resolution test pattern
    d. All of the above

97. The fluoroscopic image may be viewed or recorded using which of the following devices:
    a. Television system
    b. Cine camera
    c. Spot film camera
    d. All of the above

98. The amount of mA used for fluoroscopy is:
    a. 300 to 500
    b. 3 to 5
    c. 10 to 12
    d. 100 to 300

99. Marks on the focal track of the anode resulting from bombardment of electrons are called:
    a. Melts
    b. Bullet marks
    c. Pitting
    d. Cracks

100. Effective quality control and quality assurance programs are required for accreditation by:
    a. Joint Commission on Accreditation of Healthcare Organizations
    b. Joint Review Committee on Education in Radiologic Technology
    c. American Healthcare Radiology Administrators
    d. Starfleet Academy

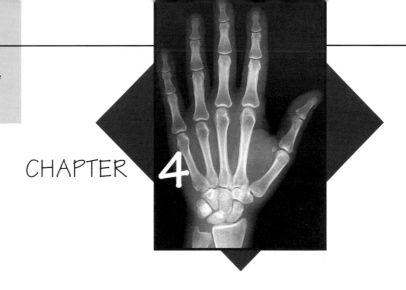

CHAPTER **4**

Review of Image Production and Evaluation

DENSITY

A. Amount of blackness on a given area of a radiograph
B. Also known as the *logarithm of opacity* or *optical density (OD)*
C. Defined as the ratio of the amount of light incident on the film to the amount of light transmitted through the film
  1. Light incident may be thought of as the light striking the radiograph from the back, coming from the view box
  2. Light transmitted may be thought of as the light that is seen coming through the radiograph while being viewed either by the human eye or a densitometer
  3. $OD = \log 10 \dfrac{\text{Light incident}}{\text{Light transmitted}}$
D. A result of exit x rays and light rays from intensifying screens striking the film's emulsion
E. Made visible when the crystals in the film's emulsion are converted to black metallic silver in the developer solution
F. Controlled by the following
  1. The number of exit rays striking the film-screen combination
  2. The speed of the film-screen combination
  3. Processing

Factors Controlling and Influencing Density

A. mAs
  1. Controls the number of electrons passing from cathode to anode in the x-ray tube
  2. Controls the quantity of x rays produced at the anode

  3. Controls the amount of radiation exiting the x-ray tube
    a. This is a directly proportional relationship
    b. As mAs is increased, density increases in the same amount
    c. As mAs is decreased, density decreases in the same amount
  4. Directly controls the number of x-ray photons that will emerge from the patient as exit rays
  5. Directly controls the number of x rays that eventually strike the film-screen system as exit rays
  6. Governed by the reciprocity law
    a. Any combinations of mA and time that produce the same mAs value will result in the same density on the radiograph
    b. Sometimes expressed by the equation: mAs = mAs
B. kVp
  1. Directly controls the energy or quality of the x rays produced
    a. As the kVp increases, a greater potential difference exists between the cathode and the anode
    b. As the potential difference increases, the electrons from the cathode strike the anode in greater numbers and with greater energy
    c. This results in an increased level of production of short-wavelength, high-energy radiation
  2. Directly affects density, although not in a directly proportional relationship
    a. As kVp increases, density increases
    b. As kVp decreases, density decreases
    c. Governed by the 15% rule (an increase in kVp of 15% will double density; a decrease in kVp of 15% will halve density)

3. Determines the penetrating ability of the x-ray beam
   a. As kVp is increased, wavelength decreases and x rays become more penetrating
   b. As kVp is decreased, wavelength increases and x rays become less penetrating
4. Penetrating ability of the x rays also determines the number of x rays exiting the patient to strike the film

C. Distance
1. Density is inversely proportional to the square of the distance
2. Governed by the inverse square law
   a. The intensity of the x-ray beam is inversely proportional to the square of the distance
   b. Density is expressed by the equation

$$\frac{\text{Old mAs}}{\text{New mAs}} = \frac{(\text{New distance})^2}{(\text{Old distance})^2}\left(\frac{\text{mAs}_o}{\text{mAs}_n} = \frac{D_n{}^2}{D_o{}^2}\right)$$

   c. If distance is doubled, density decreases four times
   d. If distance is halved, density increases four times
   e. Any other combinations can be calculated using the inverse square law equation just presented
   f. Variation in density is the result of the divergence of the x-ray beam as it travels through space

D. Film-screen combination
1. Directly proportional relationship with density
   a. As speed (sensitivity) increases, density increases
   b. As speed (sensitivity) decreases, density decreases

E. Grids
1. Decrease the amount of scatter radiation striking the film
2. Density decreases when using grids unless mAs is increased to compensate for the loss of scatter fog

F. Beam restriction
1. Decreases density by limiting the size of the x-ray beam unless mAs is increased to compensate
2. Decreases density by limiting the area of the patient being struck by x rays
3. Reduces the amount of scatter radiation being produced, which adds density to the film in the form of fog

G. Anatomy and pathology
1. Anatomy affects density through its variation of atomic number, tissue thickness, and tissue density
2. Pathology affects density by altering tissue integrity, atomic number, tissue density, and tissue thickness (see Chapter 5 for specific pathologic conditions and their effects on radiographic technique)

H. Anode heel effect
1. X-ray intensity varies along the longitudinal axis of the x-ray beam
   a. Density is greater near the cathode end of the x-ray beam
   b. Density is less near the anode end of the x-ray beam because of absorption of x rays by the "heel" of the anode

2. Thicker anatomy should be placed under the cathode side of the x-ray tube to take advantage of the anode heel effect

I. Filtration
1. Negligible effect on density; largely a radiation protection accessory
2. Some reduction in the number of soft, long-wavelength rays striking the patient, most of which would not have exited the patient to strike the film
3. Compensating filters even out density of irregular anatomy

CONTRAST

A. Differences in adjacent densities on the radiograph
B. Primary function is to make the detail visible
C. High contrast: few gray tones, mainly black and white image; may also be referred to as *short-scale contrast*
D. Low contrast: many gray tones on image; may also be referred to as *long-scale contrast*

Factors Controlling and Influencing Contrast

A. kVp
1. Directly controls contrast
2. Controls differential absorption of the x-ray beam by the body because of its control of x-ray beam energy (Figure 4-1)
   a. As kVp is increased, contrast decreases (becomes lower or longer scale) because there is more uniform penetration of anatomic parts by the shorter-wavelength rays

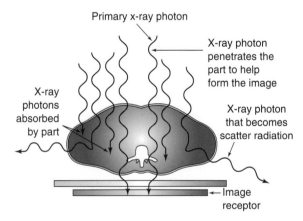

Primary x-ray photon

X-ray photon penetrates the part to help form the image

X-ray photons absorbed by part

X-ray photon that becomes scatter radiation

Image receptor

Figure 4-1 As the primary x-ray beam interacts with the anatomic part, photons are absorbed, scattered, and transmitted. The differences in the absorption characteristics of the anatomic part create an image that structurally represents the anatomic part.

b. As kVp is decreased, contrast increases (becomes higher or shorter scale) as a result of greater absorption of lower-energy rays by the anatomic parts (increased photoelectric interaction)

3. High kVp = low contrast = long-scale contrast = many gray tones

4. Low kVp = high contrast = short-scale contrast = few gray tones (mainly black and white tones)

B. Grids
1. Reduce the amount of scatter reaching the film
2. Less scatter fog results in fewer gray tones, which increases contrast

C. Beam restriction
1. Limits area being irradiated
2. Produces less scatter by reducing number of Compton's interactions taking place
3. Less scatter fog reduces the number of gray tones on the radiograph, thereby increasing contrast

D. Filtration (Figure 4-2)
1. As filtration is increased, beam becomes harder (average photon striking the patient has shorter wavelength)

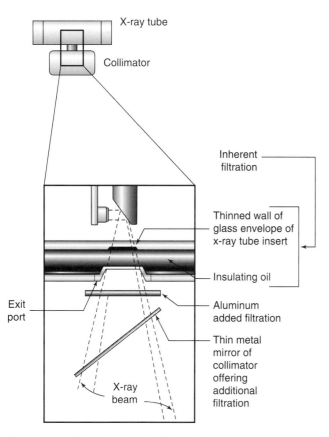

Figure 4-2 Aluminum added filtration is shown at the port of the x-ray tube. The inherent filtration of the glass envelope, the oil, and the collimator mirror are shown.

2. Contrast decreases as filtration increases

E. Anatomy and pathology
1. Also known as *subject contrast*
2. Control contrast with variations in the following
   a. Atomic number
   b. Tissue density
   c. Tissue thickness
3. Cause differential absorption of x-ray photons, which results in contrast

RECORDED DETAIL

A. Sharpness with which anatomic structures are displayed on an image receptor
B. May be described as the geometric representation of part being radiographed
C. May also be referred to as *detail sharpness, definition,* or *image resolution*

Factors Controlling and Influencing Recorded Detail

A. Object-to-image distance (OID)
1. Distance from the anatomic part being imaged to the image receptor (usually film)
2. Shortest possible OID should be used
3. Increased OID causes magnification of the image, resulting in loss of recorded detail

B. Source-to-image distance (SID)
1. Distance from the source of radiation (usually anode in the x-ray tube) to the image receptor (usually film)
2. Longest practical SID should be used
3. Shorter SID causes magnification of the image, resulting in loss of recorded detail

C. Focal spot size (Figure 4-3)
1. Use small focal spot when possible
2. Use of large focal spot decreases sharpness of recorded detail
3. Decreased sharpness is caused by x rays emanating from a larger area of the anode; accentuates beam divergence

D. Film-screen combination
1. Use of slower-speed film-screen system results in increased sharpness of recorded detail
2. Use of faster-speed film-screen system results in decreased sharpness of recorded detail
3. Film-screen system speed primarily affected by size of phosphor crystals in the active layer of the intensifying screen and to a lesser degree the size of the silver bromide crystals in the emulsion of the film
   a. The larger the crystals, the poorer the recorded detail (resolution)
   b. The smaller the crystals, the greater the recorded detail (resolution)

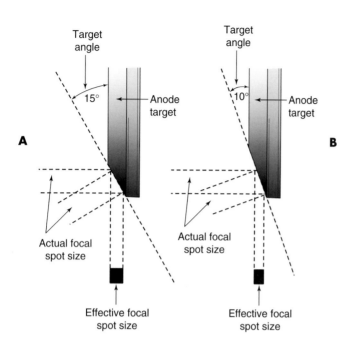

Figure 4-3 The line focus principle states that a large target angle will produce a large effective focal spot size **(A)** and that a small target angle will produce a small effective spot size **(B).** Both actual focal spot sizes are the same, meaning that they can withstand the same heat loading from the same exposure factors.

E. Motion
  1. Any motion results in image blur and subsequent loss of recorded detail
  2. Motion may be caused by the following
    a. Patient motion
    b. X-ray tube motion
    c. Excessive motion from reciprocating grid

DISTORTION

A. Any misrepresentation of an anatomic structure on an image receptor that alters its size and/or shape
B. Two types of distortion: size and shape

Factors Controlling Distortion

A. Size
  1. Magnification
  2. Caused by excessive OID
  3. Caused by insufficient SID
  4. Causes anatomic structure to appear larger on film than in reality
B. Shape (Figure 4-4)
  1. Elongation

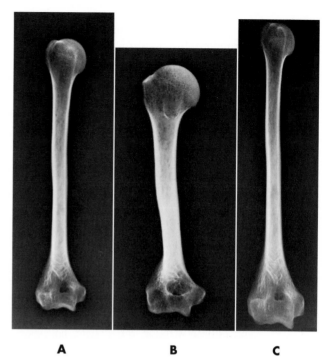

Figure 4-4 **A,** No distortion. **B,** Foreshortened. **C,** Elongated.

    a. Causes anatomic structure to appear longer than in reality
    b. Caused by improper tube, part, or film angulation or alignment
    c. Caused by angulation along the long axis of the part
  2. Foreshortening
    a. Causes anatomic structure to appear shorter than in reality
    b. Caused by improper tube, part, or film angulation
    c. Caused by angulation against the main axis of the part

RADIOGRAPHIC FILM

A. Base
  1. Made of polyester
  2. Approximately 0.008 inch thick
  3. Blue dye added
    a. To enhance contrast
    b. To reduce glare
B. Emulsion (Figure 4-5)
  1. Double-emulsion film (also called *duplitized film*): coated on both sides of base
  2. Single-emulsion film: coated on one side of base
  3. Consists of silver halide crystals suspended in gelatin
    a. Gelatin: easily suspends crystals and expands and contracts in processing solutions

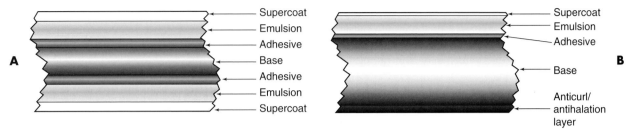

Figure 4-5   Cross section of double-emulsion **(A)** and single-emulsion **(B)** film.

b. Silver halide crystals: primarily silver bromide, most of which have sensitivity specks on the surface
   c. Sensitivity specks serve as centers for making the latent image visible; made of an impurity (silver sulfite)
   d. Latent image: image contained in the silver halide crystals after exposure but before development
4. Approximately 0.0003 inch thick per coating
C. Film characteristics
1. Speed (sensitivity)
   a. Determined by the size and/or number of the silver halide crystals and the thickness of the emulsion
   b. The larger the crystals and/or the thicker the emulsion, the faster the film
2. Contrast
   a. Determined by the size of the silver halide crystals and the thickness of the emulsion
   b. A function of speed
   c. The faster the film, the higher the contrast (shorter scale, more black and white image)
   d. The slower the film, the lower the contrast (longer scale, grayer image)
3. Latitude
   a. Determined by the inherent contrast of the film
   b. The lower the inherent contrast, the wider the latitude of the film
   c. The higher the inherent contrast, the narrower the latitude of the film
   d. Latitude may be thought of as the range of exposures over which the film will produce diagnostically useful densities
4. Exposure latitude
   a. Wider exposure latitude at higher kVp levels
   b. Narrower exposure latitude at lower kVp levels

Sensitometry

A. H & D curves (Figure 4-6)
1. Also called *sensitometric curves, characteristic curves,* and *D log E curves*
2. Compare exposure (plotted on x-axis) with density (plotted on y-axis) (Figure 4-7)

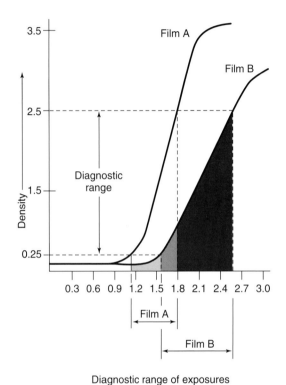

Figure 4-6   A higher-contrast film, Film A, has a narrower range of exposures available to produce optical densities within the straight-line region compared with a lower-contrast film, Film B.

3. Curve always assumes some form of S or sigmoid shape
4. Toe
   a. Portion of curve representing low exposure and density; base plus fog
   b. Portion of curve from 0 to 0.25 density
5. Body
   a. Also called *straight-line portion, gamma,* or *slope*
   b. Portion of curve from 0.25 to 2.5 density
   c. Measures usable densities
   d. Indicates overall gray scale (contrast) of the film

6. Shoulder
   a. Portion of curve from 2.5 to maximum density (also called *D-max*)
   b. Measures unusable densities on the radiograph (blackest portion)
7. Use of H & D curves
   a. May be used to determine the characteristics of a certain film
   b. May be used to compare the characteristics of several films
8. Film characteristics as plotted on H & D curves
   a. Speed (sensitivity): the closer the curve to the y-axis, the faster the film
   b. Contrast: the steeper the curve, the higher the contrast; the more shallow the curve, the lower the contrast
   c. Latitude: the steeper the curve, the more narrow the latitude; the shallower the curve, the wider the latitude
   d. Recorded detail (based on film speed): the steeper the curve, the poorer the recorded detail; the shallower the curve, the better the recorded detail
   e. When several films are compared, the curves to the left are faster and have higher contrast and more narrow latitude
   f. When several films are compared, the curves to the right are slower and have lower contrast and wider latitude

Film Storage and Handling

A. Storage
   1. Temperature no greater than 68° to 70° F
   2. Humidity from 40% to 60%
   3. Protected from the following to prevent increased density and fog
      a. Radiation
      b. Fumes
      c. Outdating
      d. Light
   4. Boxes stored on end, never flat; storing the boxes flat causes pressure mark artifacts (areas of increased density caused by excessive pressure applied to the film)
B. Handling
   1. Pressure marks
   2. Static
      a. Caused by static electricity discharge on film
      b. Static buildup on loading tray
      c. Static buildup on loading bench
      d. Rapidly pulling film from cassette as it rubs against intensifying screens
      e. Low humidity in film-handling area
   3. Crinkle or half-moon marks
      a. Bending film over fingernail during handling
      b. Other rough handling

INTENSIFYING SCREENS

A. Base or backing (Figure 4-8)
   1. Made of polyester
   2. Mounted inside the cassette in pairs for use with double-emulsion film
B. Reflective layer
   1. Between base and active layer
   2. Reflects light from crystals toward film, increasing the speed of the system
C. Active layer
   1. Also called the *phosphor layer*

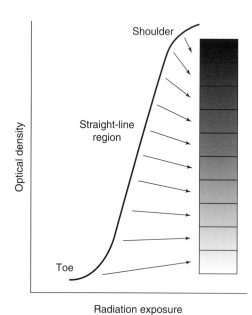

Figure 4-7 Plotting optical densities corresponding to the change in intensity of exposure results in a curve characteristic of the type of the film.

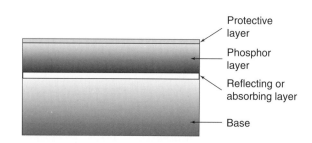

Figure 4-8 Cross section of an intensifying screen.

2. Adheres to the base
3. Contains phosphors (crystals that glow with visible light when struck by radiation)
4. As phosphor size or active layer thickness decreases, the resolution of the screen increases
   a. Resolution is measured in line pairs per millimeter
   b. Resolution quality control test uses a device called a *resolution grid*, which is radiographed, and the image is evaluated
D. Protective layer
1. Thin coating placed on top of active layer to provide protection from scratching or other damage
E. Screen speed (sensitivity)
1. Primarily controlled by the following
   a. Phosphor used
   b. Phosphor size (larger phosphors are faster)
   c. Active layer thickness (thicker layer is faster)
   d. Efficiency of reflective layer (higher efficiency makes screen faster)
   e. kVp used (higher kVp increases screen speed)
   f. Presence of yellow dye in active layer (yellow dye absorbs some of the phosphors' light and reduces speed)
   g. Conversion efficiency: ability of phosphors to absorb x-ray energy and convert it to visible light rays
F. Film-screen combination summary (speed primarily controlled by screens; contrast primarily controlled by film)
1. Faster-speed system
   a. Higher contrast
   b. Narrower latitude
   c. Less recorded detail
   d. Increased density
2. Slower-speed system
   a. Lower contrast
   b. Wider latitude
   c. Greater recorded detail
   d. Decreased density

3. Single-emulsion films
   a. Used with one intensifying screen
   b. Slower
   c. Lower contrast
   d. Wider latitude
   e. Better recorded detail
   f. Decreased density
4. Double-emulsion films
   a. Used with two intensifying screens
   b. Faster
   c. Higher contrast
   d. Narrower latitude
   e. Poorer recorded detail
5. Identified by relative speed numbers; 100 speed is the "base speed"
   a. Based on intensification factor: ratio of exposure in mAs needed to produce image without screens to exposure in mAs needed to produce image with screens

$$IF = \frac{\text{Exposure without screens}}{\text{Exposure with screens}}$$

   b. Example: a 200-speed system is twice as fast as a 100-speed system, so half the mAs would be needed to produce the same density
   c. Relative speed numbers allow for exposure calculations and modifications when moving from one film-screen system to another, eliminating guesswork
   d. Generally, slower systems are used for extremity radiography; faster systems are used for spine, abdomen, trauma, and pediatric radiography
6. Spectral matching
   a. Wavelength of light emitted by screens must be matched with wavelengths to which film is most sensitive
   b. Example: green-emitting screens must be used with green-sensitive film
7. Film-screen contact
   a. Must be perfect
   b. Poor contact results in localized loss of recorded detail
   c. Tested by radiographing a wide mesh screen

Table 4-1 summarizes the effect of screen construction factors on screen speed, recorded detail, and patient dose.

GRIDS

A. Use
1. Reduces the amount of scatter radiation reaching the film
   a. Scatter travels in divergent paths compared with image-producing rays (Figure 4-9)
   b. More likely to be absorbed in the grid

TABLE 4-1 **Summary of Effect of Screen Factors on Screen Speed, Recorded Detail, and Patient Dose**

Screen factor	Screen speed	Recorded detail	Patient dose
Thicker phosphor layer	↑	↓	↓
Larger phosphor crystal size	↑	↓	↓
Reflective layer	↑	↓	↓
Absorbing layer	↓	↑	↑
Dye in phosphor layer	↓	↑	↑

From Fauber TL: *Radiographic imaging & exposure*, St Louis, 2000, Mosby.

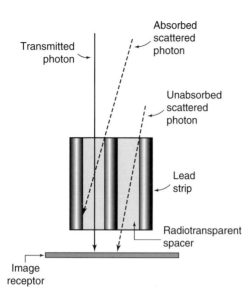

Figure 4-9 Ideally, grids would absorb all scattered radiation and allow all transmitted photons to reach the film. In reality, however, some scattered photons are allowed to pass through to the film, and some transmitted photons are absorbed.

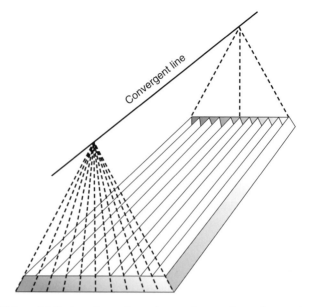

Figure 4-10 Imaginary lines drawn above a linear focused grid from each lead line meet to form a convergent line.

2. Generally used when part thickness is 10 cm or greater
B. Construction
  1. Lead strips separated by aluminum interspacers
  2. Grid ratio
    a. Grid ratio is the height of the lead strips divided by the distance between the lead strips: grid ratio = H/D
    b. Ratios range from 4:1 to 16:1
  3. Grid frequency
    a. Number of lead strips per inch (or centimeter)
    b. As grid frequency increases, lead strip thickness decreases and becomes less visible
    c. Ranges from 60 to 150 lines per inch
C. Grid types
  1. Linear (Figure 4-10)
    a. Lead strips are parallel to one another
    b. X-ray tube may be angled along the length of the grid without cutoff
    c. Grid cutoff: decreased density along the periphery of the film caused by absorption of image-forming rays
    d. Used primarily with large SID or small field
  2. Focused grids (Figure 4-11)
    a. Lead strips are angled to coincide with divergence of the x-ray beam
    b. Used within specific ranges of SID
    c. Grid radius: distance at which focused grid may be used (also called *focal distance* or *focal range*)

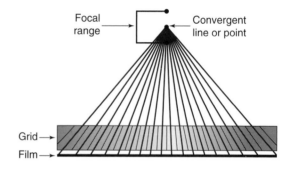

Figure 4-11 The convergent line or point of a focused grid falls within a focal range.

    d. Focal range is wide for low ratio grids
    e. Focal range is narrow for high ratio grids
    f. Focal range is stated on the front of the grid
  3. Crossed grids (Figure 4-12)
    a. Also called *crosshatch grids*
    b. Consist of two linear grids placed perpendicular to one another
    c. Superior scatter cleanup
    d. Allow for no angulation of x-ray beam
    e. Require perfect positioning and centering
    f. Primary use is biplane cerebral angiography
D. Grid characteristics
  1. Contrast improvement factor
    a. Measure of a grid's ability to enhance contrast

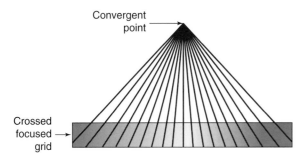

Figure 4-12   Imaginary lines drawn above a crossed focused grid from each lead line meet to form a convergent point.

b. Expressed as the ratio of the contrast with a grid to the contrast without a grid
2. Grid selectivity
   a. Expressed as the ratio of primary radiation transmitted through the grid to secondary radiation transmitted through the grid
   b. The higher the grid frequency and grid ratio, the more selective it will be
   c. High selectivity indicates high efficiency of scatter cleanup
3. Grid conversion factor
   a. Also called *Bucky factor*
   b. Amount of exposure increase necessary to compensate for the absorption of image-forming rays and scatter in the cleanup process
   c. Used to indicate the increase in mAs needed when converting from nongrid to grid status
   d. When converting from grid to nongrid status, use reciprocal of grid conversion factor
   e. Grid conversion factors increase with higher kVp because there is an increase in Compton's interactions, which produce more scatter
   f. Factors used at 120 kVp—5:1 grid, 3×; 8:1 grid, 4×; 12:1 grid 5×; 16:1, 6×
E. Grid motion
1. Stationary grids
   a. Do not move during the exposure
   b. Grid lines may be seen
2. Moving grids
   a. Reciprocate (move back and forth) during exposure
   b. Eliminate the visibility of grid lines
F. Grid errors: focused grids
1. Upside down
   a. Result will be normal density in the middle of the radiograph with decreased density on the sides
   b. Focused grid must be placed with labeled tube side facing x-ray tube
2. Off-level

a. Result will be image-forming rays absorbed all across the radiographic field, with cutoff (decreased density) visible over the entire radiograph
   b. Grid must be perpendicular to the central ray
3. Lateral decentering
   a. Central ray does not strike the grid in the center
   b. Cutoff visible, more to one side of the radiograph
4. Grid-focus decentering
   a. Violation of the grid radius when using a focused grid
   b. Normal density in the middle of the radiograph with cutoff visible on the sides
G. Air gap technique
1. Uses increased OID
2. Increased OID allows scatter (which travels in widely divergent paths) to exit the patient and miss the film
3. Example: lateral cervical spine
   a. Distance from spine to shoulder causes gap
   b. Eliminates need for grid (gap is similar to using a 10:1 grid)
   c. Use of grid serves only to increase patient dose
4. Example: cerebral angiography
   a. Distance to the rapid film changers allows for gap
   b. Biplane angiography produces large amount of scatter
   c. Air gap usually used along with grids in rapid film changers
H. Radiographic quality and grids
1. Produce higher contrast by absorbing Compton's scatter rays, which produce fog if they strike the film
2. Decrease recorded detail if used in a Potter-Bucky diaphragm because of increased OID
Table 4-2 summarizes variables and how they affect the radiographic image.

TECHNIQUE CHARTS

A. Measurement
1. Part thickness should always be measured using calipers
2. Caliper measurement is then used to consult the technique chart
B. Types of technique charts
1. Fixed kVp-variable mAs
   a. Assumes optimum kVp for the part being radiographed
   b. Except for exceptionally large patients, kVp never changes for a given projection
   c. mAs is varied according to the part thickness as measured with the calipers
   d. Based on the assumption that thicker parts will absorb more rays and therefore more rays must be placed in the primary beam
2. Variable kVp

TABLE 4-2	Variables and Their Effect on Both the Photographic and Geometric Properties of the Radiographic Image

Radiographic variables	Photographic properties		Geometric properties	
	Density	Contrast	Recorded detail	Distortion
↑ mAs*	↑	0	0	0
↓ mAs	↓	0	0	0
↑ kVp	↑	↓	0	0
↓ kVp	↓	↑	0	0
↑ SID	↓	0	↑	↓
↓ SID	↑	0	↓	↑
↑ OID†	↓	↑	↓	↑
↓ OID	↑	↓	↑	↓
↑ Grid ratio	↓	↑	0	0
↓ Grid ratio	↑	↓	0	0
↑ Film-screen speed	↑	0	↓	0
↓ Film-screen speed	↓	0	↑	0
↑ Collimation	↓	↑	0	0
↓ Collimation	↑	↓	0	0
↑ Focal spot size	0	0	↓	0
↓ Focal spot size	0	0	↑	0
↑ Central ray angle	↓	0	↓	↑

From Fauber TL: *Radiographic imaging & exposure*, St Louis, 2000, Mosby.
↑, Increased effect; ↓ decreased effect; *0*, no effect; *OID*, object-to-image distance; *SID*, source-to-image distance.
*The mAs has no significant effect on contrast as long as densities remain within diagnostic range.
†The amount of OID needed to affect contrast depends on the type of anatomic part being imaged.

a. kVp is varied according to part thickness as measured with the calipers
b. Based on the assumption that thicker parts require a beam with shorter-wavelength rays that are more penetrating
3. Variable technique
a. Provides for alteration of routine techniques because of pathology, patient age, ability to cooperate, casts, contrast media

AUTOMATIC EXPOSURE CONTROLS

A. Use fixed kVp while machine controls mAs
B. Require proper ionization chambers to be selected for part being radiographed
C. Part being radiographed must be placed exactly over ionization chamber
D. Varying kVp when using automatic exposure control (AEC) does not alter density, although contrast will change
E. Varying kVp serves to alter penetrating ability of the beam, resulting in faster or shorter exposure time
F. Changing density controls on AEC allows density to be increased or decreased; each step represents a change of 25% in density

AUTOMATIC PROCESSING AND QUALITY ASSURANCE

Chemistry

A. Developer
1. Converts exposed silver bromide crystals (latent image) to black metallic silver (visible image)
2. Reducing agents
   a. Hydroquinone: works slowly to build black tones
   b. Phenidone: works quickly to build gray tones
3. Activator
   a. Sodium carbonate
   b. Softens and swells film emulsion
4. Hardener
   a. Glutaraldehyde
   b. Controls swelling of film emulsion to allow safe transport through the processor
5. Restrainer
   a. Potassium bromide
   b. Prevents reducing agents from producing fog, which is created when unexposed silver bromide crystals develop
6. Preservative
   a. Sodium sulfite
   b. Slows oxidation of reducing agents by room air

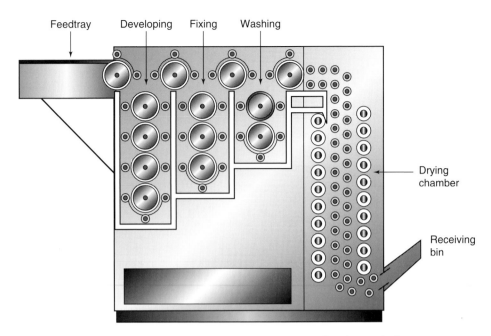

Figure 4-13 Cross section of an automatic processor showing the vertical transport system of rollers.

7. Solvent
   a. Water
   b. Medium in which chemicals are dissolved
B. Fixer
1. Fixing agent
   a. Also called *hypo*
   b. Ammonium thiosulfate
   c. Clears and removes unexposed silver bromide crystals
2. Acidifier
   a. Acetic acid
   b. Provides acid medium in which fixing agent operates
   c. Stops action of alkaline developer solution on contact
3. Hardener
   a. Aluminum chloride
   b. Shrinks and hardens emulsion in preparation for viewing and storage
4. Preservative
   a. Sodium sulfite
   b. Slows oxidation of solution by room air
   c. Chemical component common to both developer and fixer
5. Solvent
   a. Water
   b. Medium in which chemicals are dissolved
C. Washing solution
1. Water
2. Removes chemicals remaining on film

Systems
Transport (Figure 4-13)
A. Moves film through the processor
B. Agitates chemistry
C. Consists of series of 1-inch-diameter rollers with 3-inch rollers at the bottom of racks
1. Entrance roller or detector roller
   a. Rubber serrated edges grab film as it enters the processor and moves it into the developer tank
   b. Activates microswitch that turns on replenishment pump
2. Deep racks (transport racks)
   a. Move film into and through solutions in developer, fixer, and wash tanks and between drying tubes in dryer section
   b. Use turnaround assembly (with metal guide shoes) at bottom of rack to change direction of film transport upward toward top of tank
3. Crossover assembly
   a. Moves film from developer tank to fixer tank and from fixer tank to wash tank
   b. Rollers also help force solution from film back into tank it is exiting
4. Squeegee assembly
   a. Multiple roller assembly that moves film from wash tank to dryer section
   b. Uses extensive squeegee action to remove as much water as possible from film

c. Shortens drying time and reduces humidity buildup in dryer section

D. Drive system
1. Motor-driven gears that mesh with gears at the end of top rollers on racks

Replenishment

A. Adds fresh developer and fixer solution for each film fed into the processor

B. Replenishment occurs as film is being fed into processor; activated by microswitch at end of entrance roller
1. Motorized pumps send solution to the processor
2. Films should always be fed into processor by the short length to prevent overreplenishment

C. Solution is pumped from holding tanks through tubing into processor

D. Replenishment rates based on average number of 14- × 17-inch films fed through the processor in a typical workday

Recirculation

A. Agitates developer solution

B. Helps stabilize developer temperature
1. Constant agitation and circulation of developer keep temperature constant throughout the tank
2. Agitation also keeps solution in contact with heater element in bottom of tank and prevents stratification of chemicals
3. Developer temperature maintained in the range of 90° to 95° F, depending on brand of chemicals used
4. Heating element controlled by thermostat

C. Removes reaction particles by use of a filtration system

Dryer

A. Dries film after it leaves wash tank

B. Consists of thermostatically controlled heating element with blower fan

C. Film passes between tubes through which hot air is blowing

D. Film is dried at approximately 120° F

Maintenance

A. Start-up procedure
1. Close wash tank valve
2. Turn on water source
3. Turn on processor
4. Wash crossover racks
5. Put lid in place
6. Run several 14- × 17-inch films through processor
7. Check replenishment rates (also check several times throughout the day)
8. Check developer temperature after warm-up

B. Shutdown procedure
1. Turn off water source
2. Turn off processor
3. Open wash tank valve and drain tank
4. Wash crossover racks
5. Leave lid ajar several inches to prevent contamination of solutions resulting from condensation

C. Cleaning
1. Daily
   a. Wash crossover racks (start-up and shutdown or morning and evening)
   b. Drain wash tank
2. Weekly
   a. Clean deep racks
   b. Change water filters
3. Monthly
   a. Drain and clean by hand all tanks and dryer
   b. Put in fresh developer and fixer
   c. Add starter solution to developer chemicals
   d. Change developer filter

D. Sensitometric testing
1. Performed daily on every processor
2. Ensures consistent processing of films by monitoring speed, contrast, and base plus fog (routine may also include measuring developer temperature)
3. Film from control box is exposed using a sensitometer
4. Film is processed
5. Speed step on film is measured using densitometer
6. Contrast step on film is measured using densitometer and subtracted from speed step
7. Speed and contrast are plotted on sensitometric graph
8. Values must not fluctuate more than ±0.10 from baseline
9. Unexposed region of film is measured using densitometer
10. Value given is base plus fog
11. Value must not fluctuate more than 0.05 from baseline
12. Speed and contrast steps are chosen from the H & D curve for the control film
    a. Speed step is the step closest to density reading of 1
    b. Contrast step is the step near the top of the straight-line portion of the curve, just below the shoulder

Processor Malfunctions

A. Artifacts (Figures 4-14 through 4-17)
1. Unwanted, irregular mark or density on the radiograph
2. Guide shoe scratches
   a. Straight-line scratches, at regular intervals, running in direction of film travel
   b. Caused by guide shoes being out of adjustment
   c. Guide shoes must be readjusted

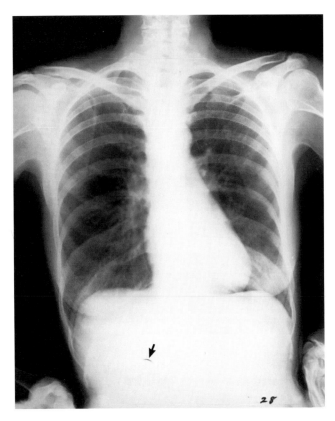

Figure 4-14 Plus-density half-moon artifacts can be caused by bending or kinking the film before exposure.

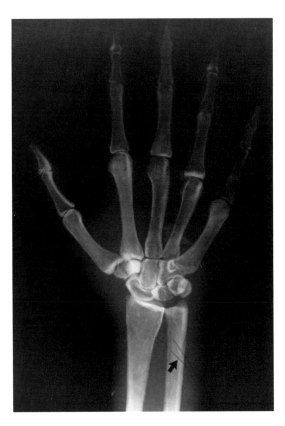

Figure 4-15 Plus-density scratch artifacts can be caused by a fingernail before exposure.

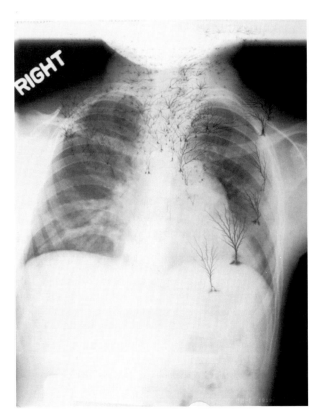

Figure 4-16 Plus-density static discharge artifact can be caused by sliding a film over a flat surface.

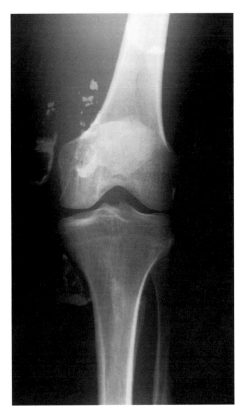

Figure 4-17 Minus-density caused by moisture on finger before exposure.

3. Pi lines
   a. Small marks on radiograph 3.1416 inches apart on 1-inch rollers
   b. Caused by raised nick on roller scratching film as it passes by
   c. Also caused by chemical stain or dirt on roller
   d. Roller must either be replaced or carefully cleaned
B. Temperature fluctuations
   1. Increased developer temperature causes chemical fog and increased density
      a. Temperature must be adjusted
      b. Thermostat must be examined for possible malfunction
   2. Decreased developer temperature causes decreased density
      a. Temperature must be adjusted
      b. Thermostat must be examined for possible malfunction
   3. Damp films emerge from processor
      a. Dryer temperature must be increased
      b. Dryer thermostat must be examined for possible malfunction
   4. Damp films may also exist during times of high humidity when air within dryer compartment is saturated
      a. Dryer temperature may be increased
      b. Front of the processor may be temporarily removed to allow humidity to escape
C. Contamination
   1. Fixer solution splashing into developer tank in amount as small as 1 ml will cause contamination
   2. Verified by checking for odor of ammonia in developer solution
   3. Will cause increased density on films
   4. May occur when fixer deep rack is put back in place too rapidly and chemicals pour over divider
   5. May occur secondary to film jam if films splash around and spray fixer back into developer
   6. Processor must be immediately shut down; developer tank must be drained, completely cleaned, and refilled with fresh solution
D. Jamming (Figure 4-18)
   1. Films caught during transport
   2. Rollers out of alignment
      a. May be caused by tension springs on the end of the racks breaking, which releases rollers from proper position
      b. May be caused by inadequate replenishment rate, depriving the film of hardener, which allows the emulsion to swell to the point where it will not pass between the rollers
E. Photographic anomalies: causes and corrections
   1. Dark films
      a. Developer temperature too high: adjust
      b. Developer overreplenishment: correct

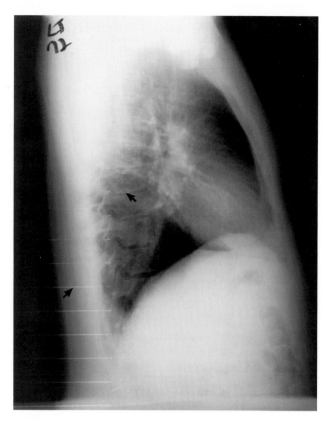

Figure 4-18 Minus-density scratch artifacts can be caused by transport rollers.

   c. Fixer contamination of developer: clean and replace
   d. White light leak: find and correct
   e. Crack in safelight filter: replace
   2. Light films
      a. Developer temperature too low—adjust
      b. Underreplenishment—correct
   3. Films appear milky: poor fixer replenishment—correct
   4. Films appear greasy: inadequate washing—check water flow rate and level of water in tank
   5. Dark flakes: algae from wash water—drain tank, clean rollers
   6. Film fog
      a. Developer contamination—drain and clean tank; add fresh solution
      b. Developer overreplenishment—correct
      c. White light leak—find and correct
      d. Crack in safelight filter—replace
      e. Developer temperature too high—correct
      f. Outdated film—verify with date on box, discard if outdated

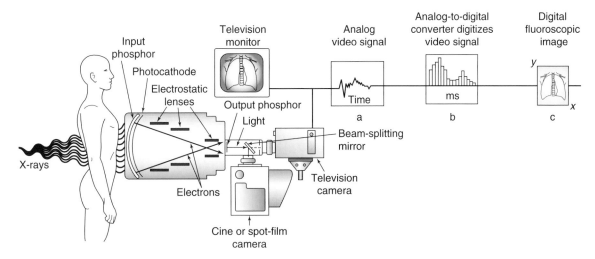

Figure 4-19 Analog and digital signals in fluoroscopy. The video signal from the television camera is analog, where the voltage signal varies continuously. This analog signal is sampled *(a)*, producing a stepped representation of the analog video signal *(b)*. The numerical values of each step are stored *(c)*, producing a matrix of digital image data. (Courtesy Eastman Kodak Company.)

Digital Imaging Units

A. Digital fluoroscopy (Figure 4-19)
  1. Initial image is obtained in a manner similar to technique of conventional fluoroscopy and sent to monitor
  2. The analog signal is sent through an analog-to-digital converter (ADC) to convert information into numerical data
  3. Viewing should take place on a high-resolution monitor to take advantage of the digital capabilities
  4. Postprocessing manipulation of the image is possible because the image is in digital format
B. Computed radiography (Figure 4-20)
  1. Radiographer selects exposure factors, as in conventional radiography
  2. Accurate positioning remains critical
  3. Image receptor is an imaging plate (IP)
     a. Made of a photostimulable phosphor that absorbs the photon energies exiting the patient
     b. Energy in the IP is released by scanning with a laser beam inside the reader unit
     c. Energy is then converted from analog to digital form and sent to the computer for processing
  4. IP can store the image for several hours, but after that the energy slowly dissipates and the latent image fades
  5. The correct algorithm (mathematical formula) must be chosen so that the computer can reconstruct the image specific to the examination that was performed
C. Image characteristics
  1. Wider exposure latitude than with conventional radiography
  2. Exhibits better visualization of soft tissue and bone
  3. Conversion of the image into data allows for postprocessing image enhancement
     a. Subtraction, edge enhancement, contrast enhancement, and black/white reversal
     b. Subtraction: removal of superimposed or unwanted structures from the image
     c. Contrast enhancement: altering of image to display varying brightnesses
     d. Edge enhancement: improves visibility of small high-contrast areas
     e. Black/white reversal: reversal of the gray scale in the image
  4. Digital image is composed of rows and columns called a matrix
     a. Smallest component of the matrix is the pixel (picture element)
     b. Each pixel corresponds to a shade of gray representing an area in the patient called a *voxel* (volume element)
  5. Postprocessing can compensate for overexposures or underexposures of considerable degrees
     a. Because radiographers comply with the ALARA (as low as reasonably achievable) concept, the patients should never be overexposed with the intention of correcting the resultant images in the postprocessing mode
  6. Image may be printed onto film with a laser camera
  7. At present, resolution is limited to approximately 2.5 line pairs per millimeter
  8. Changing the window level (midpoint of densities) adjusts the image brightness throughout the range of densities

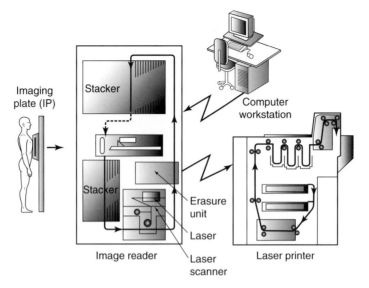

Figure 4-20 The exposed imaging plate is placed in a reader unit to release the stored image, convert the analog image to a digital image, and send the data to a computer monitor or a laser printer. The reader unit also erases the exposed imaging plate in preparation for the next exposure. (Courtesy Fuji Medical Systems.)

9. Changing the window width adjusts the radiographic contrast in postprocessing mode
10. Quantum mottle is a source of noise in the image, as in conventional radiography
11. Artifacts may be present in computed radiography
    a. May be caused by dust on the imaging plate
    b. Improper use of grids may cause a moiré pattern
    c. Scatter radiation is easily imaged with the sensitive IP
12. Computed radiography may be part of an integrated system of images and written data called *PACS*
    a. PACS: picture archiving and communications system
    b. May be combined with radiology information systems (RIS) and hospital information systems (HIS)
    c. Network links images, patient data, radiologist reports, and so forth into one seamless system

REVIEW QUESTIONS

For each of the following questions, choose the single best answer.

1. Density may be defined as:
   a. Differences in opacities on a radiograph
   b. The logarithm of opacity
   c. The darkness on a radiograph
   d. b and c

2. Most of the latent image is formed by:
   a. Exit rays striking the film's emulsion
   b. Light from intensifying screen phosphors responding to scatter radiation
   c. Cosmic rays
   d. Light from intensifying screen phosphors produced in response to exit rays

3. The primary controlling factor of density is:
   a. kVp
   b. mAs
   c. SID
   d. OID

4. Which of the following describes the relationship between mAs and density?
   1. Density is directly proportional to mAs
   2. Density is inversely proportional to mAs
   3. Density is directly proportional to mAs^2
   4. mAs controls the number of electrons boiled off the anode and therefore the number of x rays produced
   5. The number of electrons boiled off the cathode and consequently the number of x rays produced are controlled by mAs
   a. All of the above
   b. 1, 4
   c. 2, 5
   d. 1, 5

5. The law stating that any combinations of mA and time that produce the same mAs value will produce the same radiographic density is the:
a. Inverse square law
b. mAs-density law
c. Reciprocity law
d. 15% law

6. $\dfrac{\text{Light incident}}{\text{Light transmitted}}$ is best described as:
a. The ratio of light being seen from the radiograph divided by the light from the view box striking the radiograph
b. Radiographic contrast
c. The latent image
d. The ratio of the light striking the radiograph from the view box divided by the light transmitted through the radiograph

7. mAs directly controls:
a. The energy of the x-ray emission spectrum
b. The quality and quantity of x rays produced at the cathode
c. The quality and quantity of x rays produced at the anode
d. The quantity of x rays produced

8. Differences in densities on a radiograph describe:
a. Density
b. Recorded detail
c. Log relative exposure
d. Contrast

9. The primary controlling factor of contrast is:
a. mAs, which controls the energy of the x rays produced
b. kVp, which controls the quantity of x rays produced at the target
c. Focal spot size, which controls the quantity and quality of x rays produced
d. kVp, which controls the quality of x rays produced at the anode

10. The relationship between kVp and density may be described as:
a. Directly proportional
b. Direct, although not proportional
c. Governed by the 15-50 rule
d. Controlled by x-ray tube current

11. The 15% rule states that:
a. Density may be halved by decreasing kVp by 15%
b. kVp should be 15% of the mAs selected
c. Density may be doubled by increasing kVp by 15%
d. More than one but not all of the above

12. Which of the following is (are) true concerning the role of kVp in radiograph production?
1. As kVp is increased, penetrating ability of the x rays increases
2. As kVp is increased, more x rays exit the patient to strike the film-screen system
3. As kVp is decreased, wavelength and density decrease
4. As kVp increases, radiographic density increases
5. As kVp decreases, radiographic density remains constant because mAs controls density
a. 1, 2, 4
b. 1, 2, 3
c. 1, 3, 4
d. 5

13. Given an original technique of 30 mAs and 80 kVp, which of the following will produce a radiograph with double the density?
a. 60 mAs, 90 kVp
b. 30 mAs, 92 kVp
c. 60 mAs, 80 kVp
d. More than one but not all of the above

14. Which of the following describes the relationship between SID and density?
a. Reciprocity law
b. 15% rule
c. Inverse square law
d. $\dfrac{\text{Old mAs}}{\text{New mAs}} = \dfrac{\text{New distance}}{\text{Old distance}}$

15. If SID is doubled, what may be said about radiographic density?
a. Density doubles
b. Density is reduced by half
c. Density is reduced by new mAs^2
d. Density is reduced to one fourth

16. If SID is reduced by half, what must be done to mAs to maintain a constant density?
a. Reduce mAs to one fourth its original value
b. Reduce mAs to half its original value
c. Increase mAs by four times its original value
d. Increase mAs by two times its original value

17. Which of the following describes the relationship between film-screen system speed and density?
a. System speed is inversely proportional to density
b. Density is inversely proportional to system speed
c. Density is directly proportional to system speed
d. There is no relationship between system speed and density

18. As film-screen system sensitivity decreases:
   a. Radiographic density decreases
   b. Radiographic density increases
   c. Radiographic contrast increases
   d. Recorded detail decreases

19. As film-screen system speed increases:
   a. Radiographic density decreases
   b. Radiographic contrast decreases
   c. Radiographic density increases
   d. a and b

20. Which of the following describes the relationship between radiographic density and the use of grids?
   a. Grids always reduce density
   b. Grids reduce density unless mAs is increased to compensate
   c. Grids reduce density by absorbing scatter radiation
   d. Density increases as grid ratio increases

21. The use of filtration:
   a. Greatly reduces radiographic density because of the absorption of short-wavelength x rays
   b. Greatly reduces radiographic density because of the absorption of high-energy x rays
   c. Increases radiographic density by removing long-wavelength x rays
   d. Has little effect on density because x rays removed from beam are not image-producing rays

22. As beam restriction increases (tighter):
   a. Density increases
   b. Density increases as a result of focusing of x rays
   c. Density decreases
   d. Density is not affected

23. Which of the following affect radiographic density?
   a. Atomic number of anatomic structures
   b. Tissue density of anatomic structures altered by pathology
   c. Tissue thickness
   d. All of the above

24. The variation of x-ray intensity along the longitudinal axis of the x-ray beam describes:
   a. Beam collimation
   b. Positive beam limitation
   c. Anode heel effect
   d. X-ray emission spectrum

25. The thicker part of anatomy should be placed under which aspect of the x-ray tube?
   a. Central ray
   b. Cathode
   c. Anode
   d. Collimator

26. Contrast may be defined as:
   a. The slope of the characteristic curve of a film
   b. Difference in densities on a radiograph
   c. The radiographic quality that makes detail visible
   d. All of the above

27. A radiograph with few gray tones, primarily exhibiting black and white, would be described as having what type of contrast?
   1. Long scale
   2. Short scale
   3. Low
   4. High
   a. 2 and 4
   b. 1 and 3
   c. 1 and 4
   d. 2

28. The primary controlling factor of contrast is:
   a. mAs
   b. Focal spot size
   c. OID
   d. kVp

29. High kVp produces which of the following?
   1. High contrast
   2. Few gray tones
   3. Long-scale contrast
   4. Short-scale contrast
   5. Low contrast
   6. Many gray tones
   a. 1, 2, 4
   b. 3, 5, 6
   c. 5
   d. 1

30. Low kVp produces which of the following?
   1. High contrast
   2. Few gray tones
   3. Long-scale contrast
   4. Short-scale contrast
   5. Low contrast
   6. Many gray tones
   a. 1, 2, 4
   b. 3, 5, 6
   c. 5
   d. 1

31. More uniform penetration of anatomic structures occurs when using what level of kVp?
   a. Low
   b. High
   c. kVp does not affect penetration
   d. Level at which photoelectric interaction predominates

32. Differential absorption of the x-ray beam is a function of:
   a. Photoelectric interaction
   b. Atomic number of anatomic structures
   c. kVp
   d. All of the above

33. Beam restriction has the following effect on contrast:
   a. Decreases contrast by focusing x-ray beam
   b. Decreases contrast because of higher kVp level used
   c. Increases contrast because of reduction in the number of Compton's interactions that occur
   d. All of the above

34. The adjustment in technical factors required when using beam restriction is:
   a. Increase kVp
   b. Decrease kVp to reduce the number of Compton's interactions taking place
   c. Decrease mAs to reduce the number of Compton's interactions taking place
   d. Increase mAs to compensate for the number of rays removed from the primary beam

35. The use of radiographic grids has the following effect on contrast:
   a. Decreases contrast
   b. Increases contrast
   c. No effect on contrast
   d. Increases contrast by absorbing scatter radiation

36. As the amount of beam filtration is increased:
   a. Contrast increases
   b. There is no effect on contrast
   c. Contrast decreases
   d. Contrast increases because beam is harder

37. The portion of contrast that is caused by variations in the anatomy or is secondary to pathologic changes is called:
   a. Radiographic contrast
   b. Anatomic contrast
   c. Pathologic contrast
   d. Subject contrast

38. Recorded detail is:
   a. Definition of the image
   b. Sharpness with which structures are imaged
   c. Geometric representation of the part being radiographed
   d. All of the above

39. Poor recorded detail may be caused by which of the following factors?
   1. Long SID
   2. Long OID
   3. Short SID
   4. Short OID
   5. Large focal spot
   6. Small focal spot
   7. Patient motion
   8. Magnification
   9. High-speed film-screen combination
   10. Low-speed film-screen combination
   11. X-ray tube motion
   a. 2, 3, 5, 7, 8, 9, 11
   b. 1, 4, 6, 8, 10
   c. 1, 4, 6, 10
   d. 2, 3, 6, 9

40. Optimum recorded detail may be caused by which of the following factors?
   1. Long SID
   2. Long OID
   3. Short SID
   4. Short OID
   5. Large focal spot
   6. Small focal spot
   7. Patient motion
   8. Magnification
   9. High-speed film-screen combination
   10. Low-speed film-screen combination
   11. X-ray tube motion
   a. 2, 3, 5, 7, 8, 9, 11
   b. 1, 4, 6, 8, 10
   c. 1, 4, 6, 10
   d. 2, 3, 6, 9

41. Film-screen system effect on recorded detail is controlled by:
   a. Size of the screen's phosphors
   b. Size of the film's silver halide crystals
   c. Thickness of the screen's active layer
   d. All of the above

42. Distortion may be described as:
   a. Misrepresentation of an anatomic structure on film
   b. Foreshortening
   c. Elongation
   d. Magnification

43. Elongation and foreshortening are examples of:
   a. Size distortion
   b. Shape distortion
   c. Motion
   d. Distortion caused by short SID and long OID

44. Magnification is caused by:
1. Short SID
2. Long SID
3. Short OID
4. Long OID
5. Long SOD
6. Short SOD
a. 2, 3, 5
b. 1, 4, 5
c. 1, 3, 6
d. 1, 4, 6

45. Distortion that occurs when the x-ray beam is angled against the long axis of a part is:
a. Elongation
b. Magnification
c. Minification
d. Foreshortening

46. Distortion that occurs when the x-ray beam is angled along the long axis of a part is:
a. Elongation
b. Magnification
c. Minification
d. Misrepresentation

47. The purpose of adding blue dye to the base of radiographic film is to:
a. Reduce glare when viewing the image
b. Enhance radiographic contrast
c. Reduce exposure to the patient
d. a and b

48. The emulsion of radiographic film consists of:
a. Silver halide crystals suspended in plastic
b. Sensitivity specks attached to silver halide crystals
c. Gelatin in which silver halide crystals are suspended
d. b and c

49. Sensitivity specks on silver halide crystals serve as:
a. Focus centers for x rays
b. Development centers for building the manifest image
c. Crystals that allow the gelatin to expand and contract
d. Gatekeepers for photon-crystal interactions

50. Characteristics associated with high-speed film are:
1. Small silver halide crystals
2. Thick emulsion layer
3. Low film contrast
4. Large silver halide crystals
5. High film contrast
6. Thin emulsion layer
7. Wide latitude
8. Long-scale contrast
9. Narrow latitude
10. Short-scale contrast
a. 1, 3, 6, 7, 8
b. 1, 2, 5, 7, 10
c. 2, 4, 5, 9, 10
d. 3, 4, 6, 7, 8

51. Characteristics associated with slow-speed film are:
1. Small silver halide crystals
2. Thick emulsion layer
3. Low film contrast
4. Large silver halide crystals
5. High film contrast
6. Thin emulsion layer
7. Wide latitude
8. Long-scale contrast
9. Narrow latitude
10. Short-scale contrast
a. 1, 3, 6, 7, 8
b. 1, 2, 5, 7, 10
c. 2, 4, 5, 9, 10
d. 3, 4, 6, 7, 8

52. A film's response to radiation exposure may be plotted using a graph known as the:
a. H & D curve
b. Sensitometric curve
c. Characteristic curve
d. All of the above

Use Figure 4-21 to answer questions **53-63:**

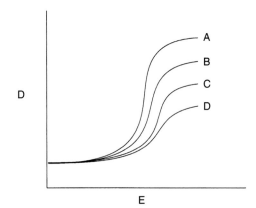

Figure 4-21

53. Which film is slowest?

54. Which film has the highest contrast?

55. Which film has the thinnest emulsion?

56. Which film has the narrowest latitude?

57. Which film has the lowest contrast?

58. Which film is fastest?

59. Which film has the thickest emulsion?

60. Which film provides the best recorded detail?

61. Which film has the widest latitude?

62. Which film has the poorest recorded detail?

63. Which film would most student radiographers prefer to use because of latitude?

For each of the following questions, choose the single best answer.

64. Which of the following best describes ideal storage conditions for x-ray film?
   a. Protected from radiation, fumes, outdating
   b. 68% to 70% humidity, 40° to 60° F
   c. 68° to 70° F, 40% to 60% humidity
   d. a and c

65. Characteristics associated with high-speed intensifying screens are:
   1. Poor contrast
   2. Poor recorded detail
   3. Thin active layer
   4. Good contrast
   5. Yellow dye incorporated into phosphor layer
   6. Small phosphors
   7. Good recorded detail
   8. Thick active layer
   9. Large phosphors
   10. Lower conversion efficiency
   11. Higher relative speed number
   12. Lower relative speed number
   13. Low intensification factor
   14. High intensification factor
   15. Higher conversion efficiency
   a. 2, 4, 5, 8, 9, 10, 11, 15
   b. 1, 3, 5, 6, 7, 10, 12, 13
   c. 2, 8, 9, 11, 14, 15
   d. 1, 2, 3, 6, 11, 14

66. Characteristics associated with slower-speed intensifying screens are:
   1. Poor contrast
   2. Poor recorded detail
   3. Thin active layer
   4. Good contrast
   5. Yellow dye incorporated into phosphor layer
   6. Small phosphors
   7. Good recorded detail
   8. Thick active layer
   9. Large phosphors
   10. Lower conversion efficiency
   11. Higher relative speed number
   12. Lower relative speed number
   13. Low intensification factor
   14. High intensification factor
   15. Higher conversion efficiency
   a. 2, 4, 5, 8, 9, 10, 11, 15
   b. 3, 5, 6, 7, 10, 12, 13
   c. 2, 4, 8, 9, 11, 14, 15
   d. 1, 2, 3, 6, 11, 14

67. Grid ratio is defined as:
   a. The ratio of the lead strips to the space between them
   b. The thickness of the lead strips divided by the thickness of the aluminum interspacers
   c. The ratio of the height of the lead strips over the distance between the lead strips
   d. The ratio of the distance between the lead strips over the height of the lead strips

68. Grid frequency is defined as:
   a. The same as grid ratio
   b. The amount of lead in the grid (expressed in terms of focusing distance)
   c. How often a grid is used
   d. The amount of lead in the grid (expressed as the number of lead strips per inch)

69. Which of the following statements concerning grids are true?
1. Contrast improvement factor is the measure of a grid's ability to enhance contrast
2. Grid selectivity is the ratio of primary radiation transmitted through the grid to secondary radiation transmitted through the grid
3. Grids are used when part thickness is less than 10 cm
4. Grid conversion factor is the amount of increase in kVp necessary when converting from nongrid to grid technique
5. Their primary purpose is radiation protection
6. Their main function is to prevent Compton's scatter from reaching the film
7. Grids prevent the production of scatter
   a. 1, 2, 6
   b. 1, 2, 4, 6
   c. 1, 2, 3, 5, 7
   d. 1, 2, 6, 7

70. A grid with lead strips and aluminum interspacers that are angled to coincide with the divergence of the x-ray beam is called a:
   a. Parallel grid
   b. Focused grid
   c. Crosshatch grid
   d. Rhombic grid

71. The range of SIDs that may be used with a focused grid is called:
   a. Grid ratio
   b. Objective plane
   c. Anticutoff distances
   d. Grid radius

72. The best scatter cleanup is achieved with the use of:
   a. Air gap technique
   b. Focused grids
   c. Crosshatch grids
   d. Parallel grids

73. Grid cutoff may be described as:
   a. Decreased density in the middle of the radiograph caused by the use of a parallel grid inserted upside down
   b. Decreased density on a radiograph as a result of absorption of image-forming rays
   c. Increased density in the center of a radiograph caused by the use of a focused grid inserted upside down
   d. Decreased density on the edges of a radiograph only

74. When changing from a nongrid technique using 10 mAs and 75 kVp to a 12:1 grid using 75 kVp, what new mAs must be used to maintain the same density as the original film?
   a. 50 mAs
   b. 2 mAs
   c. 40 mAs
   d. 120 mAs

75. The use of air gap technique:
   a. Works because x rays are absorbed in the air between the patient and the film
   b. Should occur when possible
   c. May cause some magnification because of decreased OID
   d. Works because scatter radiation travels in divergent paths and misses the film as a result of increased OID

76. The use of technique charts:
   a. Is unnecessary for any exam because of AECs
   b. Requires the part thickness to be measured using calipers
   c. Is usually based on fixed kVp and variable mAs
   d. Some of the above

77. When AEC is used, increasing the kVp will:
   a. Increase density proportionately
   b. Increase radiographic contrast
   c. Increase exposure time
   d. Have no effect on density

78. The function of automatic processing is to:
   a. Make the latent image visible
   b. Convert exposed silver halide crystals to black metallic silver
   c. Prepare the radiograph for viewing and storage
   d. All of the above

79. Which of the following are contained in the developer solution?
   1. Activator
   2. Hypo
   3. Hardener
   4. Preservative
   5. Reducing agents
   6. Water
   7. Acidifier
   8. Restrainer
   a. 2, 3, 4, 6, 7
   b. 5, 6, 8
   c. 1, 3, 4, 5, 6, 8
   d. 1, 2, 5, 6

80. Which of the following are contained in the fixer solution?
1. Activator
2. Hypo
3. Hardener
4. Preservative
5. Reducing agents
6. Water
7. Acidifier
8. Restrainer
a. 2, 3, 4, 6, 7
b. 5, 6, 8
c. 1, 3, 4, 5, 6, 8
d. 1, 2, 5, 6

81. Which of the following statements is true concerning developer solution?
1. The reducing agents convert all silver halide crystals to black metallic silver
2. A hardener is added to the developer to control the swelling of the emulsion
3. The activator keeps the chemicals at full strength
4. The reducing agents convert all silver halide crystals with sensitivity specks to black metallic silver
5. Rapid oxidation of the reducing agents is prevented by mixing them in water
6. The preservative keeps the finished radiograph from yellowing while in storage
a. All are true
b. 2
c. None are true
d. 4, 5, 6

82. Which of the following statements are false concerning the fixer solution?
1. Fixing agent clears all silver halide crystals from the emulsion
2. Water keeps the fixer solution neutral
3. Rapid oxidation of the solution is prevented by the use of a preservative
4. The hardener shrinks and hardens the emulsion
5. Hypo removes all unexposed silver halide crystals
a. 3, 4, 5
b. All are true
c. 1, 2, 5
d. 1, 2

83. Which of the following statements is true concerning automatic processing chemistry?
1. Developer is kept at 90° to 95° C
2. Fixer is an acidic solution
3. The preservative helps prevent rapid oxidation by room air
4. Developer is an alkaline solution
5. The restrainer prevents the reducing agents from developing the unexposed silver halide crystals
6. Water is the solvent in which chemicals are mixed
7. The activator softens and swells the film's emulsion so that chemistry can come in contact with the silver halide crystals
8. The hardener in the developer controls the swelling of the emulsion so that silver halide crystals do not escape into solution
a. All are true
b. 1, 2, 3, 4, 5, 6, 7
c. 2, 3, 4, 5, 6, 7
d. 1, 2, 3, 4, 5, 6

84. The function of the wash tank is to:
a. Neutralize all chemistry
b. Stop development
c. Rinse away unexposed silver halide crystals
d. Remove chemistry from film

85. Which of the following statements best describes the transport system of an automatic processor?
a. Moves film through processor with a series of rollers and racks and agitates chemistry
b. Moves film through the processor and maintains solution strength
c. Moves film through the developer and fixer and agitates chemistry
d. Moves film through the processor, maintains solution strength, and activates replenishment system

86. Which of the following statements best describes the replenishment system of an automatic processor?
a. Adds fresh developer, fixer, and water each time a film is fed into the processor
b. Adds fresh developer and fixer each time a film is fed into the processor
c. Adds fresh developer as film is being fed into the processor
d. Maintains solution strength and temperature as film is fed into the processor

87. Which of the following statements best describes the recirculation system of an automatic processor?
   a. Adds fresh chemistry and maintains temperature
   b. Maintains developer temperature at 90° to 95° F
   c. Agitates developer solution, maintains temperature, removes by-products of chemical reactions
   d. Maintains chemistry temperature and concentration

88. Which of the following statements best describes the dryer system of an automatic processor?
   a. Helps seal emulsion with heat, dries film, works at approximately 120° C
   b. Dries film as it passes between tubes blowing hot air
   c. Dries film after it leaves fixer and seals emulsion with hot air
   d. Helps seal emulsion with heat, dries film, works at approximately 120° F

89. Which of the following statements describe the maintenance schedule for an automatic processor?
   1. Wash tank should be drained at the end of each workday
   2. Entire processor should be cleaned weekly
   3. Fresh developer should be added daily after cleaning developer tank
   4. Lid on processor should be left open after shutdown to allow chemical evaporation to escape
   5. Several 14- × 17-inch films should be run through the processor at start-up
   6. Crossover racks should be cleaned at start-up and shutdown
   7. All tanks, racks, and rollers should be thoroughly cleaned monthly
   8. Starter solution should be added to developer and fixer when refilling after cleaning
   a. 1, 4, 5, 6, 7, 8
   b. 1, 2, 4, 5, 6, 7
   c. 1, 3, 4, 6, 7
   d. 1, 4, 5, 6, 7

90. When sensitometric testing is performed on an automatic processor, the acceptable range of variation for speed and contrast is:
   a. ±0.05
   b. ±0.10
   c. ±0.01
   d. ±0.25

91. When sensitometric testing is performed on an automatic processor, the acceptable range of variation for base plus fog is:
   a. ±0.05
   b. ±0.10
   c. ±0.01
   d. ±0.25

92. Sensitometric testing of automatic processors should be performed:
   a. Weekly
   b. Monthly
   c. Daily
   d. Several times each day

93. Emulsion scratches that run the length of the film in the direction of film travel are usually caused by:
   a. Pi lines
   b. Improper cleaning of rollers
   c. Inadequate replenishment
   d. Guide shoes out of adjustment

94. Contamination of developer by fixer will cause:
   a. Decreased contrast
   b. A chemical reaction that will release the odor of ammonia
   c. Increased fog on the radiograph
   d. All of the above

95. Jamming of films in the processor may be caused by:
   a. All of the below
   b. Rollers out of alignment
   c. Racks improperly seated in place
   d. Inadequate replenishment

Figure 4-22 provides H & D curves for the same film processed under varying conditions. Use it to answer questions **96-100**:

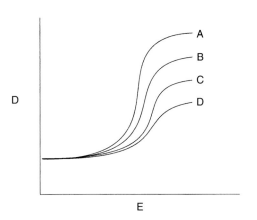

Figure 4-22

96. Which curve represents the film's response to inadequate drying?
a. A
b. B
c. C
d. None of the curves indicates this condition

97. Which curve represents the film's response to extended development time?
a. A
b. B
c. C
d. D

98. Which curve represents the film's response to developer under replenishment?
a. A
b. B
c. C
d. D

99. Which curve represents the film's response to chemical contamination?
a. A
b. B
c. C
d. D

100. Which curve represents the film's response to decreased developer temperature?
a. A
b. B
c. C
d. D

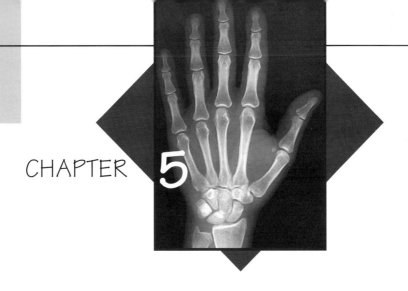

Some people dream of worthy accomplishments, while others stay awake and do them.

Review of Radiographic Procedures: Anatomy, Positioning, Procedures, Pathology

BASIC PRINCIPLES OF POSITIONING AND PROCEDURES

A. Body part placement
1. Body part should be placed on the cassette in a position that allows imaging of all anatomic features required for the procedure
2. Allow for tight collimation

B. Alignment: the long axis of the body part should correspond to the long axis of the film, except when the cassette must be rotated to fit the entire part on the film

C. Two or more projections on the same film
1. Lead strip should always be used to mask unexposed portion of cassette
2. Using only collimation may cause overlap of images; radiograph not as easy to view
3. Long axis of the bone should be oriented in the same direction for both projections

D. Precise visualization
1. Positioning must be absolutely accurate
2. No rotation of image present

E. Patient identification
1. Identification marker on cassette should not obstruct view of relevant anatomy
2. Patient information should include name and date of exam

F. Anatomic markers
1. Right or left markers must always appear on the radiograph; use a radiopaque marker placed on the cassette

2. Stickers, grease pencil writing, or felt-tip writing on the radiograph after processing are not considered legal markings; these should be used only in rare circumstances
3. Radiopaque markers must be placed just inside the collimation field and should not obstruct relevant anatomy

G. Other markers
1. Time: time indicators should always be used when radiographs are taken at specifically timed intervals
2. Direction: if the radiograph was taken erect, the lead marker indicating erect or upright must appear on the radiograph
3. Inspiration/expiration: must be used for comparison studies of the chest
4. Internal/external: must be used when both forms of rotation constitute part of an examination
5. Numeric markers: must be used when taking a series of radiographs in sequence (e.g., during trauma or surgical cases when follow-up is required in a short time)

H. Routines
1. Minimum of two views per examination except for certain cases in which a single survey radiograph suffices (e.g., kidney, ureter, bladder [KUB])
2. A minimum of two projections, 90 degrees from one another, must always be taken
    a. Superimposition of structures may prevent the visualization of some pathologic conditions

b. Lesions or foreign bodies require precise localization
c. Fractures must be seen from two points precisely 90 degrees from each other
d. Minimum of three projections (anteroposterior [AP] or posteroanterior [PA], lateral, and oblique) required for proper visualization of joints

POSITIONING TERMINOLOGY

Anterior or ventral　forward or front
Caudal, inferior　away from the head
Central　midarea
Cranial, cephalic, superior　toward the head
Distal　farthest from the origin or point of reference
Lateral　away from the median plane of the body or the middle of a part
Medial　toward the median plane of the body or the middle of a part
Posterior, dorsal　back of a part (not used to describe foot)
Proximal　nearer origin or point of reference
Dorsal recumbent　supine, lying on back
Ventral recumbent　prone, lying face down
Right lateral recumbent　lying on right side
Left lateral recumbent　lying on left side
Projection　path of the central ray
Position　placement of the body or part
View　image as seen by the image receptor (opposite of projection)
Oblique　body rotated from supine, prone, or lateral
RAO　oblique angle that places right anterior portion of the body closest to the film
LAO　oblique angle that places left anterior portion of the body closest to the film
LPO　oblique angle that places left posterior part of the body closest to the film
RPO　oblique angle that places right posterior portion of the body closest to the film
Decubitus position　patient lying down; central ray parallel to the floor (horizontal)
Left or right lateral decubitus　patient lying on left or right side; central ray parallel to the floor (horizontal); AP or PA projection
Dorsal decubitus　patient lying on back; central ray parallel to the floor (horizontal), lateral projection
Ventral decubitus　patient lying on abdomen; central ray parallel to the floor (horizontal), lateral projection
Tangential　central ray skims between body parts or skims body surface; shows profile of body part, free of superimposition
Axial　longitudinal angulation of the central ray with the long axis of the body part; projection that refers to images obtained with central ray angled 10 degrees or more along long axis of part

TOPOGRAPHY

A. Cervical region
　1. C1: mastoid tip
　2. C2, C3: gonion
　3. C5: thyroid cartilage
　4. C7: vertebra prominens
B. Thoracic region
　1. T1: 2 inches above sternal notch
　2. T2, T3: level of manubrial notch and superior margin of scapula
　3. T4, T5: level of sternal angle
　4. T7: level of inferior angle of scapula
　5. T10: level of xiphoid tip
C. Lumbar region
　1. L3: costal margin
　2. L3, L4: level of umbilicus
　3. L4: level of most superior aspect of iliac crest
D. Sacrum and pelvic region
　1. S1: level of anterior superior iliac spine (ASIS)
　2. Coccyx: level of pubic symphysis and greater trochanters
E. Lines
　1. Orbitomeatal line (OML)
　　a. Line from outer canthus of the eye to the auricular point
　　b. Seven-degree angle with infraorbitomeatal line (IOML)
　　c. Eight-degree angle with the glabellomeatal line
　　d. Also called the *radiographic baseline*
　2. Infraorbitomeatal line (also called *Reid's baseline*)
　　a. Line from just below the eye to the auricular point
　　b. Seven-degree angle with the OML
　3. Glabellomeatal line
　　a. Line from the glabella to the auricular point
　　b. Eight-degree angle with the OML
　4. Acanthiomeatal line (AML)
　　a. Line from acanthion to the auricular point

MOTION CONTROL

A. Involuntary motion (controlled with short exposure time and high-speed film-screen combination)
　1. Cardiac motion
　2. Peristalsis
　3. Muscular spasm
　4. Chills
　5. Pain
B. Voluntary motion
　1. Belligerence
　2. Excitement
　3. Fear

4. Nervousness
5. Painful discomfort
6. Age (children, elderly)
7. Controlled by the use of the following
   a. Clear communications
   b. Sandbags
   c. Sponges
   d. Tape
   e. Short exposure time
   f. Patient comfort
   g. Compression bands
   h. Pigg-o-stat (for infants)
   i. Sheets for mummification techniques (for children)
   j. Instructions: clearly explain the examination to the patient
   k. Obtain signature on consent form if required
   l. Ask patient if there are any questions to be answered, ensuring informed consent
   m. Describe examination in terminology the patient will understand
   n. Describe exactly what will be done to the patient, including the approximate number of radiographs to be taken and the duration of the exam
   o. Explain the reasons for removal of clothing and the extent of gowning
   p. Explain the reason for removal of all radiopaque objects in the area of interest
   q. Describe the required breathing pattern and the reasons for its use

EXPOSURE MODIFICATION

A. Use of optimal radiographic technique will ensure proper visualization of body parts
B. Exposure technique may need to be modified because of certain factors
   1. Pathologic conditions
   2. Age
   3. Conditions under which the radiographs are being taken (e.g., mobile radiography, crosstable projections)
   4. Body habitus

GONADAL SHIELDING

A. Used when gonads are within the primary beam or within 5 cm of the primary beam
B. Used if the shielding does not interfere with the purpose of the exam
C. Used on patients of reproductive age and younger

BODY HABITUS

A. Hypersthenic
   1. Massive build
   2. Represents 5% of the population
   3. Thorax is broad and deep
   4. Ribs are almost horizontal
   5. Thoracic cavity is shallow
   6. Lungs are short; narrow above and broad at the base
   7. Heart is short and wide
   8. Diaphragm is high
   9. Upper abdominal cavity is broad; lower part is small
   10. Stomach and gallbladder are high, horizontal
   11. Colon is high
B. Sthenic
   1. Slight modification of hypersthenic
   2. Most common body habitus
   3. Present in 50% of the population
C. Hyposthenic
   1. Between asthenic and sthenic
   2. Present in 35% of the population
D. Asthenic
   1. Slender build
   2. Present in 10% of the population
   3. Thorax is narrow and shallow
   4. Ribs slope sharply downward
   5. Thoracic cavity is long
   6. Lungs are long; broader above than at the base
   7. Heart is long and narrow
   8. Diaphragm is low and abdominal cavity is short
   9. Stomach and gallbladder are low, vertical, and near the midline
   10. Colon is low; median position

PEDIATRIC RADIOGRAPHY: GENERAL PRINCIPLES

A. Appropriately introduce radiographer to child and parent
B. Radiographer should demonstrate positive attitude toward the child
C. Maintain clear communication with child and parent
D. Determine extent of parental involvement
E. Report suspected child abuse (nonaccidental trauma) to the appropriate radiologist, attending physician, radiology supervisor, or nurse
F. Determine type of immobilization to be used for the examination
   1. Immobilization board
   2. Pigg-o-stat
   3. Sandbags
   4. Tape
   5. Compression bands
   6. Sheets and towels

G. Practice as low as reasonably achievable (ALARA) principle
  1. Gonadal shielding of children
  2. Tight collimation
  3. Pieces of lead used as contact shields
  4. Low mAs techniques
  5. No repeat radiographs
  6. High-speed film-screen combinations
H. Determine whether patient preparation was adequately carried out
I. Interview the parent and write down the appropriate history
J. Briefly discuss case with radiologist to determine specifically which projections are needed and the extent of gonadal shielding that should be used in cases in which this may be in doubt

TRAUMA: GENERAL PRINCIPLES

A. Do no additional harm to the patient
B. Work quickly and confidently, observing standard precautions
C. Be prepared to modify conventional positions in response to patient condition
D. If patient is immobilized, transfer to the x-ray table with as much help as possible
E. Skull and cervical spine injuries
  1. A crosstable lateral cervical spine radiograph must be obtained before moving the patient in any way
  2. The radiograph must be approved by a physician before moving the patient or removing a cervical collar or sandbags
F. Each body part requires at least two radiographs taken at 90-degree angles to one another
G. Projections should approach routine positioning (as the patient's condition permits), with the cassette placed as close to the body part as possible
H. Central ray entrance and exit points should be as close to routine as possible
I. Long bone radiography
  1. Always include the joint nearest the trauma
  2. The joint farthest from the trauma should also be included if possible; otherwise, separate radiographs should be taken of that joint
J. Splints or bandages
  1. Should not be removed unless permission has been obtained from the physician
  2. Exposure technique may need to be modified to compensate for splints and bandages
K. Allow the patient as much control over movement as possible
L. Whether the patient is conscious or unconscious, explain your movements clearly to encourage possible cooperation

M. Be prepared to perform several examinations at once
  1. Example: all AP projections should be taken in an uninterrupted sequence, then all lateral projections, etc.
  2. Reduces the number of times the x-ray tube must be moved
  3. Allows the overall procedure to be completed more quickly
N. Provide lead aprons for anyone who may need to be in the room caring for a critically injured patient
O. Move extremities carefully to prevent further displacing fractures or causing internal hemorrhage
P. Maintain a cooperative spirit
  1. Cooperate with other health care professionals who are attempting to care for the patient at the same time: medical technologists, respiratory therapists, physicians, nurses; may need to be caring for the patient simultaneously during the radiographic examinations in cases of severe trauma
  2. Radiographer is a vital part of a trauma team and needs to work in harmony with the other health care professionals present for the proper care of the patient
Q. Inability of the patient to move and difficulty obtaining routine projections must never be used as an excuse to submit radiographs of poor quality
  1. Severely traumatized patients need fully diagnostic radiographs to receive optimal care
  2. Radiographer must be proficient in radiographic exposure and positioning so that high-quality radiographs may be obtained under difficult conditions

REVIEW OF ANATOMY RELEVANT TO RADIOGRAPHY

Planes of the Body

A. Median sagittal plane (MSP or midsagittal plane)
  1. Passes vertically through the midline of the body from front to back
  2. Divides body into equal right and left portions
  3. Any plane parallel to the MSP is called a *sagittal plane*
B. Midcoronal plane
  1. Passes vertically through the midaxillary region of the body and the coronal suture of the cranium at right angles to the MSP
  2. Divides body into anterior and posterior portions
  3. Any plane passing vertically through the body from side to side is called a *coronal plane*
C. Transverse plane (axial plane)
  1. Passes crosswise through the body at right angles to its longitudinal axis and the MSP and coronal planes
  2. Divides body into superior and inferior portions

Clinical Divisions of the Abdomen

A. Divided into four quadrants by a transverse plane and the MSP intersecting at the umbilicus
B. Quadrants
   1. Right upper quadrant
   2. Right lower quadrant
   3. Left upper quadrant
   4. Left lower quadrant

Anatomic Divisions of the Abdomen

A. Abdomen is divided into nine regions using four planes
   1. Two transverse planes
   2. Two sagittal planes
B. Planes are called *Addison's planes*
C. Transverse planes are drawn
   1. At the levels of the tip of the ninth costal cartilage
   2. At the superior margin of the iliac crest
D. Two sagittal planes are drawn
   1. Each midway between the anterior superior iliac spines of the pelvis and the MSP of the body
E. Nine regions of the body
   1. Superior
      a. Right hypochondrium
      b. Epigastrium
      c. Left hypochondrium
   2. Middle
      a. Right lumbar
      b. Umbilical
      c. Left lumbar
   3. Inferior
      a. Right iliac
      b. Hypogastrium
      c. Left iliac

Skeletal System

Functions

A. Provides a rigid support system
B. Protects delicate structures
C. Bones supply calcium to the blood and are involved in the formation of blood cells
D. Bones serve to provide attachment of muscles and form levers in the joint spaces allowing movement

Ossification

A. Cartilage is covered with perichondrium that is converted to periosteum
B. Diaphysis: central shaft
C. Epiphysis: located at both ends of the diaphysis
D. Growth in the length of the bone is provided by the metaphyseal plate located between the epiphyseal cartilage and the diaphysis
E. An osseous matrix is formed in the cartilage
F. Bone appears at the site where cartilage existed
G. Ossification is completed as the proximal epiphysis joins with the diaphysis between 20 and 25 years of age

Marrow

A. Fills spaces of spongy bone
B. Contains blood vessels and blood cells in various stages of development
C. Red bone marrow
   1. Site of formation of red blood cells and some white blood cells
   2. Found in spongy bone of adults
      a. Sternum
      b. Ribs
      c. Vertebrae
      d. Proximal epiphysis of long bones
D. Yellow bone marrow
E. Fatty marrow: replaces red bone marrow in the adult except in areas previously mentioned

Types of Bones

A. Long bones (e.g., femur, humerus)
B. Short bones (e.g., wrist, ankle bones)
C. Flat bones (e.g., ribs, scapulae)
D. Irregular bones (e.g., vertebrae, sesamoids [patella])

Descriptive Terminology for Bones

A. Projections
   1. Process: prominence
   2. Spine: sharp prominence
   3. Tubercle: rounded projection
   4. Tuberosity: larger rounded projection
   5. Trochanter: very large bony prominence
   6. Crest: ridge
   7. Condyle: round process of an articulating bone
   8. Head: enlargement at end of bone
B. Depressions
   1. Fossa: pit
   2. Groove: furrow
   3. Sulcus: synonymous with *groove*
   4. Sinus: cavity within a bone
   5. Foramen: opening
   6. Meatus: tubelike

Division of the Skeleton

A. Axial skeleton
   1. Composed of 74 bones
   2. Upright axis of the skeleton
   3. Components
      a. Skull
      b. Hyoid bone
      c. Vertebral column
      d. Sternum
      e. Ribs

B. Appendicular skeleton
1. Composed of 126 bones
2. Bones attached to the axial skeleton
   a. Upper and lower extremities
   b. Auditory ossicles: six bones

Articulations

A. Classification basis
1. Structure
2. Composition
3. Mobility
B. Fibrous joints (synarthroses)
1. Surfaces of bones almost in direct contact, with limited movement
2. Generally immovable
3. No joint cavity or capsule
4. Examples: skull sutures
C. Cartilaginous joints (amphiarthroses)
1. No joint cavity; contiguous bones united by cartilage and ligaments
2. Slightly movable
3. Examples: intervertebral disks, pubic symphysis
D. Synovial joints (diarthroses)
1. Approximating bone surfaces covered with cartilage
2. Freely movable
3. Bones held together by a fibrous capsule lined with synovial membrane and ligaments
4. Examples of movement
   a. Hinge: permits motion in one plane only (elbow)
   b. Pivot: permits rotary movement in which a ring rotates round a central axis (proximal radioulnar articulation)
   c. Saddle: opposing surfaces are concavoconvex, allowing flexion, extension, adduction, and abduction (carpometacarpal joint of thumb)
   d. Ball and socket: capable of movement in an infinite number of axes; rounded head of one bone moves in a cuplike cavity of the approximating base (hip)
   e. Gliding: articulation of contiguous bones allows only gliding movements (wrist, ankle)
   f. Condyloid: permits movement in two directions at right angles to one another; circumduction occurs, rotation does not (radiocarpal joints)
E. Bursae
1. Sacs filled with synovial fluid; located where tendons or muscles slide over underlying parts
2. Some bursae communicate with a joint cavity
3. Prominent bursae found at the elbow, shoulder, hip, and knee
F. Movements
1. Gliding
   a. Simplest kind of motion in a joint
   b. Motion of a joint that does not involve any angular or rotary movements

2. Flexion: decreases the angle formed by the union of two bones
3. Extension: increases the angle formed by the union of two bones
4. Abduction: occurs by moving part of the appendicular skeleton away from the median plane of the body
5. Adduction: occurs by moving part of the appendicular skeleton toward the median plane of the body
6. Circumduction
   a. Occurs in ball-and-socket joints
   b. Circumscribes the conic space of one bone by the other bone
7. Rotation: turning on an axis without being displaced from that axis

Skull Morphology

A. Mesocephalic skull
1. Considered the "typical" skull
2. Petrous ridge forms 47-degree angle with MSP
B. Brachycephalic skull
1. Petrous ridge forms 54-degree angle with MSP
2. Short from front to back
3. Broad side to side
4. Shallow from vertex to base
C. Dolichocephalic
1. Petrous ridge forms 40-degree angle with MSP
2. Long from front to back
3. Narrow side to side
4. Deep from vertex to base

Axial Skeleton

Skull

A. Cranium (Figures 5-1 and 5-2)
1. Superior portion formed by the frontal parietal and occipital bones
2. Lateral portions formed by the temporal and sphenoid bones
3. Cranial base formed by the temporal, sphenoid, and ethmoid bones
4. Fontanelles: soft spots at birth in which ossification is incomplete
B. Frontal bone
1. Forms the forehead
2. Contains the frontal sinuses
3. Forms the roof of the orbits
4. Union with the parietal bones forms the coronal suture
C. Parietal bones
1. Union with the occipital bone forms the lambdoid suture
2. Union with the temporal bone forms the squamous suture
3. Union with the sphenoid bone forms the coronal suture

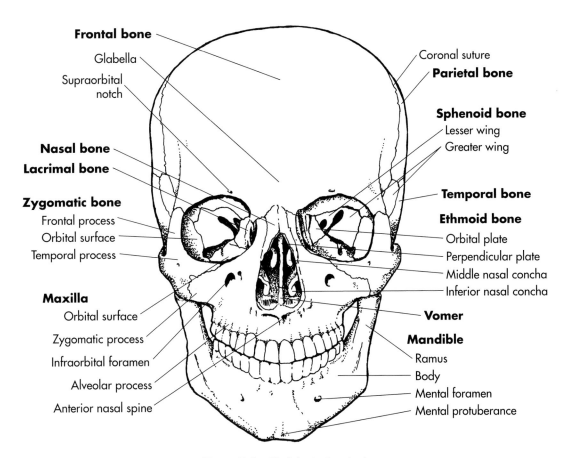

Figure 5-1 Skull (anterior view).

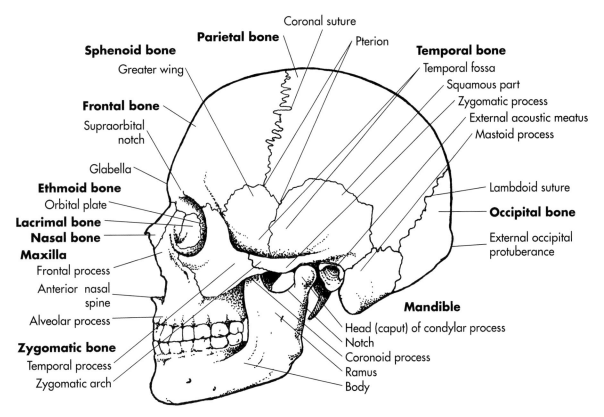

Figure 5-2 Skull (lateral view).

D. Temporal bones
  1. Contain the external auditory meatus and middle and inner ear structures
  2. Squamous portion: above the meatus; zygomatic process: articulates with the zygoma to form the zygomatic arch
  3. Petrous portion
     a. Contains organs used for hearing and equilibrium
     b. Prominent elevation on the floor of the cranium
  4. Mastoid portion
     a. Protuberance behind the ear
     b. Mastoid process
  5. Mandibular fossa: articulates with the condyle on the mandible
  6. Styloid process: anterior to the mastoid process; several neck muscles attach here
  7. Jugular foramen: located between the petrous portion and the occipital bones; opening from which cranial nerves IX, X, and XI exit
E. Sphenoid bone
  1. Bounded by the ethmoid and frontal bones anteriorly and the temporal and occipital bones posteriorly
  2. Greater wings: lateral projections (Figure 5-3)
     a. Form outer wall and floor of the orbits
     b. Foramen rotundum: round; located horizontally in the anteromedial portion of the greater wing adjacent to the lateral wall of the sphenoid sinus; maxillary division of cranial nerve V exits
     c. Foramen ovale: oval; located laterally and posteriorly to foramen rotundum; mandibular division of cranial nerve V exits
     d. Foramen spinosum: located near posterior angle of the greater wing; lateral and posterior to foramen ovale; transmits an artery to the meninges
     e. Foramen lacerum: contains the internal carotid artery

  f. Superior orbital fissure: transmits cranial nerves III and IV and part of the cranial nerve V
  3. Lesser wings
     a. Posterior part of the roof of the orbits
     b. Optic foramen: cranial nerve II exits
  4. Body
     a. Sella turcica: holds the pituitary gland (hypophysis)
     b. Contains the sphenoid sinuses
     c. Medial and lateral pterygoid processes located here
F. Ethmoid bone
  1. Contributes to the formation of the base of the cranium, orbits, and roof of the nose
  2. Perpendicular plate: forms the superior part of the nasal septum
  3. Horizontal plate (cribriform plate)
     a. Located at right angles to the perpendicular plate
     b. Olfactory nerves pass through
     c. Contains the crista galli; meninges of the brain attached to this process
  4. Lateral masses
     a. Form the orbital plates
     b. Contain the superior and middle conchae (lateral walls of the nose)
     c. Contain the ethmoid sinuses
G. Occipital bone
  1. Forms the posterior part of the cranium
  2. Foramen magnum: spinal cord enters to attach to the brainstem
  3. Condyles (two)
     a. On both sides of the foramen magnum
     b. Articulate with depressions on the C1 vertebrae
  4. External occipital protuberance: located on the posterior surface

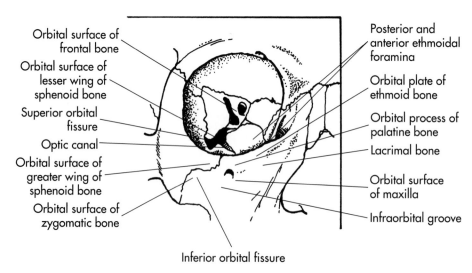

Figure 5-3 Right orbit.

Facial bones

A. Appear suspended from the middle and anterior parts of the cranium

B. Ethmoid and frontal bones also contribute to the framework of the face

C. All the facial bones except the mandible touch the maxilla
1. Alveolar process: forms the upper jaw containing the maxillary teeth
2. Forms the floor of the orbits; infraorbital foramen is inferior from the orbit
3. Forms the walls of the nasal cavities and the hard palate (palatine process)
4. Maxillary sinus: large air space

D. Mandible (Figure 5-4)
1. Body: central horizontal portion
   a. Chin: symphysis in midline
   b. Alveolar process: contains the mandibular teeth
   c. Mental foramen
      (1) Below the first bicuspid on the outer surface
      (2) Transmits nerves and blood vessels
2. Ramus: upward process on both sides of the posterior body of the mandible
   a. Condyle: articulates with the mandibular fossa
   b. Coronoid process: attachment site for the temporalis muscle
   c. Mandibular foramen: located on the inner surface

E. Zygomatic bone
1. Prominence of cheek: attaches to the zygomatic process of the temporal bone to form the zygomatic arch
2. Other margin of the orbit

F. Lacrimal: medial part of the wall of the orbit

G. Nasal bones: upper bridge of the nose

H. Inferior nasal concha
1. Horizontally placed along the lateral wall of the nasal fossa
2. Inferior to the middle and superior conchae of the ethmoid

I. Palatine bones
1. Horizontal plates form the posterior part of the hard palate
2. Perpendicular plates form the sphenoid palatine foramen

J. Vomer
1. Plowshare-shaped
2. Forms the lower part of the nasal septum

K. Hyoid
1. U-shaped bone
2. Body
3. Greater horn
4. Lesser horn
5. Suspended by ligaments from the styloid process

Vertebral column

A. Part of the axial skeleton
1. Supports the head
2. Gives base to the ribs
3. Encloses the spinal cord

B. Vertebrae
1. Consist of the following 34 bones that make up the spinal column
   a. Cervical: 7 bones
   b. Thoracic: 12 bones

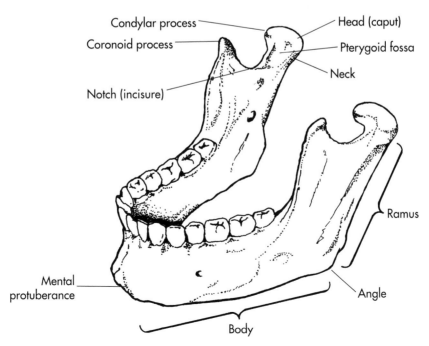

Figure 5-4 Mandible (anterolateral superior view).

Condylar process
Coronoid process
Notch (incisure)
Head (caput)
Pterygoid fossa
Neck
Ramus
Mental protuberance
Angle
Body

Atlas (C1): superior view

Anterior arch

Articular facet for dens

Transverse process

Lateral mass

Transverse foramen

Vertebral foramen

Superior articular facet for occipital condyle

Posterior arch

Tubercle for transverse ligament

Axis (C2): anterior view

Dens

Superior articular facet for atlas

Anterior articular facet for atlas

Pedicle

Body

Lateral mass

Inferior articular facet for C3

Transverse process

Atlas (C1): inferior view

Transverse process

Posterior arch

Vertebral foramen

Transverse foramen

Inferior articular facet for axis

Anterior arch

Axis (C2): posterosuperior view

Superior articular facet for atlas

Dens

Posterior articular facet for transverse ligament

Lateral mass

Inferior articular process

Transverse process

Spinous process

Cervical vertebra: superior view

Body

Anterior tubercle

Transverse process

Posterior tubercle

Transverse foramen

Vertebral foramen

Pedicle

Lamina

Superior articular facet

Spinous process

Inferior articular facet

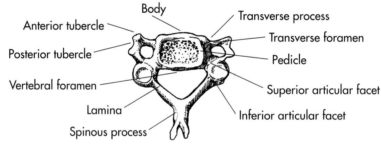

Figure 5-5 Distinguishing features of cervical vertebrae.

c. Lumbar: 5 bones
d. Sacral: 5 bones
e. Coccygeal: 4 to 5 bones

2. In the adult, the vertebrae of the sacral and coccygeal regions are united into two bones: the sacrum and the coccyx

C. Curvatures: from a lateral view, there are four curves, alternately convex and concave ventrally
1. Two convex curves are the cervical and lumbar
2. Two concave curves are the thoracic and sacral

D. Vertebrae morphology
1. Each vertebra differs in size and shape but has similar components
2. Body: central mass of bone
  a. Weight bearing
  b. Forms anterior part of vertebrae
3. Pedicles of the arch: two thick columns that extend

backward from the body to meet the laminae of the neural arch

4. Processes: seven (one spinous [except C1], two transverse, two superior articular, and two inferior articular)
  a. Spinous process extends backward from the point of the union of the two laminae
  b. Transverse processes project laterally on both sides from the junction of the laminae and the pedicle
  c. Articular processes arise near the junction of the pedicle and the laminae; superior processes project upward, inferior processes project downward
  d. Surfaces of the processes are smooth
  e. Inferior articular processes of the vertebrae fit into the superior articular processes below

Superior view **Lateral view**

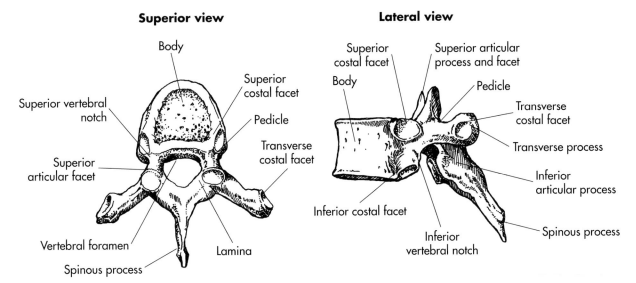

Figure 5-6 Thoracic vertebra.

f. Form true joints but the contacts established serve to restrict movement

E. Distinguishing features
1. Cervical region: triangular shape
   a. All have foramina in the transverse processes (upper six transmit the vertebral artery)
   b. Spinous processes are short
      (1) C3 to C5 are bifurcated
      (2) C7 is long prominence felt at the back of the neck
   c. Have small bodies (except for C1 vertebra)
   d. C1 vertebra (atlas) (Figure 5-5)
      (1) No body
      (2) Anterior and posterior arches and two lateral masses
      (3) Superior articular processes join with the condyles of the occipital bone
   e. C2 vertebra (axis): process on the upper surface of the body (dens or odontoid) forms a pivot about which the axis rotates
2. Thoracic region (Figure 5-6)
   a. Presence of facets for articulation with the ribs
   b. Processes are larger and heavier than those of the cervical region
   c. Spinous process is projected downward at a sharp angle
   d. Circular vertebral foramen
3. Lumbar region (Figure 5-7)
   a. Large and heavy bodies
   b. Four transverse lines separate the bodies of the vertebrae on the pelvic surface
   c. Triangular shape: fitted between the halves of the pelvis
   d. Four pairs of dorsal sacral foramina communicate with four pairs of pelvic sacral foramina

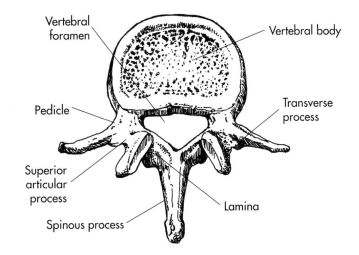

Figure 5-7 Lumbar vertebra (superior view).

4. Sacral vertebrae
   a. Formed by fusion of five sacral segments in curved, triangular bone
   b. Base directed obliquely, superiorly, anteriorly
   c. Apex directed posteriorly, inferiorly
   d. Longer, narrower, more vertical in males than in females
   e. Body of sacrum has sacral promontory, a prominent ridge at upper anterior margin
5. Coccygeal vertebrae
   a. Four to five modular pieces fused together
   b. Triangular, with the base above and apex below
6. Defects
   a. Lordosis: exaggerated lumbar concavity
   b. Scoliosis: lateral curvature of any region
   c. Kyphosis: exaggerated convexity in the thoracic region

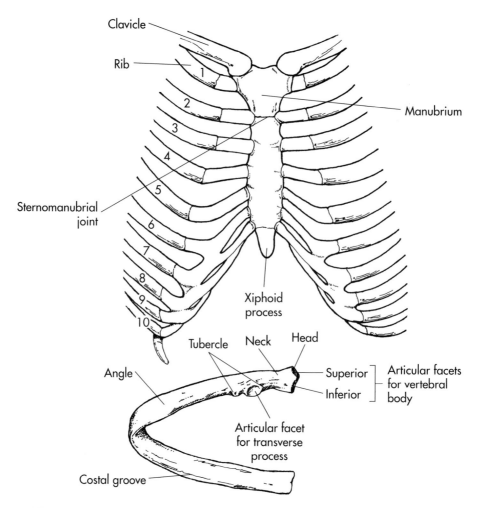

Figure 5-8   Sternocostal articulations (anterior view); middle rib (posterior view).

Bones of the thorax

A. Sternum
1. Forms the medial part of the anterior chest wall
2. Manubrium (upper part): clavicle and first rib articulate with the manubrium; contains notch on superior border called *jugular (manubrial) notch*
3. Body (middle blade): ribs articulate with the body via the costal cartilages
4. Xiphoid (blunt cartilaginous tip)

B. Ribs: 12 pairs (Figure 5-8)
1. Each rib articulates with both the body and the transverse process of its corresponding thoracic vertebra
2. Second to ninth ribs articulate with the body of the vertebra above
3. Ribs curve outward, forward, and then downward
4. Anteriorly, each of the first seven ribs joins a costal cartilage that attaches to the sternum
5. Next three ribs (eighth to tenth) join the cartilage of the rib above
6. Eleventh and twelfth ribs do not attach to the sternum and are called *floating ribs*

Appendicular Skeleton

Upper extremity

A. Shoulder: clavicle and scapula (Figure 5-9)
1. Clavicle
   a. Articulates with the manubrium at the sternal end
   b. Articulates with the scapula at the lateral end
   c. Slender S-shaped bone that extends horizontally across the upper part of the thorax
2. Scapula (see Figure 5-9)
   a. Triangular bone with the base upward and the apex downward
   b. Lateral aspect contains the glenoid cavity (fossa) that articulates with the head of the humerus
   c. Spine extends across the upper part of the posterior surface; expands laterally and forms the acromion (point of shoulder)

Posterior view

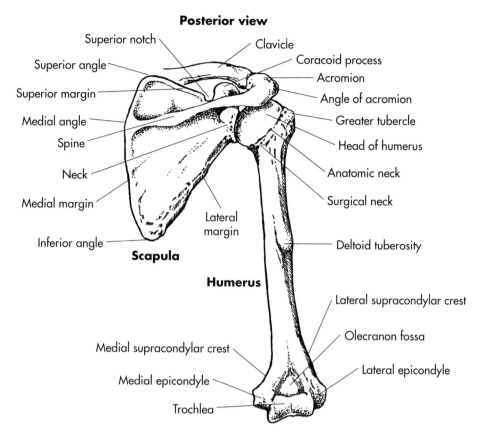

Anterior view

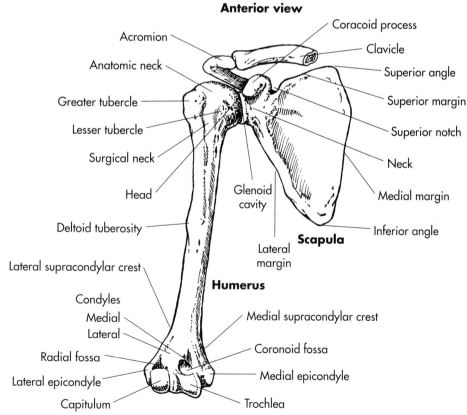

Figure 5-9 Humerus and scapula.

d. Coracoid process projects anteriorly from the upper part of the neck of the scapula

B. Humerus

1. Consists of a shaft (diaphysis) and two ends (epiphyses)
2. Proximal end has a head that articulates with the glenoid cavity (fossa) of the scapula
3. Greater and lesser tubercles lie below the head
   a. Intertubercular groove (bicipital groove) is between them; long tendon of the biceps attaches here
   b. Surgical neck is below the tubercles
4. Radial groove runs obliquely on the posterior surface; radial nerve is here
5. Deltoid muscles attach in a V-shaped area in the middle of the shaft called the *deltoid tuberosity*
6. Distal end has two projections
   a. Capitulum: lateral, articulates with the radius; expanded area just superior is called the *lateral epicondyle*
   b. Trochlea: medial, articulates with the ulna; expanded area just superior is called the *medial epicondyle*

C. Forearm (Figure 5-10)

1. Radius
   a. Lateral bone of the forearm
   b. Radial tubercle (tuberosity) is located below the head on the medial side
   c. Proximal end has disklike head
   d. Neck is just inferior to head
   e. Distal end is broad for articulation with the wrist
   f. Has styloid process on its lateral side
2. Ulna
   a. Medial bone of the forearm
   b. Conspicuous part of the elbow joint (olecranon)
   c. Curved surface that articulates with the trochlea of the humerus is the trochlear notch
   d. Lateral side is concave (radial notch); articulates with the head of the radius
   e. Distal end contains the styloid process

D. Hand and wrist (Figure 5-11)

1. Carpal bones: eight
   a. Arranged in two rows of four
   b. From lateral to medial, proximal row: scaphoid, lunate, triquetrum, and pisiform
   c. From lateral to medial, distal row: trapezium, trapezoid, capitate, and hamate
2. Metacarpal bones: five
   a. Framework of the hand
   b. Numbered 1 through 5, beginning on the lateral side
   c. Phalanges: 14
      (1) Form the fingers
      (2) Three phalanges in each finger; two phalanges in the thumb

Radius and ulna in supination: anterior view

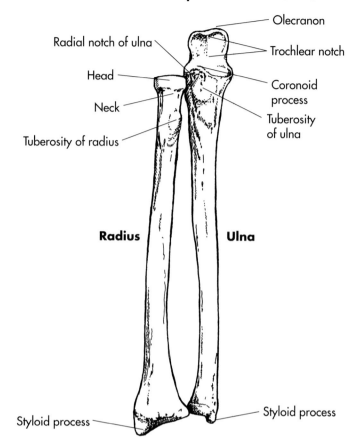

Figure 5-10   Forearm.

Lower extremity

A. Hip (os coxae or innominate) (Figure 5-12)

1. Constitutes the pelvic girdle
2. United with the vertebral column
3. Union of three parts that is marked by a cup-shaped cavity (acetabulum)
4. Ilium
   a. Prominence of the hip
   b. Superior border is the crest
   c. ASIS: projection at the anterior tip of the crest; just inferior to the ASIS is the anterior inferior iliac spine
   d. Corresponding projections on the posterior part are the posterior superior and posterior inferior iliac spines
   e. Greater sciatic notch: located beneath the articular surface
   f. Most is a smooth concavity (iliac fossa)
   g. Posteriorly it is rough and articulates with the sacrum in the formation of the sacroiliac joint
5. Pubic bone
   a. Anterior part of the innominate bone

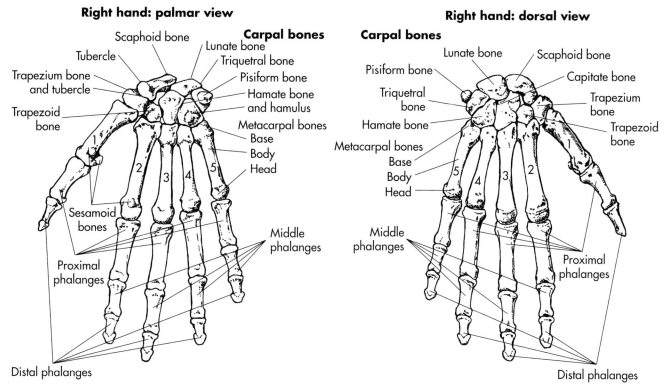

Figure 5-11 Wrist and hand.

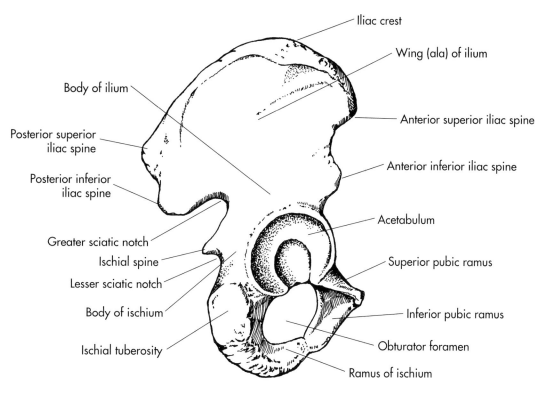

Figure 5-12 Coxal bone (lateral view).

b. Symphysis pubis: joining of the right and left pubic bones at the midline

c. Body and two rami

(1) Body forms one fifth of the acetabulum

(2) Superior ramus extends from the body to the median plane; superior border forms the pubic crest

(3) Inferior ramus extends downward and meets with the ischium

(4) Pubic arch is formed by the inferior rami of both pubic bones

6. Ischium

a. Forms the lower and back part of the innominate bone

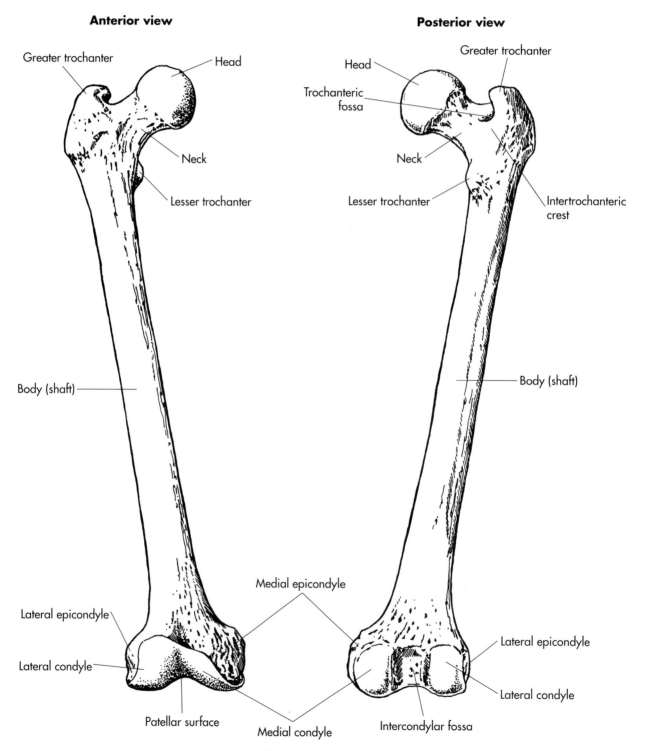

Figure 5-13   Femur.

b. Body
   (1) Forms two fifths of the acetabulum
   (2) Ischial tuberosity supports the body in a sitting position
c. Ramus: passes upward to join the inferior ramus of the pubis
d. Opening created by this ring is known as the *obturator foramen*

B. Pelvis
1. Formed by the right and left hip bones, sacrum, and coccyx

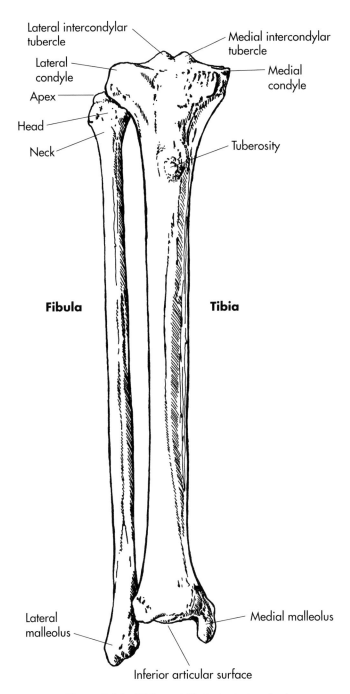

Lateral intercondylar tubercle
Medial intercondylar tubercle
Lateral condyle
Medial condyle
Apex
Head
Neck
Tuberosity
Fibula
Tibia
Lateral malleolus
Medial malleolus
Inferior articular surface

Figure 5-14 Tibia and fibula (anterior view).

2. Greater pelvis
   a. Bounded by the ilia and lower lumbar vertebrae
   b. Gives support to the abdominal viscera
3. Lesser pelvis
   a. Brim of the pelvis corresponds to the sacral promontory
   b. Inferior outlet is bounded by the tip of the coccyx, ischial tuberosities, and inferior rami of the pubic bones
4. Female pelvis
   a. Shows adaptations related to functions as a birth canal
   b. Wide outlet
   c. Angle of the pubic arch is obtuse
5. Male pelvis
   a. Shows adaptations that contribute to power and speed
   b. Heart-shaped outlet
   c. Angle of the pubic arch is acute
C. Femur (Figure 5-13)
1. Longest and strongest bone of the body
2. Proximal end has a rounded head that articulates with the acetabulum
3. Constricted portion: neck
4. Greater and lesser trochanters connected by intertrochanteric crest
5. Slightly arched shaft: is concave posteriorly
6. Distal end has two condyles separated on the posterior side by the intercondyloid fossa
D. Patella
1. Sesamoid bone
2. Embedded in the tendon of the quadriceps muscle
3. Articulates with the femur
E. Leg (Figure 5-14)
1. Tibia: medial bone
   a. Proximal end has two condyles that articulate with the femur
   b. Triangular shaft
      (1) Anterior: shin
      (2) Posterior: soleal line
      (3) Distal: medial malleolus articulates with the lattice that forms the ankle joint
2. Fibula: lateral bone
   a. Articulates with the lateral condyle of the tibia but does not enter the knee joint
   b. Distal end projects as the lateral malleolus
F. Ankle, foot, and toes (Figure 5-15)
1. Adapted for supporting weight but similar in structure to the hand
2. Talus
   a. Occupies the uppermost and central portion of the tarsus
   b. Distributes the body weight from the tibia above to the other tarsal bones
3. Calcaneus (os calcis, heel): located beneath the talus

Dorsal view

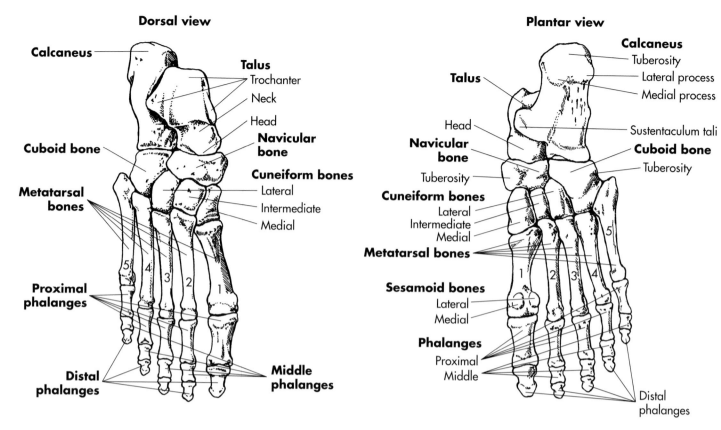

Calcaneus

Talus
- Trochanter
- Neck
- Head

Navicular bone

Cuboid bone

Cuneiform bones
- Lateral
- Intermediate
- Medial

Metatarsal bones

5 4 3 2 1

Proximal phalanges

Distal phalanges

Middle phalanges

Plantar view

Calcaneus
- Tuberosity
- Lateral process
- Medial process

Talus

Sustentaculum tali

Head

Navicular bone

Cuboid bone
- Tuberosity

Tuberosity

Cuneiform bones
- Lateral
- Intermediate
- Medial

Metatarsal bones

1 2 3 4 5

Sesamoid bones
- Lateral
- Medial

Phalanges
- Proximal
- Middle

Distal phalanges

Lateral view

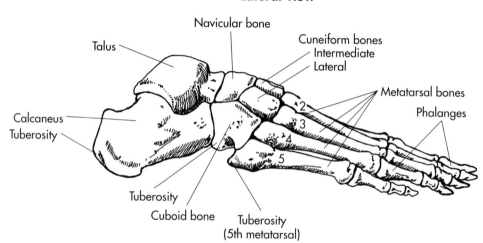

Navicular bone

Cuneiform bones
Intermediate
Lateral

Talus

Metatarsal bones

Phalanges

Calcaneus
Tuberosity

2
3
4
5

Tuberosity

Cuboid bone

Tuberosity
(5th metatarsal)

Medial view

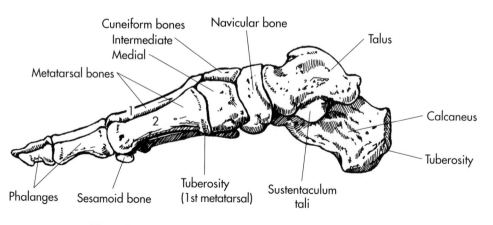

Cuneiform bones
Intermediate
Medial

Navicular bone

Talus

Metatarsal bones

Calcaneus

1

2

Tuberosity

Phalanges

Sesamoid bone

Tuberosity
(1st metatarsal)

Sustentaculum tali

Figure 5-15 Foot.

4. Navicular: located in front of the talus on the medial side; articulates with three cuneiform bones distally
5. Cuboid: lies along the lateral border of the navicular bone
6. Metatarsals
   a. First, second, and third metatarsals lie in front of the three cuneiform bones
   b. Fourth and fifth metatarsals lie in front of the cuboid bone
7. Phalanges
   a. Distal to the metatarsals
   b. Two in the great toe; three in each of the other four toes
8. Longitudinal arches of the foot: two
   a. Lateral: formed by the calcaneus, talus, cuboid, and fourth and fifth metatarsal bones
   b. Medial: formed by the calcaneus; talus; navicular; cuneiform; and first, second, and third metatarsal bones
9. Transverse arches: formed by the tarsal and metatarsal bones

Nervous System

A. Adapts to environmental influences
   1. By stimulating skeletal, cardiac, and smooth muscles
   2. Adaptation by the muscular system is almost immediate
B. Organized into various systems
   1. Central nervous system (CNS)
      a. Consists of the brain and spinal cord
   2. Peripheral nervous system (PNS)
      a. Contains the nerves to and from the body wall that connect to the CNS
      b. Also known as the *somatic division* because it is under voluntary control
   3. Autonomic nervous system (ANS)
      a. Not under conscious control (involuntary)
      b. Provides stimulus for the viscera and smooth and cardiac muscles
      c. Sympathetic division includes motor (afferent) nerves from the ANS
      d. Parasympathetic division involves motor (efferent) nerves from the ANS
C. Nerve cell: neuron
   1. Dendrite carries impulse toward the cell body under normal conditions
   2. Axon carries impulse away from the cell body and makes contact with the next cell; release of chemicals starts impulse in the next neuron
   3. Myelin sheath: fatty substance around some cell axons provides insulation
   4. Neurons can carry impulses in different directions
      a. Afferent neurons carry the sensory information to the CNS
      b. Efferent neurons carry the motor information away from the CNS
   5. Central neurons are found entirely within the CNS; relay information within the system
      a. Spinal cord is approximately 45.8 cm long; occupies the upper two thirds of the vertebral canal
      b. There are 31 pairs of spinal nerves; each has a dorsal (afferent) route and a ventral (efferent) route
D. Brain: consists of four regions
   1. Cerebrum
      a. Seat of conscious activities
      b. Largest portion of the brain
      c. Located most superiorly
      d. Cerebral cortex: thin outside layer; gray color; consists of several layers of cells; convoluted surface
      e. Longitudinal fissure: divides into two hemispheres
      f. Corpus callosum: heavy band of white fibers; forms the floor of the longitudinal fissure
      g. Central fissure: posterior to the midline
      h. Frontal lobe: anterior to the central fissure
      i. Parietal lobe: posterior to the central fissure
      j. Temporal lobe: below the lateral fissure
      k. Occipital lobe: posterior part of the brain
      l. Broca's area: controls the muscular part of speech
      m. Somatesthetic area: interprets body sensations
      n. Visual area: fibers from the medial part of the retina cross to opposite sides in the brain; fibers from the lateral portion do not cross
      o. Auditory area: superior central portion of the temporal lobe
      p. Prefrontal area: personality characteristics
   2. Cerebellum: coordinates balance and equilibrium
   3. Medulla oblongata
      a. Bulb of the spinal cord located inside the foramen magnum
      b. White on the outside, gray on the inside
      c. Controls three vital functions: cardiac, respiratory, and basal motor
      d. Also controls chewing, salivation, swallowing, emesis, lacrimation, blinking, coughing, and sneezing
      e. Pons: ropelike mass of white fibers; connects the halves of the cerebellum
   4. Mesencephalon
      a. Short part of the brainstem
      b. Above the pons
      c. Mostly white matter
E. Meninges: membranous coverings of the brain and spinal cord
   1. Dura mater
      a. Double layer around the brain

b. Single layer around the spinal cord, including the cauda equina
2. Arachnoid
a. Membrane just inside the dura mater
b. Relatively thin
3. Pia mater
a. Soft covering that fits against the brain and spinal cord
b. Contains an enormous amount of blood
4. Subarachnoid space
a. Threadlike structure through which cerebrospinal fluid circulates
b. Located between the pia mater and arachnoid
F. Cranial nerves
1. Part of the PNS
2. Originate at the base of the brain
3. Twelve pairs of cranial nerves
4. Referred to by name or roman numerals
5. Provide motor impulses, sensory impulses, or mixed impulses

Heart

A. Composed of cardiac muscle and serves to pump the blood through the circulatory system
B. Located behind the sternum
C. The size of a human fist
D. The apex of the heart points down and to the left
E. Located in a space between the lungs and the thoracic cavity, known as the *mediastinum*
F. Consists of four chambers: two atria and two ventricles
1. Blood from the superior and inferior vena cavae fills the right atrium and passes into the right ventricle through the tricuspid valve
2. The unoxygenated blood moves from the right ventricle to the lungs through the semilunar valve and the pulmonary artery
3. Oxygenated blood is sent from the lungs to the left atrium through the pulmonary veins; the left semilunar valve separates the left atrium from the pulmonary veins
4. From the left atrium, blood flows through the mitral valve into the left ventricle
5. Blood enters circulation by passing through the left semilunar valve into the aorta
G. Heart wall consists of three layers
1. Visceral pericardium or epicardium
2. Myocardium: heaviest covering
3. Endocardium: smooth continuous covering
4. All valves and chambers are lined by endothelium
H. Heartbeat
1. Averages 70 to 72 beats per minute
2. Cannot contract without nerve impulses
3. Nerves regulate the rate of the beat

I. Cardiac cycle
1. Consists of a relaxation-contraction cycle
2. Lasts for approximately 0.8 second
J. Electrocardiogram is a record of the action current as it travels across the heart

Circulatory System

A. Overview
1. The connection of the heart to the arteries, arterioles, capillaries, venules, and veins
2. The lymphatic system, which also interacts with the circulatory system
B. Arteries
1. Thick-walled elastic vessels
2. End in arterioles
C. Arterioles
1. The smallest branch of an artery
2. Connected to venules by capillaries
D. Capillaries
1. Connect arterioles to venules
2. Are lined by a thin layer of endothelium
3. Capillaries can dilate or constrict depending on the tissue's needs
4. Red blood cells go through capillaries one cell at a time
E. Venules
1. Connected to veins that carry blood toward the heart and carry unoxygenated blood (except in the pulmonary vein)
F. Veins
1. Have the same layers as arteries but are thinner
2. Veins will collapse without blood
3. Valves in the veins help resist the forces of gravity
G. Arteriovenous shunt (anastomosis)
1. A large blood vessel that connects an artery and vein directly
2. Skin color is caused by blood in the capillaries and anastomosis; important for heat distribution
3. Found only in the hands, face, and toes, where the body is exposed to weather

Arterial Systemic Circulation

A. Aorta
1. Arises from the left ventricle of the heart
2. First 5 cm is called the *ascending aorta*
3. Two left and right coronary arteries branch off directly above the left semilunar valve and supply blood to the cardiac muscle
B. Aortic arch
1. Loops back over the top of the heart and left of the trachea
2. Continues down in back of the heart
3. Three arteries come off the arch

a. Brachiocephalic
   (1) Only a few centimeters in length
   (2) Right subclavian artery arises from brachiocephalic artery and supplies blood to the right shoulder
   (3) Right common carotid artery arises from brachiocephalic artery and supplies blood to the right side of the head
   b. Left common carotid artery supplies blood to the left side of the head
   c. Left subclavian artery supplies branches to the upper chest and scapula

C. Carotid arteries
   1. Supply the head
   2. Right carotid artery originates from the brachiocephalic artery
   3. Left carotid artery originates from the aortic arch

D. Subclavian arteries
   1. Provide blood to the shoulder and arm
   2. Left one comes from the aortic arch
   3. Right one comes from the brachiocephalic artery
   4. Pass over the first rib and under the clavicle
   5. Become the axillary arteries as they pass through the shoulder region
   6. First branch off the subclavian artery is the vertebral artery

E. Vertebral artery
   1. Passes up the neck through the transverse foramen of the cervical vertebrae
   2. Enters the skull through the foramen magnum
   3. The two paired arteries join on the ventral side of the medulla and become the basilar artery; this artery joins branches from the internal carotid artery to form the circle of Willis, also called the *cerebral arterial circle*

F. Axillary artery
   1. Becomes the brachial artery at the humerus
   2. Moves along the medial surface across the elbow region and then divides into radial and ulnar arteries

G. Radial artery
   1. Moves along the radius and crosses it at the distal end
   2. A pulse can be felt at the distal end
   3. Moves across the metacarpals and deep into the palm
   4. Forms a loop that connects with the ulnar artery

H. Ulnar artery
   1. Travels down the medial surface of the forearm
   2. Becomes the superficial palmar artery that joins with the radial artery
   3. Digital arteries supply the fingers and branch off from the palmar loop

I. Descending aorta: consists of the thoracic and abdominal sections of the aorta
   1. Thoracic aorta
      a. Starts after the left subclavian artery branches off the aortic arch
      b. Extends from T4-T5 to T12-L1
      c. Passes down and in front of the vertebral column and through the diaphragm
      d. Gives off several branches supplying the ribs, lungs, and diaphragm
      e. After it passes through the diaphragm, it is called the *abdominal aorta*
   2. Abdominal aorta
      a. Extends to the L4 vertebra
      b. Gives rise to the visceral and parietal arteries
      c. Celiac artery: visceral artery that is 1.5 cm long; it divides into several branches
         (1) Left gastric artery: smallest branch to the stomach
         (2) Hepatic artery: supplies most of the blood to the liver; divides at the liver
            (a) Cystic artery: serves the gallbladder
            (b) Gastric duodenal artery: divides to serve the stomach, pancreas, and duodenum
         (3) Splenic artery: largest branch to the spleen
      d. Superior mesenteric artery: supplies all of the small intestine except the duodenum and superior ascending and transverse portion of the colon; comes off the front of the aorta below the celiac artery
      e. Inferior mesenteric artery: supplies blood for part of the transverse colon and all of the descending and sigmoid colon, rectum, and bladder
      f. Renal artery: supplies the kidneys; located below the superior mesenteric artery
         (1) Right renal artery slightly longer and lower because the aorta is slightly left of the midline
         (2) Enters the kidney at the hilus
      g. Suprarenal artery: branches off the aorta above the renal artery (may be branches of the renal arteries)
      h. Aorta then bifurcates and becomes the right and left common iliac arteries

J. Common iliac arteries: bifurcate
   1. Internal iliac artery supplies the pelvic wall and viscera
   2. External iliac artery goes into the thigh
      a. Passes over the pelvic brim and under the inguinal ligament
      b. Becomes the femoral artery

K. Femoral artery
   1. Supplies thigh
   2. Becomes the popliteal artery just above the knee and goes behind the knee to bifurcate
      a. Anterior tibial artery
      b. Posterior tibial artery
      c. Anterior and posterior tibial arteries spread out at the ankle and become the dorsal artery of the foot

Venous Systemic Circulation

A. Consists of one set of superficial veins and one set of deep veins

B. Veins have a higher blood capacity than the arteries but have lower blood pressure and velocity

C. Three sets of veins connect to the heart
  1. Vena cavae: superior and inferior
     a. Serve the body
     b. Return unoxygenated blood
  2. Coronary sinus
     a. Serves the heart
     b. Returns unoxygenated blood
  3. Pulmonary veins
     a. Serve the lungs (two per lung)
     b. Return oxygenated blood to the left atrium

D. Superior vena cava
  1. Begins at the level of the first rib
  2. Is formed by two veins
     a. Left and right brachiocephalic veins (return blood from the head, shoulders, and arms)
     b. Each brachiocephalic vein is a union of the internal jugular vein with the subclavian vein

E. Jugular veins drain blood from the head
  1. External jugular vein
     a. Drains the face and the scalp
     b. Is the union of three main veins that unite just below the ear and empty into the subclavian vein
  2. Internal jugular vein
     a. Returns from the internal carotid vein
     b. Originates in the skull

F. Vertebral veins
  1. Arise outside of the skull at the level of the atlas
  2. Pass through the transverse foramen to the subclavian artery

G. Arms and shoulders are drained by the deep veins that run alongside the arteries

H. Inferior vena cava
  1. Formed by two common iliac veins at the L5 vertebra in front of the vertebral column

I. Azygos vein
  1. Branches off the inferior vena cava at the level of the renal veins
  2. Goes through the aortic hiatus of the diaphragm just below the heart
  3. Empties into the superior vena cava
  4. Picks up veins from the esophagus and bronchi

J. Other veins serving the abdomen and thorax are named for the region or organs that they serve

K. Veins of the lower extremities
  1. Deep veins have the same names as the arteries
  2. Superficial veins
     a. Great saphenous vein: drains the dorsalis pedis of the foot
     b. Small saphenous vein: drains the lateral side of the foot
     c. Popliteal vein: drains the lateral side of the leg

Lymphatic System

A. Carries lymph

B. Involved in the maintenance of fluid pressure

C. Contains lymph glands that filter foreign particles
  1. Tissue fluid is located in the intracellular spaces and is derived from the blood
  2. Is constantly moving
  3. Similar to plasma without large proteins

D. Lymph is tissue fluid that has been reabsorbed into lymphatic vessels

E. Valves are necessary in the lymphatic system
  1. To keep fluid flowing in the right direction
  2. Most valves are located in the arms and legs, where gravity is a problem

F. Lymph nodes
  1. Spongy masses of tissue through which lymph filters
  2. Have more afferent vessels coming to the node than efferent vessels leaving the node

G. Lymphocytes are small white blood cells that originate from stem cells

H. Right lymphatic duct
  1. Drains the upper right quadrant of the thorax, right arm, and right side of the head
  2. Empties into the right subclavian vein

I. Thoracic duct
  1. Drains the rest of the body
  2. Begins at the cisterna chyli
  3. Passes up the left side of the vertebral column, through the aortic hiatus of the diaphragm, and into the left subclavian vein

J. Lymphoidal tissue is found in various anatomic structures
  1. Spleen: the graveyard of red blood cells
  2. Thymus: atrophies after puberty but is involved in the cell-mediated immune system
  3. Tonsils: located in the oral cavity

Respiratory System

A. Respiratory tract: begins at the nostril opening and extends to the alveoli of the lungs

B. Air is drawn in through the nose, where it is warmed, humidified, and cleansed

C. Nasal cavity is lined with olfactory epithelium in the sphenoethmoid recess and by respiratory epithelium in the lower part

D. Superior, middle, and inferior turbinates are located on the lateral surface of the nasal cavity

E. Frontal, ethmoidal, maxillary, and sphenoidal sinuses empty into the nasal cavity
F. Pharynx
   1. Second part of the respiratory tract
   2. Starts at the base of the skull and extends to the esophagus
   3. Divided into three parts
      a. Nasopharynx: behind the nasal cavity
         (1) Eustachian tube (auditory tube): connects the middle ear with the pharynx; open only during swallowing; equalizes pressure
         (2) Pharyngeal tonsils (adenoids): on the upper back wall of the nasopharynx; a mass of lymphoid tissue
      b. Oropharynx: extends from the soft palate to the base of the tongue; separated from the oral cavity by the palatine arches
      c. Laryngopharynx: extends from the hyoid bone to the larynx
G. Larynx
   1. Located at the base of the tongue
   2. Made up of nine cartilages
H. Vocal chords
   1. Folds of mucous membranes
   2. Elastic connective tissue at the edges
I. Trachea
   1. Approximately 12 cm long
   2. In front of the esophagus
   3. Composed of 16 to 20 C-shaped rings that prevent its collapse
   4. At the end of the T4 vertebra, the trachea divides into left and right branches known as the *primary bronchi*
J. Primary bronchi
   1. Left primary bronchus is longer than the right and forms a sharp angle
   2. Right primary bronchus has a larger diameter than the left and comes off almost forming a straight line
K. Secondary bronchi branch off the primary bronchi
   1. Three secondary bronchi for the right lung, one per lobe
   2. Two secondary bronchi for the left lung, one per lobe
L. Tertiary bronchi
   1. Branch off the secondary bronchi
   2. Each lung has 10 tertiary bronchi because there are 10 segments per lung
M. Bronchioles: smaller branches of the tertiary bronchi
   1. Terminal bronchiole: not involved in gaseous exchange
   2. Respiratory bronchiole: branch off terminal bronchiole; first site of diffusion of oxygen into the blood
N. Alveolar ducts
   1. Branch off respiratory bronchiole
   2. Alveolar sacs attach to the alveolar ducts

O. Two cone-shaped lungs in the thoracic cavity
   1. Base rests on the diaphragm
   2. Apex is located at the level of the clavicle
   3. Right lung
      a. Has three lobes: superior, middle, and inferior
      b. Larger than the left lung
   4. Left lung
      a. Smaller than the right lung because two thirds of the heart is located on the left side
      b. Contains only two lobes
   5. Ten bronchopulmonary segments per lung
      a. Each has a branch from the tertiary bronchi
      b. Used as points of reference for surgery
P. Cardiac notch: depression on the medial surface of the left lung
   1. Hilus
      a. Point of attachment to a lung
      b. Blood vessels, bronchial tree, and nerves enter at the hilus
Q. Pleura: serous membrane surrounding the visceral and parietal layers of each lung
   1. Space between the two layers is the pleural cavity
   2. Lungs are not located in the pleural cavity
R. Mechanics of respiration
   1. Involve changing the pressure in the lungs to cause inspiration or expiration
   2. Inspiration
      a. Occurs when the air pressure in the lungs is decreased
      b. Causes the volume of the lungs to increase
      c. External intercostal muscles cause the ribs to elevate and increase the size of the chest cavity
      d. Dome-shaped diaphragm between the thoracic and abdominal cavities pulls downward when contracted
      e. Also increases the size of the chest cavity
   3. Expiration
      a. Basically a passive movement
      b. Ribs fall down
      c. Diaphragm is pushed up by the abdominal viscera
      d. Abdominal muscles force the abdominal contents up
      e. Internal intercostal muscles pull the ribs down

Digestive System

A. Digestive or alimentary tract
   1. Consists of a tube 6 m long from the mouth to the anus
   2. Selectively absorbs nutrients and water for the body
B. Mouth
   1. Site where food processing and digestion begin
   2. Secondary teeth tear and grind the food

C. Tongue
  1. Fibromuscular organ
  2. Contains the taste buds
  3. Transmits the sensation of taste to the brain
  4. Rolls the food into a bolus for swallowing
D. Saliva
  1. Added to help food become a bolus for easier passage down the esophagus

2. Produced by three major paired glands and many minor glands
E. Salivary glands
  1. Parotid glands
    a. Located in the preauricular region
    b. Saliva travels down Stensen's (parotid) duct, which opens opposite the second maxillary molar

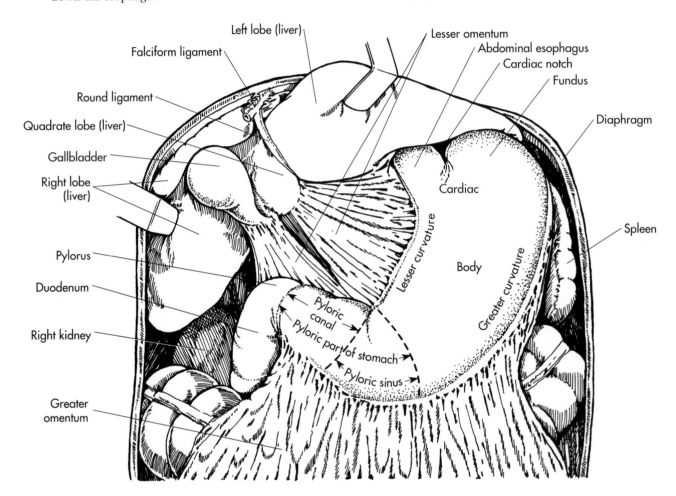

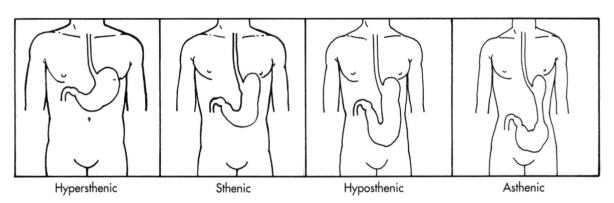

Variations in position and contour of stomach in relation to body habitus

Figure 5-16 Stomach.

2. Sublingual glands
   a. Lie under the tongue and rest against the mandible
   b. Saliva travels down Bartholin's duct and enters the oral cavity through Rivinus' (lesser sublingual) ducts on the sublingual fold
3. Submandibular glands
   a. Lie on the medial surface of the mandible
   b. Saliva travels down Wharton's (submandibular) duct and is released into the mouth at the sublingual caruncles

F. Swallowing
1. Bolus of food moves from the mouth and pharynx to the esophagus
2. During swallowing, the soft palate is pushed back against the posterior pharyngeal wall, closing the passage to the nasopharynx
3. Larynx is elevated; superior opening is protected by the epiglottis
4. Bolus moves into esophagus
5. Esophagus: a muscular tube located posterior to the trachea and connected to the stomach
6. Bolus moved through esophagus by peristalsis and gravity

G. Stomach: dilated portion of the alimentary canal lying in the upper abdomen just under the diaphragm (Figures 5-16 and 5-17)
1. Functions
   a. Stores food
   b. Digests: secretes pepsin, renin, and gastric lipase
   c. Produces hydrochloric acid
2. Shaped like the letter J: internal surface is wrinkled (rugae)
   a. Cardiac portion: esophagus entrance
   b. Body: main part

c. Fundus: bulge at the upper end, left of the esophageal area
d. Pyloric portion: narrow distal end that connects with the small intestine

H. Small intestine: thin-walled muscular tube
1. Three portions
   a. Duodenum (horseshoe-shaped): bile and pancreatic secretions are added to the small intestine
   b. Jejunum (1.5 m long): greatest amount of absorption
   c. Ileum (2.5 m long): connects with the large intestine
2. Secretes several enzymes and substances

I. Large intestine: approximately 1.5 m long and divided into several divisions
1. Cecum
   a. Blind pouch in the lower right quadrant
   b. Appendix attaches to the cecum
   c. Ileocecal sphincter separates the ileum from the cecum
2. Colon
   a. Ascending: from the cecum to the hepatic flexure
   b. Transverse: from the hepatic flexure to the splenic flexure
   c. Descending: from the splenic flexure to the level of the pelvic bone on the left side of the body
3. Sigmoid: S-shaped curve
4. Rectum: from the sigmoid colon down to the pelvic diaphragm
5. Anus: 3 cm in length

J. Pancreas: endocrine and exocrine gland
1. Exocrine
   a. Produces pancreatic juice that is collected by the pancreatic (Wirsung's) duct and carried away

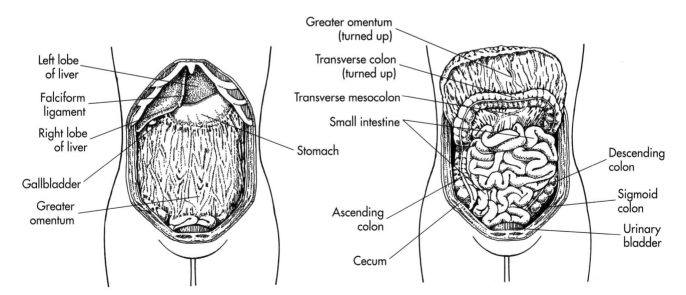

Figure 5-17   Abdominal viscera.

Anterior surface

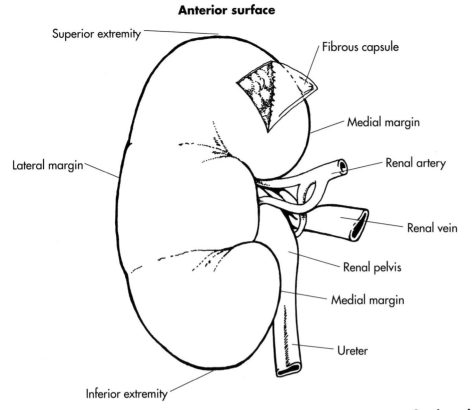

Superior extremity

Fibrous capsule

Medial margin

Renal artery

Renal vein

Renal pelvis

Medial margin

Ureter

Lateral margin

Inferior extremity

Sectioned

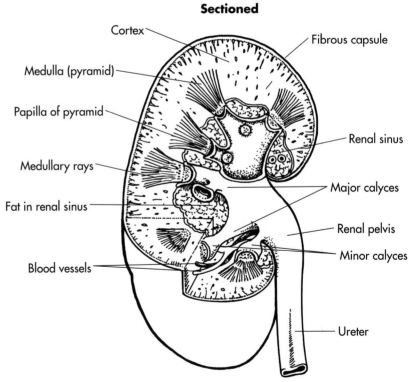

Cortex

Fibrous capsule

Medulla (pyramid)

Papilla of pyramid

Renal sinus

Medullary rays

Major calyces

Fat in renal sinus

Renal pelvis

Minor calyces

Blood vessels

Ureter

Figure 5-18   Kidney.

b. Joins the common bile duct to form Vater's (hepatopancreatic) ampulla, which penetrates the walls of the abdomen

2. Endocrine: releases insulin that controls blood glucose levels; also releases glucagon and somatostatin

K. Liver
1. Largest and most active gland in the body
2. Two main lobes and several lobules
3. Lobules produce bile that is carried away and stored in the gallbladder
4. Stores glycogen
5. Detoxifies waste
6. Plays major role in metabolism

L. Bile ducts
1. Two main hepatic ducts join to form common hepatic duct
2. Common hepatic duct unites with cystic duct (attached to the gallbladder) to form common bile duct
3. In some cases, common bile duct joins pancreatic duct to enter hepatopancreatic ampulla
4. Hepatopancreatic ampulla opens into descending duodenum
5. In other cases, common bile duct and pancreatic duct enter duodenum directly and separately
6. Distal end of common bile duct controlled by hepatopancreatic sphincter (sphincter of Oddi)

M. Gallbladder
1. Thin-walled sac with capacity of approximately 2 oz
2. Concentrates and stores bile and evacuates bile during digestion
3. Contraction of gallbladder is controlled by hormone cholecystokinin

Urinary System

A. Kidneys (Figure 5-18)
1. Paired bean-shaped organs on both sides of the vertebral column
2. Renal artery and vein and the ureter (which leads to the bladder) are attached to the center of the kidney at the hilus
3. Outer part of the kidney is called the *cortex*, and inner part is called the *medulla*
    a. Medulla consists of several pyramids
    b. Apices of the pyramids project into the calices
    c. Nephron is the functional unit of the kidney
4. Kidney connected to the bladder by the ureters

B. Ureters
1. Approximately 27 cm long
2. Urine flows down the ureters via peristalsis

C. Bladder
1. Lies behind the symphysis pubis
2. Serves as a reservoir for the urine

D. Urethra
1. Connects the bladder to the exterior
2. Female urethra is approximately 4 cm long
3. Male urethra is approximately 20 cm long

E. Blood is filtered first in the glomeruli
1. Passed through the glomerular membrane into Bowman's capsule and then into the proximal tubules
2. Filtration rate is determined by the filtration pressure
3. Modified as it passes through the tubules by means of reabsorption and secretion
    a. Proximal convoluted tubule
    b. Loop of Henle
    c. Distal collecting tubule
4. Waste products are not reabsorbed

REVIEW OF RADIOGRAPHIC POSITIONING, PROCEDURES, AND PATHOLOGY*

Skeletal System

Pathologies Imaged

NOTE: Designation of *harder to penetrate* or *easier to penetrate* does not necessarily signify that alteration of exposure technique is required.

A. Acromegaly
1. Endocrine disorder that causes bones to become thick and coarse
2. Harder to penetrate

B. Ankylosing spondylitis
1. Inflammatory disease of the spine and adjacent structures that causes severe pain and fusion of the joints involved

C. Bony cyst
1. Fluid-filled sacs in fibrous tissue
2. Easier to penetrate

D. Bursitis
1. Inflammation of bursa; causes severe pain
2. Harder to penetrate if calcium has deposited

E. Callus
1. New bony deposit surrounding healing fractures
2. Harder to penetrate

F. Clubfoot (talipes)
1. Congenital malformation of the foot that causes foot to turn in at the ankle

G. Congenital hip anomaly
1. Caused by a malformation of the acetabulum in which the femoral head displaces superiorly and posteriorly

H. Disk herniation
1. Protrusion of an intervertebral disk

---

*Positioning routines vary from text to text and from department to department. The following is a general review of common routines.

I. Ewing's sarcoma
  1. Malignant destructive tumor of bone marrow
  2. Easier to penetrate
J. Fractures: disruption of bone tissue
  1. Complete fracture: discontinuity between two or more fragments
  2. Incomplete fracture: partial discontinuity; portion of the cortex is intact
  3. Closed fracture: overlying skin is intact
  4. Compound fracture: overlying skin is broken; bony fragments
  5. Transverse fracture: runs at right angle to the long axis of the bone
  6. Oblique fracture: runs approximately 45 degrees to the long axis of the bone
  7. Spiral fracture: encircles the shaft of the bone
  8. Avulsion fracture: small fragments of bone torn off bony prominences
  9. Comminuted fracture: produces more than two fragments
  10. Compression fracture: causes compaction of the bone, resulting in decreased length or width
  11. Stress fracture: results from repeated stresses placed on the bone
  12. Pathologic fracture: occurs as a result of bone disease
  13. Greenstick fracture: incomplete fracture with cortex intact on opposite side of the bone from the fracture
  14. Bowing fracture: occurs when stress applied to the bone causes the bone to bow but not quite fracture
  15. Undisplaced fracture: lack of angulation or separation of fractured bone
  16. Displacement: separation of bone fragments
  17. Angulation: deformity between the axis of major fragments of bone
  18. Dislocation: displacement of a bone from its normal site of articulation
  19. Subluxation: partial loss of continuity in a joint
  20. Fracture healing: characterized radiographically by calcium deposits across the fracture line that unite the fracture fragments
  21. Battered child syndrome: multiple fractures at various stages of healing located in long bones and the skull; also characterized by fractures at unusual sites (e.g., ribs, scapula, sternum, spine, clavicles)
  22. Colles' fracture: transverse fracture through the distal radius with posterior angulation and over-riding of the distal fracture fragment
  23. Boxer's fracture: transverse fracture of the neck of the fifth metacarpal with palmar angulation of the distal fragment
  24. Elbow fractures: in addition to bony involvement, radiograph will show dislocation of elbow fat pads; this necessitates the use of appropriate radiographic exposure
  25. Pott's fracture: fracture of medial and lateral malleoli of the ankle with ankle joint dislocation
  26. Bimalleolar fracture: fracture of both medial and lateral malleoli
  27. Trimalleolar fracture: fracture of the posterior portion of the tibia and the medial and lateral malleoli
  28. Jefferson's fracture: comminuted fracture of the ring of the atlas involving both anterior and posterior arches and causing displacement of the fragments
  29. Hangman's fracture: caused by acute hyperextension of the head on the neck; characterized by a fracture of the arch of C2 and anterior subluxation of C2 onto C3; primarily caused by motor vehicle accidents
  30. Seat belt fracture: transverse fracture of lumbar vertebrae in addition to substantial abdominal injuries
K. Hydrocephalus
  1. Abnormal accumulation of cerebrospinal fluid in the brain
  2. Harder to penetrate
L. Giant cell myeloma
  1. Benign or malignant tumor arising on bone with large bubble appearance
  2. Easier to penetrate
M. Gout
  1. Metabolic disorder in which urate crystals are deposited in the joints, most commonly the great toe, and cause extreme swelling
  2. Harder to penetrate
N. Multiple myeloma
  1. Malignancy of plasma cells resulting in destruction of bone, failure of bone marrow, and impairment of renal function
  2. Easier to penetrate
O. Osteoarthritis
  1. Form of arthritis characterized by degeneration of one or several joints
  2. Easier to penetrate
P. Osteoblastic metastases
  1. Dense, sclerotic tumors in bone
  2. Harder to penetrate
Q. Osteochondroma
  1. Benign projection of bone in the young
  2. Harder to penetrate
R. Osteogenic sarcoma
  1. Destructive cancer at the end of long bones
  2. Easier to penetrate (except for sclerotic area)
S. Osteoma
  1. Benign, small, round tumor
  2. Harder to penetrate

T. Osteogenesis imperfecta
1. Inherited condition causing poor development of connective tissue and brittle and easily fractured bones
2. Easier to penetrate

U. Osteomyelitis
1. Bacterial infection of bone and bone marrow
2. Easier to penetrate

V. Osteolytic metastases
1. Arise in medullary canal to destroy bone
2. Easier to penetrate

W. Osteomalacia
1. Abnormal softening of bone
2. Easier to penetrate

X. Osteopetrosis
1. Inherited condition causing increased bone density
2. Harder to penetrate

Y. Osteoporosis
1. Abnormal demineralization of bone
2. Easier to penetrate

Z. Paget's disease (osteitis deformans)
1. Nonmetabolic bone disease causing bone destruction and unorganized bone repair
2. Difficult to image properly because some areas that are easier to penetrate are adjacent to structures that are harder to penetrate

AA. Rheumatoid arthritis
1. Destructive collagen disease with inflammation and joint swelling
2. Harder to penetrate

BB. Rickets
1. Soft pliable bones resulting from deficiency of vitamin D and sunlight
2. Easier to penetrate

CC. Scoliosis: abnormal lateral curvature of the spine

DD. Spina bifida: defect of posterior aspect of spinal canal caused by failure of vertebral arch to form properly

EE. Spondylolisthesis: spondylolysis with displacement

FF. Spondylolysis
1. Defect in pars articularis, which is between the superior and inferior articular processes of a vertebra
2. No displacement present

Digits (Fingers)

A. PA
1. Patient position: seated
2. Part position: separate and center extended digit of interest with palmar surface of hand firmly against cassette
3. Central ray: perpendicular, entering proximal interphalangeal joint

B. Lateral
1. Patient position: seated

2. Part position
   a. Digit of interest is extended
   b. Close rest of digits into a fist
   c. Adjust digit of interest parallel to film plane
   d. Immobilize extended digit
3. Central ray: perpendicular, entering proximal interphalangeal joint

C. Oblique
1. Patient position: seated
2. Part position
   a. Place patient's hand in lateral position, ulnar side down
   b. Center to cassette
   c. Rotate palm 45 degrees toward cassette until digits are resting on support
   d. Immobilize separated digits
3. Central ray: perpendicular, entering proximal interphalangeal joint

Thumb

A. AP, lateral, oblique
1. Patient position: seated
2. Part position
   a. AP: patient's hand is turned in extreme internal rotation, thumb resting on cassette, other fingers held out of the way
   b. Lateral: hand in natural arched position, palm down; adjust hand to put thumb in true lateral
   c. Oblique: abduct thumb, palm down
3. Central ray (all projections): perpendicular to the metacarpophalangeal joint

Hand

A. PA
1. Patient position: seated
2. Part position
   a. Patient rests forearm on table, with palmar surface firmly against cassette
   b. Spread digits slightly
3. Central ray: perpendicular to third metacarpophalangeal joint

B. Oblique
1. Patient position: seated, forearm resting on table with hand on cassette in lateral position, ulnar side down
2. Part position
   a. Rotate hand medially
   b. Place digits on a 45-degree radiolucent support to demonstrate interphalangeal joints
   c. Adjust digits parallel to cassette
3. Central ray: perpendicular to third metacarpophalangeal joint

C. Lateral
1. Patient position: seated, resting ulnar surface of forearm on table with hand in true lateral position

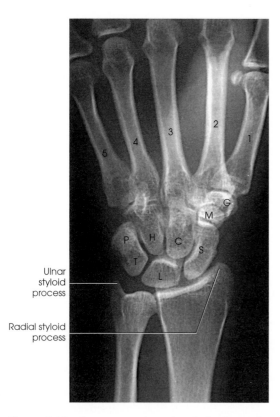

Figure 5-19 Posteroanterior wrist. *C,* Capitate; *G,* trapezium; *H,* hamate; *L,* lunate; *P,* pisiform; *S,* scaphoid; *T,* triquetrum.

2. Part position
   a. Extend digits with first digit (thumb) placed at a right angle to palm of hand
   b. As an option, patient may "fan" fingers and place on positioning sponge to reduce superimposition of phalanges
   c. Center metacarpophalangeal joints to cassette
   d. Adjust palmar surface of hand perpendicular to cassette
3. Central ray: perpendicular to second metacarpophalangeal joint

Wrist

A. PA
1. Patient position: seated, forearm resting on table
2. Part position
   a. Center carpus to cassette area
   b. Digits are flexed slightly to place wrist in contact with cassette
3. Central ray: perpendicular to midcarpal area (Figure 5-19)

B. Lateral
1. Patient position: elbow is flexed 90 degrees, with forearm and arm in contact with table
2. Part position: center carpals and adjust hand so wrist is lateral
3. Central ray: perpendicular to wrist joint (Figure 5-20)

C. Oblique
1. Patient position: seated, ulnar surface of wrist on cassette
2. Part position
   a. Center carpus to cassette area

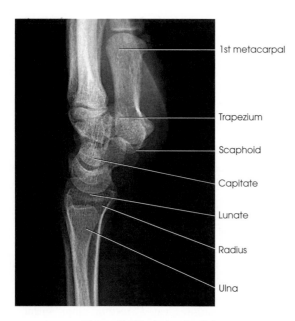

Figure 5-20 Lateral wrist.

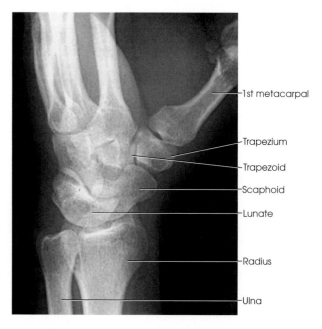

Figure 5-21 Posteroanterior oblique wrist.

    b. From true lateral, rotate part approximately 45 degrees medially and support on sponge

  3. Central ray: perpendicular to cassette, entering midcarpal area just distal to radius (Figure 5-21)

D. Scaphoid (navicular)

  1. Patient position: elbow is flexed 90 degrees, with forearm and arm in contact with table

  2. Part position

    a. Center carpals to cassette area

    b. Place patient's wrist in extreme ulnar flexion

  3. Central ray: perpendicular to scaphoid; option to delineate fracture may require angulation of 10 to 15 degrees proximally (toward elbow) or distally; another approach is to elevate distal end of cassette approximately 20 degrees

Forearm

A. AP

  1. Patient position: seated

  2. Part position: supinate hand and center forearm to cassette to include joint(s) of interest

  3. Central ray: perpendicular to midpoint of forearm (Figure 5-22)

B. Lateral

  1. Patient position: seated, with humerus and forearm in contact with table; elbow flexed

  2. Part position

    a. Elbow is flexed 90 degrees

    b. Adjust hand to lateral position (thumb up)

    c. Center forearm to cassette to include joint(s) of interest

  3. Central ray: perpendicular to midpoint of forearm (Figure 5-23)

Elbow

A. AP

  1. Patient position: seated, with arm extended

  2. Part position

    a. Extend patient's elbow

    b. Supinate hand

    c. Center elbow joint to cassette

    d. Patient may have to lean slightly laterally to ensure AP alignment

  3. Central ray: perpendicular to elbow joint (Figure 5-24)

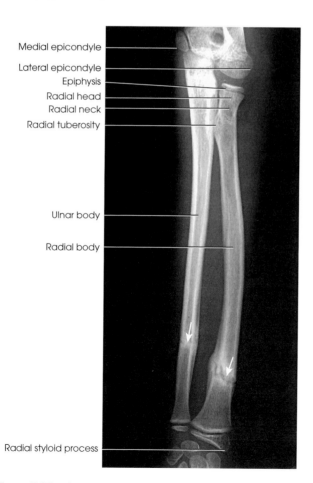

Figure 5-22   Anteroposterior forearm with fractured radius and ulna.

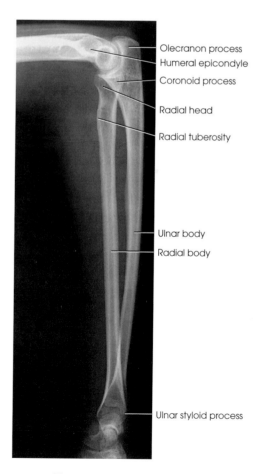

Figure 5-23   Lateral forearm.

B. Lateral
1. Patient position: seated, with elbow flexed 90 degrees; humerus and forearm resting on table
2. Part position
   a. Center 90-degree flexed elbow joint to cassette
   b. Adjust wrist and hand in lateral position
3. Central ray: perpendicular to elbow joint (Figure 5-25)

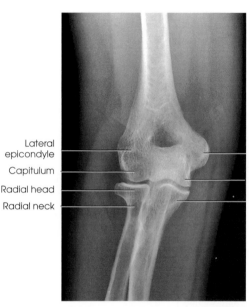

Figure 5-24   Anteroposterior elbow.

C. Medial oblique
1. Patient position: seated, with arm extended
2. Part position
   a. Pronate hand
   b. Medially rotate arm
   c. Adjust anterior surface of elbow (epicondyles) at an angle of 40 to 45 degrees
3. Central ray: perpendicular to elbow joint (Figure 5-26)

D. Lateral oblique
1. Patient position: seated, with arm extended
2. Part position
   a. Rotate patient's hand laterally
   b. Adjust posterior surface of elbow at a 40-degree angle to cassette
3. Central ray: perpendicular to elbow joint

Humerus

A. AP
1. Patient position: erect or supine
2. Part position
   a. Unless it is contraindicated, supinate patient's hand and adjust humerus with epicondyles parallel to cassette; keep humerus in neutral position if fracture is suspected or if reexamining healing fracture with a hanging cast
   b. If patient is recumbent, elevate and support opposite shoulder
   c. Center humerus to cassette

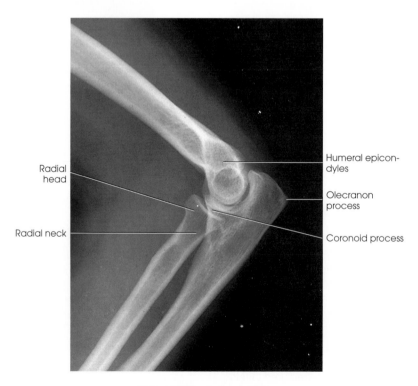

Figure 5-25   Lateral elbow.

3. Central ray: perpendicular to midpoint of humerus
B. Lateral
   1. Patient position: erect or supine
   2. Part position
     a. Unless it is contraindicated, slightly abduct the arm and center arm to cassette
     b. Medially rotate forearm until epicondyles are perpendicular to cassette
   3. Central ray: perpendicular to midpoint of humerus

Shoulder

A. AP
   1. Patient position: erect or supine
   2. Part position
     a. Center area of coracoid process to cassette
     b. Rotate patient slightly to place affected scapula parallel to cassette
     c. Adjust hand in (1) external rotation to obtain AP projection of humerus or (2) internal rotation for lateral position of humerus
     d. Respiration: suspended
   3. Central ray: perpendicular to coracoid process (Figure 5-27)
B. Transthoracic lateral
   1. Patient position: erect or supine
   2. Part position
     a. Raise uninjured arm and rest on head
     b. Elevate uninjured shoulder as much as possible
     c. Respiration: full inspiration or slow breathing
   3. Central ray: adjust patient to project humerus between vertebral column and sternum; unless it is contraindicated, adjust humeral epicondyles perpen-

dicular to cassette; central ray perpendicular to median coronal plane, exiting surgical neck of affected humerus; if patient cannot elevate unaffected shoulder, the central ray may be angled 10 to 15 degrees cephalad
C. PA oblique (scapular Y)
   1. Patient position: erect or prone oblique
   2. Part position
     a. Center anterior surface of affected shoulder to cassette
     b. Rotate patient so that midcoronal plane forms 60-degree angle from cassette
     c. Respiration: suspended
   3. Central ray: perpendicular to shoulder joint at level of scapulohumeral joint (Figure 5-28)

Acromioclavicular Articulations

A. AP
   1. Patient position: upright if condition permits
   2. Part position
     a. Adjust midpoint of cassette to level of acromioclavicular (AC) joints
     b. Center MSP of patient's body to midline of cassette, if both AC joints can be demonstrated on one radiograph
     c. Otherwise, center to each individual AC joint for two separate exposures
     d. To demonstrate AC separation, sandbags of equal weight should be attached to each wrist and a second radiograph obtained without weights
     e. Respiration: suspended
   3. Central ray: perpendicular to cassette, midway between AC joints or perpendicular to each AC joint

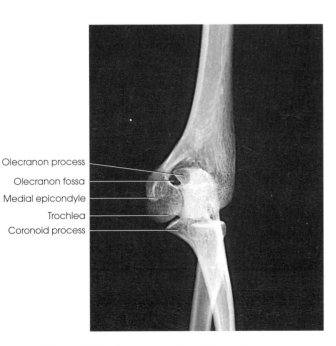

Figure 5-26 Anteroposterior oblique elbow.

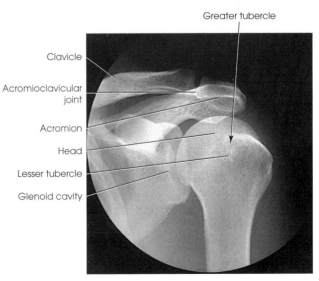

Figure 5-27 Anteroposterior shoulder.

Clavicle

A. PA

1. Patient position: erect or prone; may be AP for patient comfort
2. Part position
   a. Center clavicle to center of cassette midway between midline of body and coracoid process
   b. Head may be turned away from affected side
   c. Respiration: suspended
3. Central ray: perpendicular to midshaft of clavicle

B. PA axial

1. Patient position: erect or prone; may be supine (AP axial) for patient comfort
2. Part position
   a. Center clavicle to midline of table with cassette midway between MSP and coracoid process
   b. Head may be turned away from affected side
   c. Respiration: suspended
3. Central ray: angle 25 to 30 degrees caudad, centered to the midshaft of the clavicle (25 to 30 degrees cephalad if performed AP)

Scapula

A. AP

1. Patient position: supine or upright (upright preferred when shoulder is tender)
2. Part position
   a. Abduct arm
   b. Flex elbow
   c. Support hand near head
   d. Center palpated scapular area to cassette approximately 2 inches inferior to coracoid process
   e. Respiration: quiet breathing
3. Central ray: perpendicular to cassette at midscapular area approximately 2 inches inferior to coracoid process (Figure 5-29)

B. Lateral

1. Patient position: prone oblique or upright (upright preferred when shoulder is tender)
2. Part position
   a. Place patient in an oblique position with affected scapula centered to cassette
   b. Extend affected arm across anterior thorax
   c. Palpate axillary and vertebral borders of scapula and adjust body rotation so that scapula is lateral and will be projected free of rib cage
   d. Respiration: suspended
3. Central ray: perpendicular to medial border of protruding scapula

Toes

A. AP

1. Patient position: supine or seated on table, knees flexed with feet separated

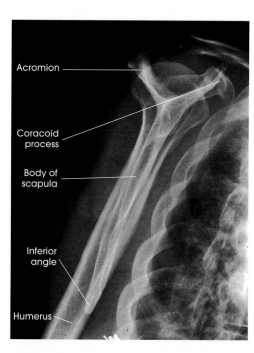

Figure 5-28 Posteroanterior oblique shoulder (scapular Y).

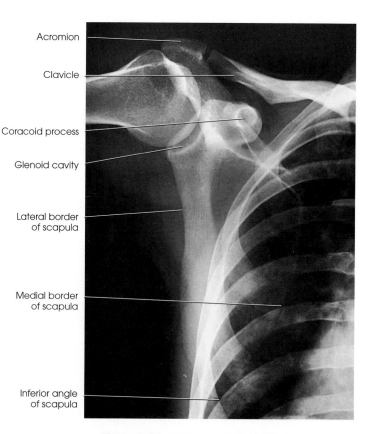

Figure 5-29 Anteroposterior scapula.

2. Part position: center toes with plantar surface flat against cassette
3. Central ray: 15 degrees cephalad, if positioning wedge is not used; enters the second metatarsophalangeal joint

B. Oblique
1. Patient position: supine or seated on table, knees flexed with feet separated
2. Part position: center patient's toes over cassette area and medially rotate leg and foot until a 30- to 45-degree angle is formed from cassette to plantar surface of foot
3. Central ray: perpendicular, entering third metatarsophalangeal joint

Foot

A. AP
1. Patient position: supine or seated on table, knees flexed with feet separated
2. Part position
   a. Plantar surface firmly resting on cassette
   b. Center foot to cassette
   c. Adjust midline of foot parallel to long axis of cassette
3. Central ray: 10 degrees toward the heel, entering base of third metatarsal

B. Medial oblique
1. Patient position: supine or seated on table, knees flexed with feet separated

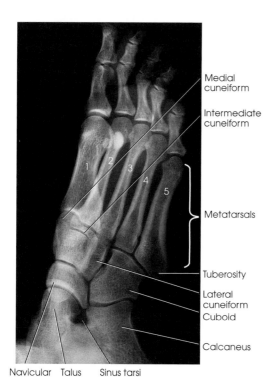

Figure 5-30 Anteroposterior oblique foot in medial rotation.

Medial cuneiform
Intermediate cuneiform
Metatarsals
Tuberosity
Lateral cuneiform
Cuboid
Calcaneus
Navicular Talus Sinus tarsi

2. Part position
   a. Center foot to cassette
   b. Rotate leg medially until plantar surface forms angle of 30 degrees to cassette
3. Central ray: perpendicular to base of third metatarsal (Figure 5-30)

C. Lateral (mediolateral)
1. Patient position
   a. With the patient lying on the affected side, adjust leg and foot in lateral position
   b. Patella perpendicular to table
2. Part position: center foot and adjust plantar surface perpendicular to cassette
3. Central ray: perpendicular to midpoint of cassette, entering base of third metatarsal

Calcaneus

A. Axial (plantodorsal)
1. Patient position: supine or seated with leg fully extended
2. Part position
   a. Center cassette to ankle
   b. Draw the plantar surface of foot perpendicular to cassette
3. Central ray: 40 degrees cephalad to long axis of foot, entering midline at level of base of fifth metatarsal

B. Lateral
1. Patient position
   a. With the patient lying on the affected side, adjust leg and foot in lateral position
   b. Patella perpendicular to table
2. Part position: center calcaneus to cassette, about 1 to 1.5 inches distal to medial malleolus
3. Central ray: perpendicular to midportion of calcaneus

Ankle

A. AP
1. Patient position: supine or seated on table with small support under knee
2. Part position
   a. Center ankle to cassette
   b. Dorsiflex foot
   c. Adjust ankle with toes pointing vertically
3. Central ray: perpendicular to ankle joint midway between malleoli (Figure 5-31)

B. Lateral
1. Patient position: supine, roll onto affected side
2. Part position
   a. Rotate patient's ankle to lateral position
   b. Adjust foot in lateral position
   c. Center ankle to cassette
3. Central ray: vertical through medial malleolus (Figure 5-32)

C. Medial oblique
1. Patient position: supine or seated on table

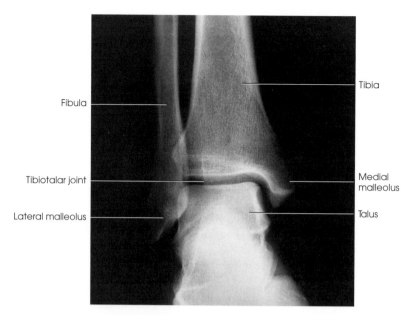

Figure 5-31   Anteroposterior ankle.

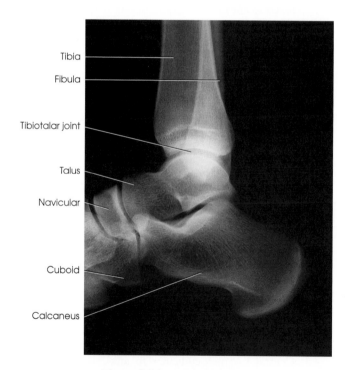

Figure 5-32   Lateral ankle.

2. Part position
  a. Rotate patient's leg and foot medially
  b. Adjust degree of medial rotation for (1) mortise joint: until malleoli are parallel with film (15 to 20 degrees); or (2) bony structure: to 45 degrees rotation
3. Central ray: vertical midway between malleoli

Leg

A. AP
  1. Patient position: supine with leg extended
  2. Part position
    a. Center leg to cassette
    b. Adjust leg to AP position
    c. Both joints should be included
  3. Central ray: vertical to midpoint of leg
B. Lateral
  1. Patient position: supine and roll onto affected side
  2. Part position
    a. Center leg to cassette
    b. Adjust leg to lateral position
    c. Patella perpendicular
    d. Both joints should be included
  3. Central ray: perpendicular to midpoint of leg (Figure 5-33)

Knee

A. AP
  1. Patient position: supine and with leg extended, adjust patient's body so that pelvis is not rotated
  2. Part position
    a. Center knee to cassette
    b. Adjust leg to AP position
  3. Central ray: 5 to 7 degrees cephalad to a point 0.5 inch inferior to patellar apex (Figure 5-34)
B. Lateral
  1. Patient position: turn patient onto affected side with knee flexed (usually 20 to 30 degrees)
  2. Part position
    a. Flex and center knee

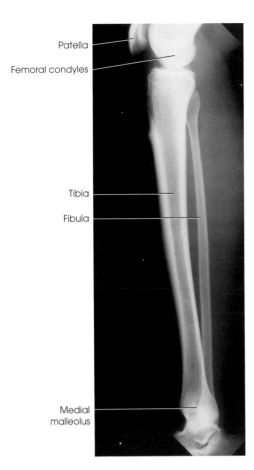

Patella
Femoral condyles
Tibia
Fibula
Medial malleolus

Figure 5-33 Lateral tibia and fibula.

b. Center cassette approximately 1 inch distal to medial epicondyle
c. Patella perpendicular to film
3. Central ray: 5 degrees cephalad, entering knee joint inferior to medial condyle

C. Intercondylar fossa (tunnel)
1. Patient position: kneeling on radiographic table with affected knee flexed 70 degrees from full extension
2. Part position
a. Center knee to cassette
b. Place at level of patellar apex
c. Flex knee 70 degrees from full extension
3. Central ray: perpendicular to long axis of lower leg, entering midpopliteal area

Patella

A. PA
1. Patient position: prone with knee extended
2. Part position
a. Center patella
b. Adjust to be parallel with cassette plane
c. Heel generally rotated 5 to 10 degrees laterally
3. Central ray: perpendicular to midpopliteal area

B. Tangential
1. Patient position: prone with foot resting on table
2. Part position: flex affected knee so that tibia and fibula form a 50- to 60-degree angle from table
3. Central ray: 45 degrees cephalad through patellofemoral joint (Figure 5-35)

C. Lateral
1. Patient position: lying on affected side
2. Part position: flex knee 5 to 10 degrees, femoral epicondyles superimposed
3. Central ray: perpendicular to patella

Femur

A. AP
1. Patient position: supine with toes up
2. Part position
a. Center affected thigh to midline of table
b. Internally rotate lower limb approximately 15 degrees
c. Both joints should be included
d. Apply gonadal shielding as appropriate
3. Central ray: perpendicular to midfemur

B. Lateral
1. Patient position: lying on affected side with knee slightly flexed
2. Part position
a. Rotate patient's unaffected hip (including hip joint) posteriorly to prevent superimposition of unaffected hip
b. Center femur to midline of table
c. Both joints should be included
d. Apply gonadal shielding as appropriate
3. Central ray: perpendicular to midfemur

Pelvis

A. AP
1. Patient position: supine
2. Part position
a. Center MSP to table
b. Adjust to AP position
c. Internally rotate feet and lower limb 15 degrees
d. Center cassette approximately 2 inches superior to level of greater trochanter
e. Use gonadal shielding as appropriate
f. Respiration: suspended
3. Central ray: perpendicular to midpoint of film 2 inches superior to symphysis pubis

Hip

A. AP
1. Patient position: supine
2. Part position
a. Rotate lower limb 15 degrees medially
b. Center hip to cassette
c. Respiration: suspended

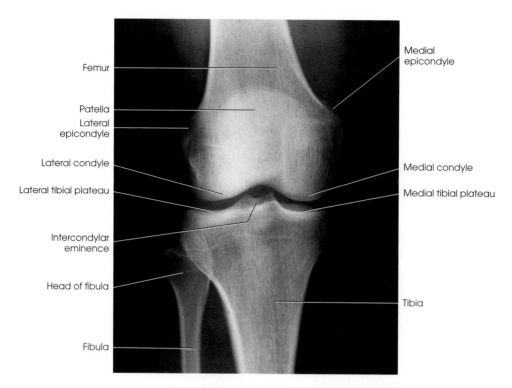

Femur

Patella

Lateral epicondyle

Lateral condyle

Lateral tibial plateau

Intercondylar eminence

Head of fibula

Fibula

Medial epicondyle

Medial condyle

Medial tibial plateau

Tibia

Figure 5-34   Anteroposterior knee.

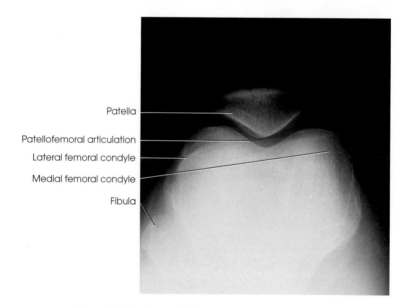

Patella

Patellofemoral articulation

Lateral femoral condyle

Medial femoral condyle

Fibula

Figure 5-35   Tangential patella (Settegast method).

3. Central ray: perpendicular to a point 2 inches medial to ASIS and at level of superior margin of greater trochanter (Figure 5-36)

B. Lateral

1. Patient position: from supine position, turn patient toward affected side to posterior oblique body position

2. Part position

a. Flex affected knee

b. Center affected hip to midline of table

c. Extend unaffected knee

d. Respiration: suspended

3. Central ray: perpendicular to a point midway between ASIS and symphysis pubis

C. Axiolateral

1. Patient position: supine with level of greater trochanter elevated to center of cassette

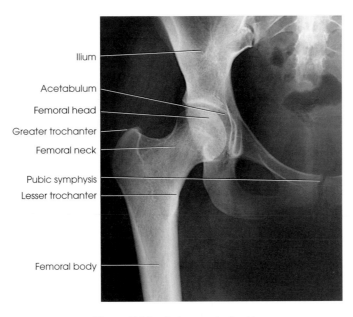

Figure 5-36 Anteroposterior hip.

2. Part position
   a. Flex knee and hip of unaffected side
   b. Elevate and rest on suitable support
   c. Adjust pelvis to supine position
   d. Unless it is contraindicated, rotate affected leg 15 to 20 degrees internally
   e. Respiration: suspended
3. Central ray: perpendicular to long axis of femoral neck and cassette

Cervical Vertebrae

A. Atlas and axis
   1. Patient position: erect or supine
   2. Part position
      a. MSP centered to cassette at level of C2
      b. Arms by sides
      c. Shoulders in same plane
      d. Have patient open mouth wide
      e. Adjust head so that line from lower edge of upper incisors to mastoid process is perpendicular to cassette
      f. Respiration: phonate "ah" during exposure
   3. Central ray: perpendicular to cassette, centered to open mouth (Figure 5-37)
B. AP
   1. Patient position: erect or supine
   2. Part position
      a. MSP centered to cassette
      b. Arms by sides
      c. Center cassette at level of C4

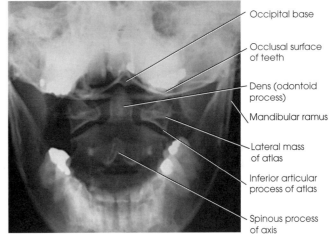

Figure 5-37 Open-mouth atlas and axis.

   d. Adjust a line between upper occlusal plane and mastoid tip, perpendicular to cassette
   e. Respiration: suspended
3. Central ray: 15 to 20 degrees cephalad, entering slightly inferior to thyroid cartilage (Figure 5-38)
C. Lateral
   1. Patient position: seated or standing in lateral position
   2. Part position
      a. Center coronal plane through mastoid tips to cassette
      b. Adjust patient's shoulders to same horizontal level and body to true lateral position

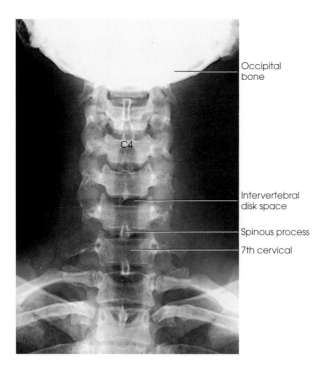

Figure 5-38   Anteroposterior axial cervical vertebrae.

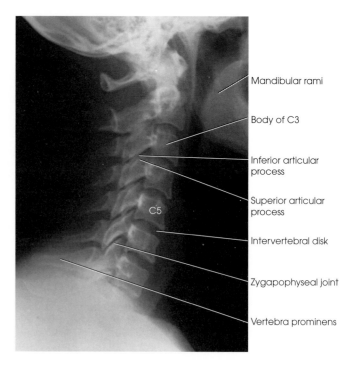

Figure 5-39   Lateral cervical vertebrae.

c. Elevate chin slightly

d. Relax shoulders

e. Weights may be attached to wrists to help lower shoulders

f. Source-to-image distance (SID) recommended: 72 inches

g. Respiration: expiration

3. Central ray: perpendicular to cassette entering C4 (Figure 5-39)

D. LPO and RPO (AP oblique projections)

1. Patient position: seated or standing

2. Part position

a. Rotate body 45 degrees

b. Place side of interest farthest from cassette

c. Have patient slightly extend chin while looking forward

d. Center spine to cassette

e. Take both obliques

f. Respiration: suspended

3. Central ray: 15 to 20 degrees cephalad, entering C4 (Figure 5-40)

Thoracic Vertebrae

A. AP

1. Patient position: supine or upright

2. Part position

a. MSP centered to cassette

b. Top of film 1.5 to 2 inches above shoulders

c. Arms by sides

d. Shoulders in same plane

e. Respiration: shallow or suspended expiration

3. Central ray: perpendicular to T7, 3 to 4 inches distal to jugular (manubrial) notch

B. Lateral

1. Patient position: lateral recumbent or erect

2. Part position

a. Elevate head to spine level

b. Extend arms forward

c. Place radiolucent support under lower thoracic region until spine is horizontal to top of table

d. Respiration: shallow or suspended expiration

3. Central ray: perpendicular to cassette, entering level of T7, approximately 3 to 4 inches below sternal angle (Figure 5-41)

C. Cervicothoracic (Twining)

1. Patient position: lateral, seated or standing

2. Part position

a. Center midcoronal plane to grid

b. Elevate arm adjacent to Bucky

c. Center film to the level of T2

d. Body in true lateral position

e. Respiration: suspended

3. Central ray: perpendicular to cassette, entering at level of T2 (Figure 5-42)

Lumbar Vertebrae

A. AP

1. Patient position: supine

2. Part position

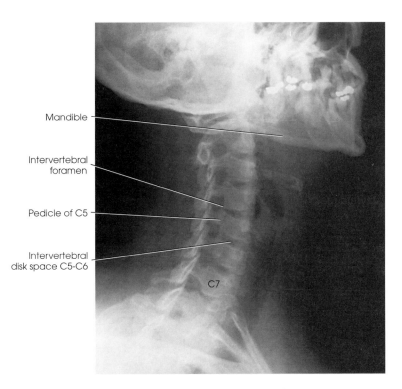

Figure 5-40 RAO showing right side.

a. MSP centered to table
b. Flex patient's knees and hips enough to place back in firm contact with table
c. Center cassette at level of iliac crest (L4)
d. Respiration: suspended
3. Central ray: perpendicular to midline, entering level of iliac crests (Figure 5-43)
B. Lateral
1. Patient position: lateral with hips and knees flexed
2. Part position
a. Center midaxillary line of body and L4 to table
b. Extend arms forward
c. Place radiolucent support under lower thorax, and adjust spine parallel to table
d. Check for true lateral position
e. Respiration: suspended
3. Central ray: perpendicular to cassette, entering midaxillary line at level of iliac crests (Figure 5-44)
C. Lateral L5 to S1
1. Patient position: lateral with hips and knees flexed
2. Part position
a. Center 1.5 inches posterior to midaxillary line and 1.5 inches below iliac crest
b. Extend arms forward
c. Place radiolucent support under lower thorax, and adjust spine parallel to table
d. Check for true lateral position
e. Collimate tightly
f. Respiration: suspended

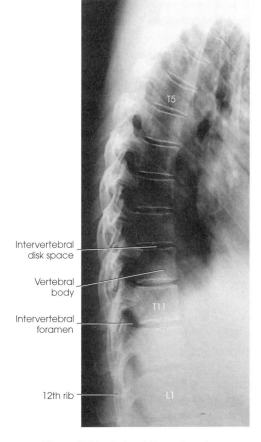

Figure 5-41 Lateral thoracic spine.

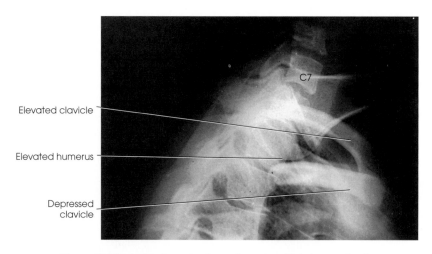

Figure 5-42 Lateral cervicothoracic region (Twining method).

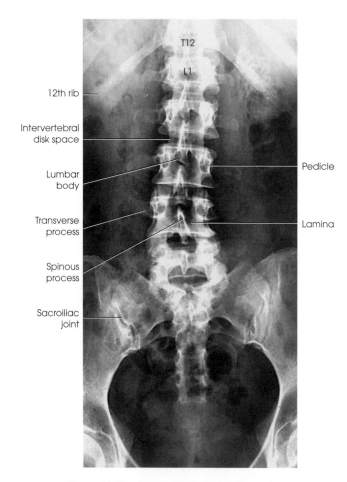

Figure 5-43 Anteroposterior lumbar spine.

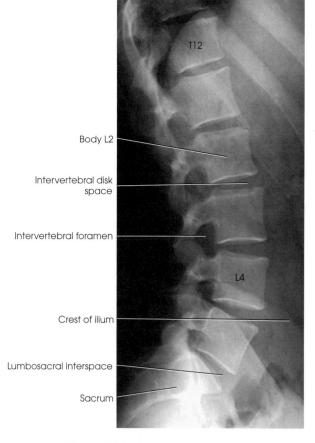

Figure 5-44 Lateral lumbar spine.

3. Central ray: perpendicular to L5 at a point 1.5 inches anterior to palpated spinous process of L5 and 1.5 inches inferior to iliac crest

D. LPO and RPO (AP obliques)

1. Patient position: posterior oblique; side closest to cassette is side of interest

2. Part position
   a. Adjust and support body obliquity to 45 degrees
   b. Adjust arms to a comfortable position
   c. Center spine to midline of table
   d. Center cassette at level of L3
   e. Take obliques of both sides

f. Respiration: suspended
3. Central ray: perpendicular to L3, 1 to 2 inches above level of iliac crest, entering elevated side 2 inches laterally from patient's midline

Sacroiliac Joints
A. LPO and RPO (AP oblique)
   1. Patient position: supine
   2. Part position
      a. Elevate and support side of interest 25 to 30 degrees from table
      b. Align sagittal plane passing 1 inch medial to ASIS of elevated side centered to film
      c. Center to table
      d. Take both obliques
      e. Respiration: suspended
   3. Central ray: perpendicular to cassette, 1 inch medial to elevated ASIS

Sacrum
A. AP
   1. Patient position: supine
   2. Part position
      a. Center MSP to center of table
      b. Respiration: suspended
   3. Central ray: 15 degrees cephalad, entering 2 inches superior to symphysis pubis
B. Lateral
   1. Patient position: lateral with hips and knees flexed
   2. Part position
      a. Support body to place long axis of spine horizontally
      b. Align coronal plane, passing 3 inches posterior to median coronal plane
      c. Center to midline of table
      d. Respiration: suspended
   3. Central ray: perpendicular to cassette, entering 3 inches posterior to median coronal plane at level of ASIS

Coccyx
A. AP
   1. Patient position: supine
   2. Part position
      a. Center MSP to center of table
      b. Respiration: suspended
   3. Central ray: 10 degrees caudad, entering 2 inches superior to symphysis pubis
B. Lateral
   1. Patient position: lateral with hips and knees flexed
   2. Part position
      a. Support body to place long axis of spine horizontally
      b. Align coronal plane passing approximately 5 inches posterior to median coronal plane

c. Center to midline of table
d. Respiration: suspended
3. Central ray: perpendicular to cassette, entering palpated coccyx located approximately 5 inches posterior to median coronal plane

Scoliosis Series
A. PA (to minimize exposure to breast tissue; AP may be performed using compensating filters)
   1. Patient position: seated or standing
   2. Part position
      a. First radiograph: MSP centered to film; film adjusted to include 1 inch of the iliac crests; arms at sides
      b. Second radiograph: MSP centered to film; elevate hip or foot of convex side of curve 3 or 4 inches on a block
   3. Central ray: perpendicular to the midpoint of the film

Thorax
Pathologies Imaged
A. Adult respiratory distress syndrome
   1. Acute life-threatening respiratory distress
   2. Large amount of fluid in interstitial and alveolar spaces
   3. Harder to penetrate
B. Asthma
   1. Pulmonary disorder with increased mucus production in bronchi, causing hyperventilation of the lungs
   2. Bronchi harder to penetrate
   3. Lungs easier to penetrate
C. Atelectasis
   1. Collapse of lung tissue
   2. Harder to penetrate
D. Bronchial adenoma
   1. Neoplasm occurring in a bronchus, causing atelectasis and pneumonitis
   2. Harder to penetrate
E. Bronchiectasis
   1. Dilatation and destruction of bronchial walls
   2. Consolidation present
   3. Harder to penetrate
F. Bronchogenic carcinoma
   1. Lung cancer arising from the bronchial mucosa
   2. Harder to penetrate
G. Chronic bronchitis
   1. Debilitating pulmonary disease with substantial increase of mucus production in the trachea and bronchi
   2. Harder to penetrate unless evolved into emphysema, which is easier to penetrate
H. Chronic obstructive pulmonary disease
   1. Progressive condition marked by diminished capabilities of inspiration and expiration
   2. Harder to penetrate

I. Croup
1. Acute viral infection of infant's respiratory system
2. Lateral soft tissue neck radiograph taken to show subepiglottic narrowing

J. Cystic fibrosis
1. Inherited pathologic condition of exocrine glands
2. Marked by increased mucus secretion in lungs and bronchi
3. Harder to penetrate

K. Emphysema
1. Overinflation of alveolar walls
2. Easier to penetrate
3. Should not be imaged using automatic exposure controls (AECs) because minimum reaction time of equipment usually results in overexposure and subsequent repeat films

L. Empyema
1. Pus in the pleural space
2. Harder to penetrate

M. Histoplasmosis
1. Infection caused by inhaling fungal spores
2. Harder to penetrate

N. Hyaline membrane disease
1. Respiratory distress syndrome of the newborn (RDS)
2. Acute lung disease in newborn; characteristics include airless alveoli and rapid respirations
3. Harder to penetrate

O. Legionnaires' disease
1. Form of acute bacterial pneumonia
2. Harder to penetrate

P. Pleural effusion
1. Accumulation of fluid in intrapleural spaces
2. Harder to penetrate

Q. Pneumoconiosis
1. Lung disease caused by inhaling dust (usually mineral dust from the environment or workplace)
2. Silicosis: caused by prolonged inhalation of silicon dioxide (sand)
3. Anthracosis: caused by prolonged inhalation of anthracite (coal dust)
4. Asbestosis: caused by prolonged inhalation of asbestos
5. Siderosis: caused by prolonged inhalation of iron dust
6. All are harder to penetrate

R. Pneumonia
1. Acute inflammation of the lungs
2. Harder to penetrate

S. Pneumothorax
1. Air in the pleural space that causes the lung to collapse
2. Easier to penetrate

T. Pulmonary metastases
1. Spread of cancer into the lungs from a primary site
2. Harder to penetrate

U. Tuberculosis
1. Chronic infection of the lungs caused by acid-fast bacillus
2. More difficult to penetrate

Chest

A. PA
1. Patient position
   a. Standing or seated erect
   b. Back of hands on hips
   c. Top of cassette 1 to 2 inches above shoulders
2. Part position
   a. MSP centered
   b. Chin extended and pointing straight ahead
   c. Roll shoulders forward
   d. SID recommended: 72 inches
   e. Respiration: full inspiration (expose at end of second inspiration)
3. Central ray: perpendicular to MSP at level of T7 (Figure 5-45)

B. Lateral
1. Patient position
   a. Standing or seated erect
   b. Left side against cassette unless otherwise specified
   c. Top of cassette 1 to 2 inches above shoulder
2. Part position
   a. MSP parallel to cassette

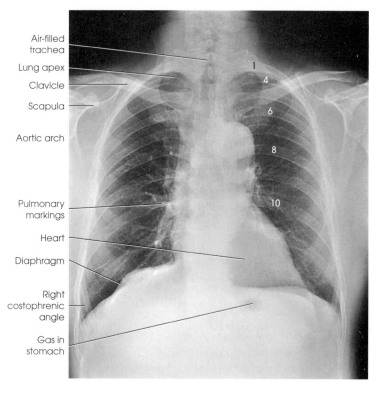

Air-filled trachea
Lung apex
Clavicle
Scapula
Aortic arch
Pulmonary markings
Heart
Diaphragm
Right costophrenic angle
Gas in stomach

Figure 5-45 Posteroanterior chest.

b. Adjacent shoulder resting against cassette holder
c. Arms raised and crossed over head
d. Center thorax to cassette
e. SID recommended: 72 inches
f. Respiration: full inspiration (expose at end of second inspiration)
3. Central ray: perpendicular to cassette, entering patient approximately 2 inches anterior to midaxillary plane at level of T7 (Figure 5-46)
C. LAO and RAO (PA obliques)
1. Patient position
a. Standing or seated
b. Adjust coronal plane 45 degrees (or 60 degrees) from plane of cassette
c. Top of cassette 2 inches above shoulders
d. Side farthest from cassette is usually side of primary interest
2. Part position
a. Shoulder nearest cassette rolled posteriorly
b. Hand placed on hip
c. Arm farthest from cassette placed on top of cassette holder
d. Thorax centered to cassette
e. SID recommended: 72 inches
f. Both 45-degree obliques (or 60-degree obliques) may be taken
g. Respiration: full inspiration
3. Central ray: perpendicular at level of T7

D. AP lordotic
1. Patient position
a. Standing approximately 1 foot in front of cassette
b. When patient is properly positioned, top of cassette should be approximately 3 inches above shoulders
2. Part position
a. MSP centered with no rotation
b. Elbows flexed
c. Hands, with palms out, on hips
d. Patient leans backward in extreme lordotic position
e. SID recommended: 72 inches
f. Respiration: full inspiration
3. Central ray: perpendicular to cassette, entering midsternum
E. Lateral decubitus
1. Patient position: lateral recumbent
2. Part position
a. Lying on affected or unaffected side, depending on existing condition
b. Elevate dependent side on firm pad
c. Extend patient's arms above head
d. Adjust thorax in true lateral position
e. Place top of cassette approximately 2 inches above shoulders
f. Respiration: full inspiration

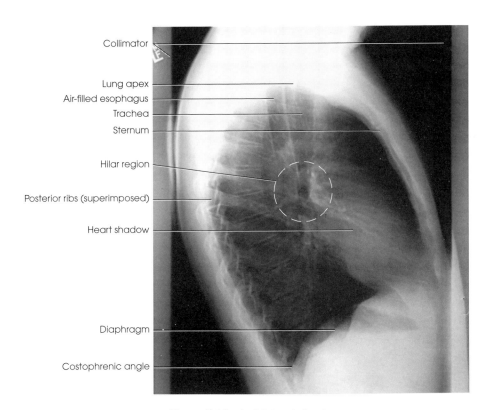

Figure 5-46 Left lateral chest.

Collimator
Lung apex
Air-filled esophagus
Trachea
Sternum
Hilar region
Posterior ribs (superimposed)
Heart shadow
Diaphragm
Costophrenic angle

3. Central ray: horizontal and perpendicular to cassette, entering T7

Ribs

A. AP
1. Patient position: erect or recumbent
2. Part position
   a. Center midsagittal plane to midline of grid
   b. Above diaphragm: center to T7; top of cassette should be 1 to 2 inches above shoulders; shoulders rotated anteriorly; respiration: full inspiration
   c. Below diaphragm: center thorax with bottom of cassette at level of iliac crests; respiration: full expiration
3. Central ray: perpendicular to T7 for upper ribs; perpendicular to T12 for lower ribs
B. LPO and RPO (AP obliques)
1. Patient position: erect or recumbent
2. Part position
   a. Rotate body 45 degrees with the affected side toward cassette
   b. Center midway between MSP and lateral surface of body to center of grid
   c. Abduct arm nearest cassette
   d. Place hand on head
   e. Abduct opposite limb

f. Place hand on hip
g. Respiration: above diaphragm, full inspiration; below diaphragm, full expiration
3. Central ray: perpendicular to cassette; above diaphragm: center at level of T7; below diaphragm: center at level of T10

Sternum

A. RAO (PA oblique)
1. Patient position: prone position for RAO (right PA oblique)
2. Part position
   a. Center sternum to cassette
   b. Rotate body 15 to 20 degrees to prevent superimposition of vertebral and sternal images
   c. Respiration: shallow breathing or suspended expiration
3. Central ray: perpendicular, exiting midsternum (Figure 5-47)
B. Lateral
1. Patient position: lateral, seated or standing
2. Part position
   a. Top of cassette 1 to 2 inches above jugular notch
   b. Shoulders and arms rotated posteriorly
   c. Center sternum to cassette
   d. Adjust to true lateral position
   e. Respiration: full inspiration
3. Central ray: perpendicular to center of midsternum

Sternoclavicular Joints

A. PA
1. Patient position: prone or upright, MSP centered to table
2. Part position
   a. Cassette centered to T3
   b. Arms on side of body, palms up, shoulders in same plane
   c. Bilateral exam: head rests on chin, MSP vertical to table
   d. Unilateral exam: turn head toward affected side, rest cheek on table
3. Central ray: perpendicular to T3
B. RAO
1. Patient position: prone or upright
2. Part position
   a. Rotate patient to an oblique position to place vertebral shadow behind sternoclavicular joint nearest film (10 to 15 degrees)
   b. Center joint to midline of film
3. Central ray: perpendicular to affected joint

Skull

Cranium

A. PA or Caldwell (Figures 5-48 and 5-49)
1. Patient position: prone or seated erect
2. Part position

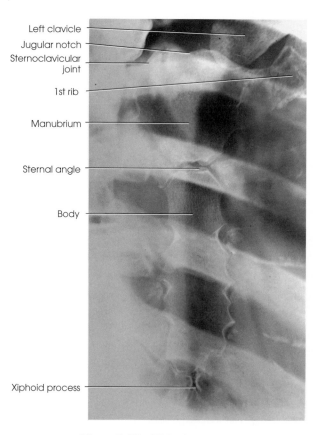

Left clavicle
Jugular notch
Sternoclavicular joint
1st rib
Manubrium
Sternal angle
Body
Xiphoid process

Figure 5-47 RAO of sternum.

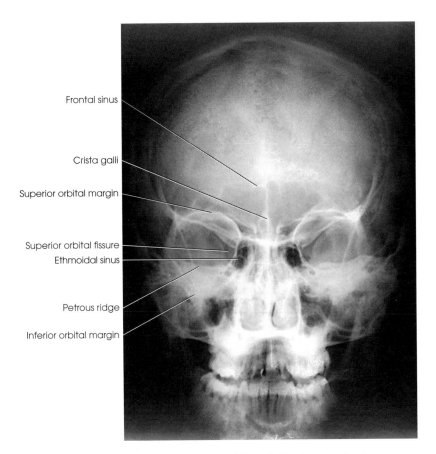

Figure 5-48 Posteroanterior axial skull (Caldwell method).

Frontal sinus
Crista galli
Superior orbital margin
Superior orbital fissure
Ethmoidal sinus
Petrous ridge
Inferior orbital margin

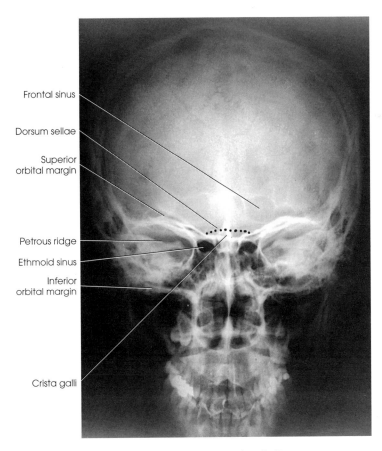

Figure 5-49 Posteroanterior skull.

Frontal sinus
Dorsum sellae
Superior orbital margin
Petrous ridge
Ethmoid sinus
Inferior orbital margin
Crista galli

a. Head resting on forehead and nose

b. MSP perpendicular to midline of grid device

c. OML perpendicular to cassette

d. Respiration: suspended

3. Central ray

   a. Caldwell method: direct central ray 15 degrees caudad to OML, exiting nasion, for survey examination

   b. PA: perpendicular to cassette, exiting nasion, to examine frontal bone

B. Lateral (Figure 5-50)

1. Patient position: seated erect or semiprone

2. Part position

   a. Center a point to the cassette that is 2 inches superior to the external auditory meatus (EAM)

   b. MSP parallel to cassette

   c. IOML parallel to transverse axis of cassette

   d. Interpupillary line (IPL) perpendicular to cassette

   e. Respiration: suspended

3. Central ray

   a. Perpendicular, entering 2 inches superior to EAM for survey exam

   b. When sella turcica is of primary interest, cassette is centered and central ray enters ¾ inch superior and ¾ inch anterior to EAM

C. AP axial (Towne) (Figure 5-51)

1. Patient position: supine or seated erect

2. Part position

   a. Center MSP to midline of grid device

   b. Adjust to be perpendicular

   c. Flex head and adjust OML perpendicular to cassette

   d. Place top of film at level of cranial vertex

   e. Respiration: suspended

3. Central ray

   a. Direct through foramen magnum with caudal angle of 30 degrees to OML or 37 degrees to IOML, entering 2 to 2.5 inches above glabella

D. Submentovertex (full basal)

1. Patient position: seated erect at head unit or supine on elevated table support

2. Part position

   a. Extend neck

   b. Rest head on vertex

   c. Center and adjust MSP perpendicular to cassette

   d. Adjust IOML parallel to plane of cassette

   e. Respiration: suspended

3. Central ray: direct perpendicular to IOML, entering between angles of mandible

Optic foramen

A. Parieto-orbital oblique (Rhese) (Figure 5-52)

1. Patient position: prone or seated erect

2. Part position

   a. Center affected orbit to cassette

   b. Rest head on zygoma, nose, and chin

   c. Adjust AML perpendicular to cassette

   d. Rotate MSP 53 degrees from cassette

   e. Respiration: suspended

3. Central ray: perpendicular, entering 1 inch superior and posterior to top of ear attachment, exiting affected orbit

Facial bones

A. Lateral (Figure 5-53)

1. Patient position: semiprone or seated erect

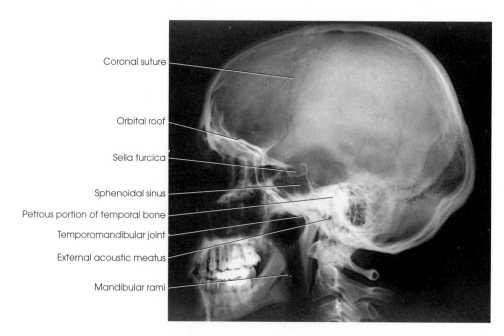

Coronal suture

Orbital roof

Sella turcica

Sphenoidal sinus

Petrous portion of temporal bone

Temporomandibular joint

External acoustic meatus

Mandibular rami

Figure 5-50   Lateral skull.

2. Part position
   a. Center zygoma
   b. Adjust MSP parallel to cassette
   c. IOML parallel to transverse axis of cassette
   d. IPL perpendicular to cassette
   e. Respiration: suspended
3. Central ray: perpendicular, entering lateral surface of zygomatic bone

B. Parietoacanthial (Waters) (Figure 5-54)
1. Patient position: prone or seated erect
2. Part position
   a. Center and adjust MSP perpendicular to cassette
   b. Rest patient's head on extended chin
   c. Adjust OML to form 37-degree angle to film plane
   d. Respiration: suspended
3. Central ray: perpendicular, exiting acanthion

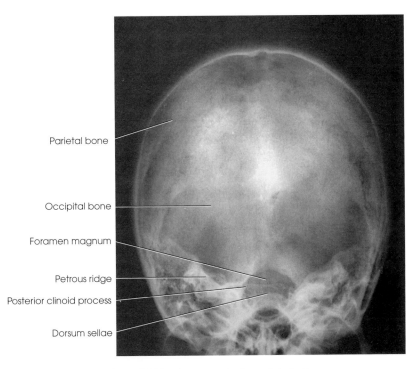

Parietal bone

Occipital bone

Foramen magnum

Petrous ridge

Posterior clinoid process

Dorsum sellae

Figure 5-51 Anteroposterior axial skull.

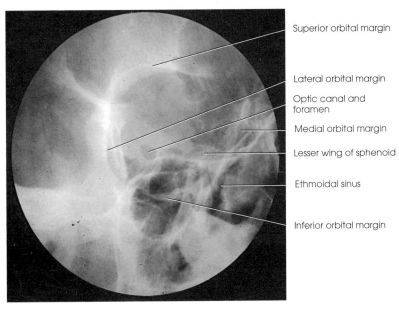

Superior orbital margin

Lateral orbital margin

Optic canal and foramen

Medial orbital margin

Lesser wing of sphenoid

Ethmoidal sinus

Inferior orbital margin

Figure 5-52 Parieto-orbital oblique optic canal (Rhese method).

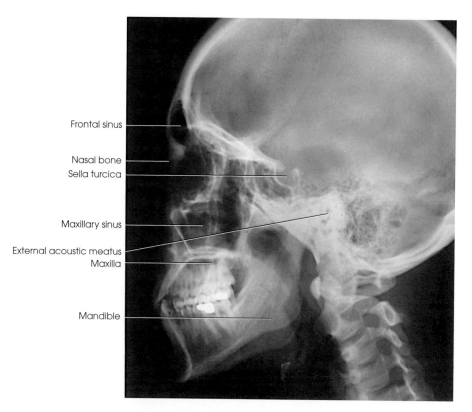

Frontal sinus

Nasal bone
Sella turcica

Maxillary sinus

External acoustic meatus
Maxilla

Mandible

Figure 5-53 Lateral facial bones.

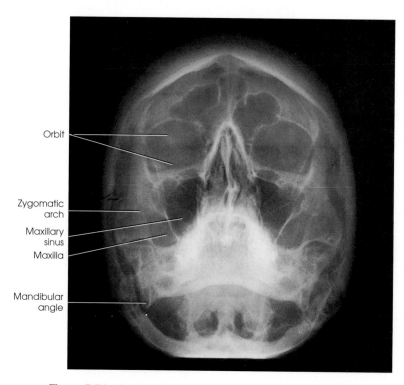

Orbit

Zygomatic
arch

Maxillary
sinus

Maxilla

Mandibular
angle

Figure 5-54 Parietoacanthial facial bones (Waters method).

Nasal bones
A. Lateral (performed as a bilateral exam)
   1. Patient position: semiprone or seated erect
   2. Part position
      a. Center nasion to cassette
      b. Adjust MSP parallel to cassette
      c. IOML parallel to transverse axis of cassette
      d. IPL perpendicular to cassette
      e. Respiration: suspended
   3. Central ray: perpendicular to the bridge of the nose, entering ¾ inch distal to nasion

Zygomatic arches
A. Bilateral tangential (basal)
   1. Patient position: seated erect or supine on elevated table support
   2. Part position
      a. Have patient extend head and rest on vertex
      b. Center and adjust MSP perpendicular to cassette
      c. Adjust IOML parallel to cassette
      d. Respiration: suspended
   3. Central ray: perpendicular to IOML, entering midway between zygomatic arches, approximately 1 inch posterior to outer canthi
B. Unilateral tangential (May)
   1. Patient position: prone or seated erect at vertical grid device
   2. Part position
      a. Extend neck and rest chin on grid device
      b. Rotate MSP 15 degrees away from side being examined
      c. Center cassette 3 inches distal to most prominent point of zygoma
      d. IOML parallel to plane of film
      e. Respiration: suspended
   3. Central ray
      a. Perpendicular to IOML
      b. Directed through zygomatic arch 1.5 inches posterior to outer canthus

Mandible
A. PA
   1. Patient position: prone or seated erect
   2. Part position
      a. Have patient rest head on nose and chin
      b. For mandibular body, center cassette at level of lips
      c. For rami and temporomandibular joint (TMJ), center to tip of nose
      d. MSP perpendicular to film
      e. Respiration: suspended
   3. Central ray
      a. For mandibular body, direct perpendicular to cassette at level of lips
      b. For rami and condylar processes, direct midway between TMJs at 30-degree cephalad angle

B. Axiolateral oblique (for mandibular body)
   1. Patient position: semiprone or seated erect
   2. Part position
      a. Adjust cassette under affected cheek
      b. Extend neck to place long axis of mandibular body parallel to cassette
      c. Center to first molar region
      d. Adjust broad surface of mandibular body parallel to cassette
      e. Respiration: suspended
   3. Central ray: direct slightly posteriorly to mandibular angle farthest from film at a 25-degree cephalad angle
C. Axiolateral oblique (for mandibular ramus)
   1. Patient position: semiprone or seated erect
   2. Part position
      a. Center cassette ½ inch anterior and 1 inch inferior to affected side EAM
      b. Extend chin
      c. Adjust broad surface of ramus parallel to cassette
      d. Respiration: suspended
   3. Central ray: direct 25 degrees cephalad, entering 2 inches distal to the mandibular angle on side farthest from film
D. Submentovertex (basal)
   1. Patient position: seated erect or supine on elevated table support
   2. Part position
      a. Extend neck and rest head on vertex
      b. Center and adjust MSP perpendicular to cassette
      c. Adjust IOML parallel to plane of film
      d. Respiration: suspended
   3. Central ray: perpendicular to IOML, entering midway between mandibular angles

Temporomandibular articulations (open- and closed-mouth laterals)
   1. Patient position: seated erect or semiprone
   2. Part position
      a. Center a point ½ inch anterior and 1 inch inferior to EAM to cassette
      b. MSP angled 15 degrees (nose toward film)
      c. AML adjusted parallel to transverse axis of cassette
      d. IPL perpendicular to cassette
      e. After first exposure (made with mouth closed and patient completely still), cassette is changed and second exposure is made with patient's mouth fully open
      f. Respiration: suspended
   3. Central ray: direct 15 degrees caudad, exiting TMJ against cassette

Paranasal sinuses
A. Lateral (Figure 5-55)
   1. Patient position: seated erect
   2. Part position

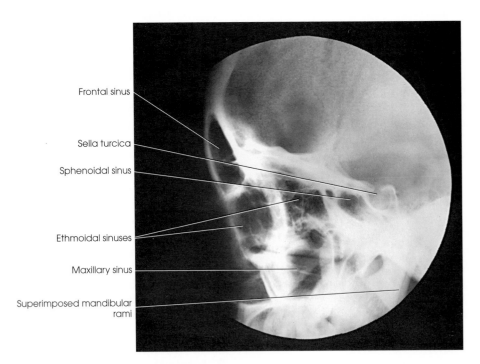

Frontal sinus

Sella turcica

Sphenoidal sinus

Ethmoidal sinuses

Maxillary sinus

Superimposed mandibular rami

Figure 5-55 Lateral sinuses.

a. Center cassette ½ to 1 inch posterior to outer canthus
b. Adjust head to true lateral position
c. MSP parallel and IPL perpendicular to cassette
d. IOML adjusted parallel to transverse axis of cassette
e. Respiration: suspended
3. Central ray: perpendicular, entering ½ to 1 inch posterior to outer canthus

B. PA axial (Caldwell)
1. Patient position: seated erect at vertical grid device
2. Part position
a. Rest head on forehead and nose
b. MSP perpendicular to midline of cassette
c. OML perpendicular to cassette
d. Respiration: suspended
3. Central ray: direct to nasion at angle of 15 degrees caudal to the OML

C. Parietoacanthial (Waters)
1. Patient position: seated erect; use horizontal central ray to demonstrate fluid level
2. Part position
a. Center and adjust MSP perpendicular to cassette
b. Rest head on extended chin
c. Adjust OML to form 37-degree angle to cassette
d. Respiration: suspended
3. Central ray: horizontal and perpendicular to cassette, exiting acanthion

D. Submentovertex (basal) (Figure 5-56)
1. Patient position: seated erect at vertical grid device

2. Part position
a. Extend head and rest on vertex
b. Center and adjust MSP perpendicular to cassette
c. Adjust IOML parallel to cassette
d. Respiration: suspended
3. Central ray: perpendicular to IOML through sella turcica, approximately ¾ inch anterior to level of EAM

Gastrointestinal System
Pathologies Imaged
A. Acute cholecystitis: inflammation of gallbladder
B. Cancer of the colon and rectum
1. Leading cause of death from cancer in the United States
2. More typical form is annular carcinoma, with classic "apple-core" pattern when imaged using barium enema
C. Cancer of the esophagus
1. Malignant neoplasm
2. Imaged during barium study
D. Cancer of the stomach
1. May appear as gross changes in the stomach wall or as a large mass
2. Imaged during barium study
3. Harder to penetrate
E. Cholelithiasis
1. Gallstones
2. Harder to penetrate

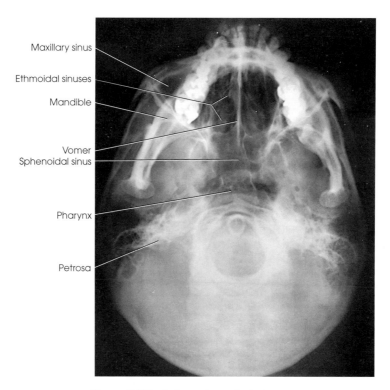

Maxillary sinus
Ethmoidal sinuses
Mandible
Vomer
Sphenoidal sinus
Pharynx
Petrosa

Figure 5-56   Submentovertical sinuses.

F. Crohn's disease
  1. Chronic inflammation of the bowel
  2. Sometimes separated by normal segments of bowel
G. Diverticulitis
  1. Inflammation of diverticula
H. Diverticulosis
  1. Presence of diverticula (pouchlike herniations through the wall of the colon)
I. Esophageal varices
  1. Varicose veins at distal end of esophagus
J. Esophagitis
  1. Inflammation of esophageal mucosal lining
K. Gastritis
  1. Inflammation of the stomach
L. Hiatus hernia
  1. Condition in which a portion of the stomach protrudes through the diaphragm
M. Ileus
  1. Intestinal obstruction
  2. Adynamic ileus (ileus caused by immobility of the bowel)
  3. Mechanical ileus (ileus caused by mechanical obstruction)
N. Intussusception
  1. Prolapse of one segment of bowel into another section of bowel
O. Irritable bowel syndrome
  1. Abnormal increase in small and large bowel motility

P. Large bowel obstruction
  1. Characterized by massive accumulation of gas proximal to obstruction
  2. Absence of gas distal to obstruction
  3. High risk of bowel perforation
  4. Extent of obstruction determines ease or difficulty of penetration
Q. Peptic ulcer disease
  1. Loss of mucous membrane in a portion of the gastrointestinal (GI) system
  2. Imaged using barium study
  3. Has craterlike appearance
R. Pyloric stenosis: narrowing of pyloric sphincter
S. Small bowel obstruction
  1. Seen as distended loops of bowel filled with gas
  2. Bowel proximal to obstruction may be filled with fluid
  3. Extent of obstruction determines ease or difficulty of penetration
T. Ulcerative colitis
  1. Severe inflammation of the colon and rectum characterized by ulceration
U. Volvulus: twisting of bowel on itself, causing an obstruction

General Survey Exams
Abdomen
A. AP (KUB)

1. Patient position: supine
2. Part position
   a. Center MSP to table
   b. Shoulders in same transverse plane
   c. Support under knees
   d. Center cassette at level of iliac crests
   e. Apply gonadal shielding as appropriate
   f. Respiration: expiration
3. Central ray: perpendicular to midline at level of iliac crests

B. AP (upright)
1. Patient position: erect
2. Part position
   a. Center MSP to table or upright grid device
   b. Shoulders in same transverse plane
   c. Center cassette 2 to 3 inches above iliac crests to include diaphragm
   d. Apply gonadal shielding as appropriate
   e. Respiration: expiration
3. Central ray: horizontal, entering MSP 2 to 3 inches superior to iliac crests

C. Lateral decubitus (Figure 5-57)
1. Patient position
   a. Lateral recumbent (usually left side down), lying on pad
   b. Arms above level of diaphragm
   c. Knees slightly flexed
2. Part position
   a. MSP centered to grid device
   b. Center cassette at level of iliac crest
   c. Apply gonadal shielding as appropriate
   d. Respiration: expiration

3. Central ray: horizontal and parallel to the MSP at level of iliac crest

Gallbladder
A. PA
1. Patient position: prone
2. Part position
   a. Center right side of abdomen to midline of table
   b. Center cassette according to patient habitus over right upper quadrant
   c. Respiration: expiration
3. Central ray: perpendicular to center of cassette

B. LAO (PA oblique)
1. Patient position: recumbent with left arm posterior, right arm by head
2. Part position
   a. Elevate right side 15 to 40 degrees to desired obliquity; thin patients require more rotation
   b. Support patient on flexed knee and elbow
   c. Center localized gallbladder area to cassette
   d. Respiration: expiration
3. Central ray: perpendicular to center of cassette

Upper Gastrointestinal System
Esophagus
A. RAO (PA oblique)
1. Patient position: recumbent with right arm posterior, left arm by head
2. Part position
   a. Elevate left side to obliquity of 35 to 40 degrees
   b. Support patient on flexed knee and elbow
   c. Align esophagus and center at level of T5 or T6

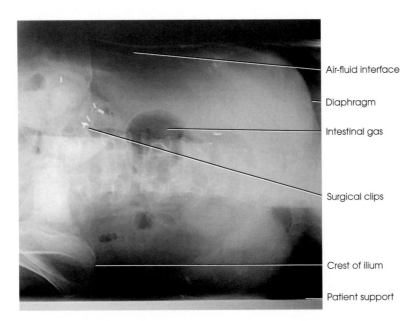

Figure 5-57 Anteroposterior abdomen. Left lateral decubitus position resulting in air marked by air-fluid interface.

d. Feed barium to patient

e. Respiration: suspended

3. Central ray: perpendicular to cassette, entering level of T5 or T6

Stomach

A. PA

1. Patient position: prone

2. Part position

a. Center at level of pylorus (approximately midway between xiphoid process and umbilicus)

b. Center halfway between midline and lateral border of abdominal cavity for 10- × 12-inch cassette or MSP for 14- × 17-inch cassette

c. Respiration: expiration

3. Central ray: perpendicular to cassette at level of pylorus (L2)

B. RAO (PA oblique) (Figure 5-58)

1. Patient position: recumbent with right arm posterior, left arm by head

2. Part position

a. Elevate left side and support patient to obliquity of 40 to 70 degrees

b. Longitudinal plane midway between vertebrae and anterior surface of elevated side is centered to cassette

c. Center at level of duodenal bulb

d. Respiration: expiration

3. Central ray: perpendicular to center of cassette midway between vertebral column and lateral border of abdominal cavity at level of L2

C. Lateral

1. Patient position: recumbent (right lateral) or erect (left lateral)

2. Part position

a. Center cassette between midaxillary plane and anterior abdominal surface

b. Center at level of pylorus

c. Adjust to true lateral

d. Respiration: expiration

3. Central ray: perpendicular to center of cassette midway between midaxillary line and anterior surface of abdomen at the level of L1 for recumbent or L3 for upright position

Small bowel

A. PA

1. Patient position: prone

2. Part position

a. MSP centered to table

b. Center cassette at level of iliac crest (may be slightly higher for early time exposures)

c. Respiration: suspended

3. Central ray: perpendicular to cassette entering midline at level of iliac crest (or slightly above)

Lower Gastrointestinal System

Colon

A. PA (Figure 5-59)

1. Patient position: prone

2. Part position

a. MSP centered to table

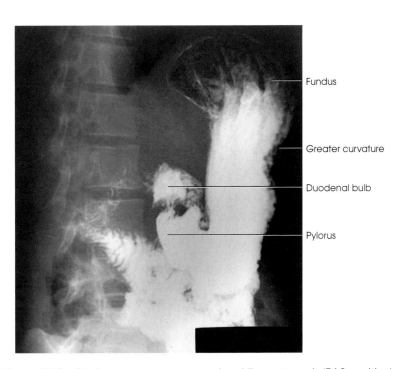

Figure 5-58 Single-contrast posteroanterior oblique stomach (RAO position).

b. Center cassette at level of iliac crest

c. Respiration: suspended

3. Central ray: perpendicular to cassette, entering level of iliac crest

B. PA axial

1. Patient position: prone

2. Part position

a. MSP centered to table

b. Center cassette at level of iliac crest

c. Respiration: suspended

3. Central ray

a. From 30 to 40 degrees caudad

b. For demonstration of rectosigmoid area using smaller cassette, central ray enters midline at level of ASIS

C. LAO and RAO (PA oblique) (Figure 5-60)

1. Patient position: PA oblique

2. Part position

a. Patient rotated 35 to 45 degrees

b. Either right or left side up

c. Center abdomen to table

d. Cassette centered at level of iliac crest

e. Respiration: suspended

3. Central ray: perpendicular to cassette, entering level of iliac crest

D. Lateral rectum

1. Patient position: lying on side

2. Part position

a. Adjust patient's body to true lateral position (right or left side down)

b. Center midaxillary plane of abdomen to center of table

c. Respiration: suspended

3. Central ray: perpendicular to cassette, entering midaxillary plane at level of ASIS

E. AP

1. Patient position: supine

2. Part position

a. MSP centered to table

b. Cassette centered at level of iliac crest

c. Respiration: suspended

3. Central ray: perpendicular to cassette, entering level of iliac crest

F. AP axial

1. Patient position: supine

2. Part position

a. MSP centered to table

b. Cassette centered 2 inches above iliac crest

c. Respiration: suspended

3. Central ray

a. Cephalad 30 to 40 degrees, entering approximately 2 inches below level of ASIS

b. When rectosigmoid is of interest, central ray enters inferior margin of symphysis pubis

G. Lateral decubitus

1. Patient position: lying on either right or left side

2. Part position

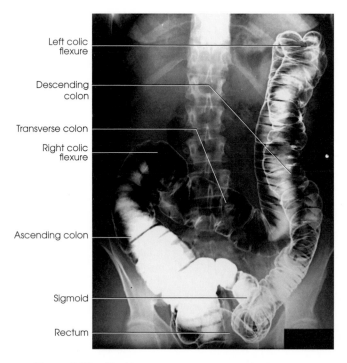

Figure 5-59 Double-contrast posteroanterior large intestine.

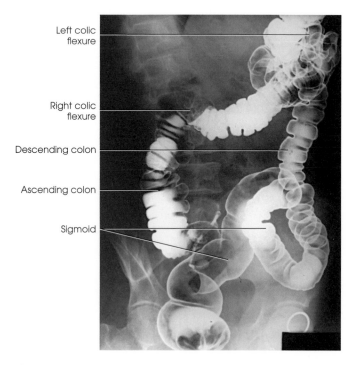

Figure 5-60 Double-contrast posteroanterior oblique large intestine.

a. Arms above head
b. Knees slightly flexed
c. Cassette centered to abdomen at level of iliac crest
d. Respiration: suspended
3. Central ray: horizontal, entering midline at level of iliac crest
H. LPO and RPO (AP oblique)
1. Patient position: AP oblique
2. Part position
a. Patient rotated 35 to 45 degrees from AP position; either right or left side up
b. Center abdomen to table
c. Cassette centered at level of iliac crest
d. Respiration: suspended
3. Central ray: perpendicular to cassette at level of iliac crest

Operative Cholangiogram

A. AP or AP oblique
1. Patient position: supine on operating table
2. Part position
a. Right upper quadrant centered to the film
b. Left side of body may be elevated into a 15- to 20-degree oblique angle to prevent bile ducts from being superimposed over the spine
3. Central ray: perpendicular to the exposed biliary tract
4. Procedure notes
a. Surgeon directs filming sequence
b. Equipment must be properly cleaned and ready to use
c. Radiographer must be in proper operating room attire
d. Appropriate radiation protection standards must

be maintained for the radiographer, as well as for the operating room staff, using distance and lead shielding
e. Exposure times must be as short as possible, with patient respiration controlled by the anesthetist
5. Exam evaluation: patency of the bile ducts, the operation of the sphincter of the hepatopancreatic ampulla, and the presence of calculi

T-Tube Cholangiogram

A. RPO (Figure 5-61)
1. Patient position: supine on fluoroscopic table
2. Part position: right upper quadrant centered to midline of table
3. Central ray: perpendicular to the biliary tract
4. Procedure notes
a. T-tube placed in common bile duct during surgery, providing for drainage and enabling postoperative evaluation of the biliary tree
b. Lower concentration, water-soluble contrast agent used to fill biliary tree
c. Spot films and radiographs may be taken during the stages of injection of the contrast medium
d. Exam continues until contrast agent is visualized entering the duodenum
e. T-tube remains clamped until end of procedure
5. Exam evaluation: patency of the bile ducts, the operation of the sphincter of the hepatopancreatic ampulla, and the presence of calculi
B. Lateral
1. Patient position: right lateral recumbent
2. Part position: centered to midline of table
3. Central ray: perpendicular to the biliary tract
4. Exam evaluation: right lateral demonstrates branch-

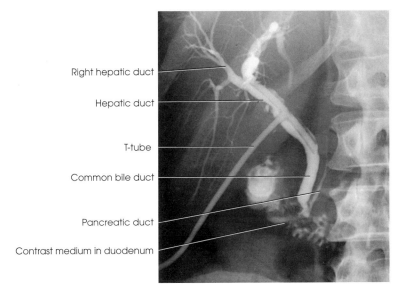

Right hepatic duct
Hepatic duct
T-tube
Common bile duct
Pancreatic duct
Contrast medium in duodenum

Figure 5-61 Anteroposterior oblique postoperative cholangiogram (RPO position).

ing of ducts and provides right-angle view to detect otherwise unseen abnormalities

Endoscopic Retrograde Cholangiopancreatography (ERCP)

A. Exam notes
1. Used to evaluate biliary and pancreatic pathologic conditions
2. Endoscope is passed into duodenum under fluoroscopic control
3. Contrast medium is injected into the common bile duct or pancreatic duct through a cannula passed through the endoscope
4. Patient is placed prone for spot films and radiographs
5. ERCP may be preceded by sonography, oral cholecystogram, or intravenous cholangiogram

Urinary System
Pathologies Imaged

A. Carcinoma of the bladder
1. Seen as solid mass arising from the bladder wall
2. Harder to penetrate
B. Cystitis: inflammation of bladder and ureters
C. Glomerulonephritis: inflammation of glomerulus of kidney

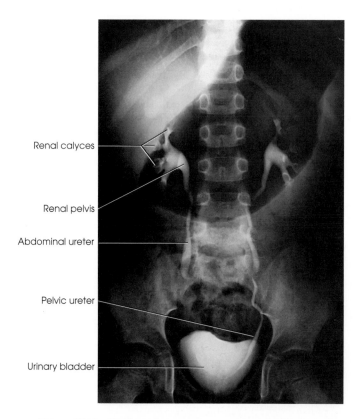

Figure 5-62 Urogram from supine position at 15-minute interval with gas-filled stomach.

Renal calyces

Renal pelvis

Abdominal ureter

Pelvic ureter

Urinary bladder

D. Polycystic kidney disease (PKD)
1. Enlarged kidneys containing numerous cysts
2. Harder to penetrate
E. Pyelonephritis: inflammation of renal pelvis and parenchyma
F. Renal calculus
1. Kidney stone
2. Harder to penetrate stone, but overall technique is not increased to compensate
G. Renal carcinoma
1. Solid mass cancer that causes renal bulging or enlargement with impact on collecting system
2. Harder to penetrate
H. Renal cysts
1. Fluid-filled masses in kidney
2. Harder to penetrate
I. Wilms' tumor
1. Malignant cancer of kidney in children
2. Harder to penetrate

Urinary System Procedures
Intravenous urography

A. KUB (AP) (Figure 5-62)
1. Patient position: supine, centered to the table
2. Part position
   a. Spine centered to the table
   b. Include entire renal outlines, bladder, and symphysis pubis, as well as the prostatic region on older male patients
3. Central ray: perpendicular to film, centered at level of iliac crest
B. Oblique (RPO, LPO) (Figure 5-63)
1. Patient position: supine
2. Part position: patient's body rotated to a 30-degree oblique angle, kidney farthest from the film will be parallel to film, and kidney nearest to the film will be perpendicular to film
3. Central ray: perpendicular to film at iliac crest
C. AP bladder
1. Patient position: supine
2. Part position: supine, centered to film
3. Central ray: perpendicular to film, centered at level of ASIS
D. Intravenous pyelogram (IVP) (intravenous urogram [IVU]) procedure notes
1. Patient should be properly prepared with a low-residue diet for 1 to 2 days before the exam and cleansing of the GI tract
2. NPO (nothing by mouth) after midnight the day of the exam but not dehydrated
3. Preliminary KUB is taken before contrast injection to verify positioning, visualize renal anatomy, or detect the presence of lesions
4. Based on patient weight, 30 to 100 ml of an iodinated contrast medium is injected; pelvocalyceal

system will appear in 2 to 8 minutes, with greatest visualization occurring in 15 to 20 minutes
5. AP and oblique radiographs are made at specific intervals after injection of the contrast medium
6. All films must be carefully identified using right, left, upright, and "postvoid" markers and numbers indicating postinjection time; stickers, felt-tip markers, and grease pencils should *not* be used to place identification on a radiograph
7. All film sizes needed for the exam should be made readily available before beginning procedure
8. AP upright positions may be used to demonstrate kidney mobility and the filled bladder
9. Oblique radiographs may be used to image kidney rotation or localize tumor masses
10. Postvoid radiographs may be taken to image tumor masses or prostatic enlargement
11. Tomography may be used during an IVP to blur gas patterns and to better image intrarenal lesions; this is termed *nephrotomography*

Cystography and cystourethrography

A. Positioning
1. AP
   a. A 5-degree caudal angle on tube
   b. Film centered at level 2 to 3 inches above symphysis pubis
2. Oblique (RPO, LPO)
   a. Patient rotated 40 to 60 degrees

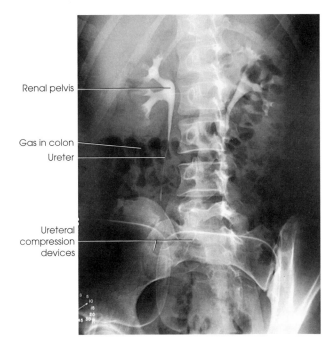

Figure 5-63 Anteroposterior oblique 10-minute postinjection urogram.

Renal pelvis

Gas in colon
Ureter

Ureteral compression devices

b. Pubic arch closest to table centered to midline of table
3. PA of bladder
   a. Patient centered
   b. Central ray enters 1 inch distal to tip of coccyx with a 10- to 15-degree cephalad angle
4. Lateral
   a. Bladder centered to film; cassette 2 to 3 inches above symphysis pubis
   b. Central ray centered and perpendicular to film

B. Procedure notes
1. Bladder is drained using catheter that has been put in place
2. Bladder is filled with contrast medium through urethral catheter
3. Once bladder is filled, clamp is closed to prevent contrast agent from draining
4. Filming follows filling of bladder
5. Cystourethrography may follow cystogram
   a. Patient is instructed to void contrast material from bladder while on fluoroscopic table
   b. Radiologist takes spot films during urination to evaluate urethra and to image reflux

Retrograde pyelography

A. Positioning
1. AP
2. RPO
3. LPO

B. Procedure notes
1. Ureters are catheterized to allow filling of the pelvocalyceal system
2. Urologist performs procedure
3. Film is placed to include both kidneys and ureters
4. Following catheterization and introduction of contrast material, urologist directs filming sequence

Refer to Table 5-1 for a list of some common additive and destructive diseases and conditions.

Other Radiologic Examinations

A. Tomography
1. Uses motion of x-ray tube and film to blur unwanted structures from the image
2. X-ray tube and film are connected by a rigid rod that pivots around a fulcrum
3. Position of fulcrum corresponds to level in the body that will appear in focus on the radiograph (called the *objective plane*)
4. Structures above and below the objective plane are blurred beyond recognition
5. Angle of arc through which the x-ray tube travels is called *exposure angle*
   a. Exposure angle determines thickness of tomographic cut
   b. Wider angles provide thin cuts

TABLE 5-1	Some Common Additive and Destructive Diseases and Conditions by Anatomic Area

Additive conditions	Destructive conditions
ABDOMEN	
Aortic aneurysm	Bowel obstruction
Ascites	Free air
Cirrhosis	
Hypertrophy of some organs (e.g., splenomegaly)	
CHEST	
Atelectasis	Emphysema
Congestive heart failure	Pneumothorax
Malignancy	
Pleural effusion	
Pneumonia	
SKELETON	
Hydrocephalus	Gout
Metastases (osteoblastic)	Metastases (osteolytic)
Osteochondroma (exostoses)	Multiple myeloma
Paget's disease	Paget's disease
Osteoporosis	
NONSPECIFIC SITES	
Abscess	Atrophy
Edema	Emaciation
Sclerosis	Malnutrition

From Fauber TL: *Radiographic imaging & exposure*, St Louis, 2000, Mosby.

    c. Narrower angles provide thick cuts
  6. Thick-section tomography is called *zonography*
  7. Blurring pattern on radiograph determines detail visibility
  8. Blurring pattern is determined by motion used
  9. Types of motions
    a. Linear
    b. Circular
    c. Elliptical
    d. Hypocycloidal
    e. Spiral
  10. Patient positioning must be extremely accurate
  11. Equipment must be kept in proper working condition to prevent unwanted stray motion in linkages connecting x-ray tube, rod, and tray
  12. Primary use of tomography is nephrotomography
  13. Tomography largely displaced by computed tomography

B. Myelography
  1. Pathologies imaged
    a. Herniated intervertebral disks
    b. Degenerative diseases of the CNS
    c. Space-occupying lesions
  2. Pathologies imaged by displacing column of contrast material in the subarachnoid space
  3. Lumbar puncture performed by physician at L3-L4

interspace allows injection of water-soluble contrast agent into subarachnoid space
  4. Small amount of spinal fluid is withdrawn for laboratory analysis
  5. X-ray table is tilted up and down to distribute contrast medium
  6. Contrast medium should not be allowed to enter cerebral ventricles; head must be kept hyperextended to compress cisterna magna when working with contrast medium in cervical region
  7. Spot films are taken under fluoroscopic control in PA and oblique positions
  8. Crosstable lateral radiographs are taken by radiographer to provide right-angle views
  9. Contrast medium is absorbed by patient's body

C. Arthrography
  1. Contrast exam of an encapsulated joint
    a. Knee
    b. Shoulder
    c. Hip
    d. Wrist
    e. TMJ
  2. Pathologies imaged
    a. Joint trauma
    b. Meniscal tears
    c. Capsular damage
    d. Deformities secondary to arthritis
    e. Rupture of articular ligaments
  3. Performed under local anesthetic using asepsis
  4. Physician injects contrast material
  5. Joint is manipulated to distribute contrast agent
  6. Fluoroscopic spot films and radiographs may be taken
  7. Arthrography gradually being replaced by magnetic resonance imaging (MRI)

D. Venography
  1. Pathologies imaged
    a. Embolism: lodging of an embolus in a blood vessel
    b. Thrombophlebitis: inflammation of a vein, accompanied by the formation of clots
    c. Thrombosis: formation of blood clot (thrombus) within a blood vessel
    d. Varicose veins: dilated veins with malfunctioning valves
    e. Vessel damage secondary to trauma
  2. Upper extremity venograms
    a. Performed to evaluate presence of thrombosis
    b. Contrast medium injected into superficial vein at elbow or wrist, by hand or with automatic injector
    c. Flow of contrast agent may be observed using fluoroscopy and spot filming; automatic film changer may be used
    d. Radiography performed using AP projection
    e. Radiograph should extend from site of injection to superior vena cava
    f. Contrast agent may be forced into deep veins by

applying a tourniquet proximal to the injection site

3. Lower extremity venograms
    a. Used to evaluate thrombosis in legs
    b. Contrast medium injected into superficial vein of foot, by hand or with automatic injector
    c. Flow of contrast agent may be observed using fluoroscopy and spot filming; automatic film changer may be used
    d. Radiography performed using AP projection of legs with 30-degree internal rotation
    e. Automatic long leg film changer may be used for serial radiography 5 to 10 seconds apart
    f. Contrast agent may be forced into deep veins by applying a tourniquet proximal to the injection site
    g. Radiographs should extend from site of injection to inferior vena cava

REVIEW QUESTIONS

Use the following list to answer questions **1-8**. Items may be used more than once.

A. Hypersthenic habitus
B. Sthenic habitus
C. Hyposthenic habitus
D. Asthenic habitus

1. Slender build D

2. Massive build A

3. Stomach and gallbladder are low, vertical, near the midline D

4. Average build, present in about 35% of the population C

5. Most common body habitus, present in about 50% of the population B

6. Stomach and gallbladder high and horizontal A

7. Thorax narrow and shallow D

8. Thorax broad and deep A

For the following questions, choose the single best answer.

9. Key points in performing pediatric radiography are:
    a. Work quickly and impersonally, use gonadal shielding, report suspected child abuse, keep parents in waiting room
    b. Work quickly, communicate clearly with child and parent(s), use gonadal shielding, report suspected child abuse
    c. Work quickly and impersonally, report suspected child abuse, keep parents in waiting room, always use Pigg-o-stat
    d. Work quickly and impersonally, use gonadal shielding only on abdominal exams, report suspected child abuse, keep parents in waiting room

10. The most important point to remember when performing trauma radiography is:
    a. Use gonadal shielding because this patient will be having many follow-up exams
    b. Work quickly because the injuries may be life threatening
    c. Do no additional harm to the patient
    d. Do only the projections ordered by the physician

11. When performing trauma radiography:
    a. Splints, bandages, and cervical collars should be removed so that they do not obstruct the anatomy that must be imaged
    b. Remove cervical collars only under the direction of a radiologist
    c. Remove cervical collars only under the direction of an emergency room physician or radiologist
    d. Splints, bandages, and cervical collars should be removed after preliminary films have been viewed by a physician so that they do not obstruct the anatomy that must be imaged

Use the following list to answer questions **12-16**. Items may be used more than once.

A. Transverse plane
B. Midcoronal plane
C. Median sagittal plane
D. Sagittal plane

12. Passes transversely across the body *A*

13. Passes vertically through the midline of the body from front to back *C*

14. Divides the body into superior and inferior portions *A*

15. Passes vertically through the midaxillary region of the body and through the coronal suture of the cranium at right angles to the midsagittal plane *B*

16. Any plane parallel to the MSP *D*

Use the following list to answer questions **17-21**. Items may be used more than once.

A. Ball-and-socket joint
B. Pivot joint
C. Hinge joint
D. Saddle joint

17. An example is the hip *A*

18. Rounded head of one bone moves in a cuplike cavity *A*

19. Permits motion in one plane only *C*

20. Opposing surfaces are convex-concave, allowing great freedom of motion *A*

21. Permits rotary movement in which a ring rotates around a central axis *B*

For the following questions, choose the single best answer.

22. Which of the following conditions would *not* be an indication for performing hysterosalpingography?
a. Determine the patency of the oviducts
b. Status of pregnancy
c. Abnormal uterine bleeding
d. Uterine polyps

23. Which of the following are true regarding venography?
1. Performed to visualize thrombophlebitis, varicose veins, or vessel damage secondary to trauma
2. Requires AP and lateral projections
3. Use of exam is limited because deep veins cannot be imaged
4. Injection is made into superficial veins
a. All are true
b. 1, 4
c. 2, 3
d. 1, 2, 4

24. Which of the following are true regarding contrast arthrography?
1. Asepsis required
2. May be performed on knee, shoulder, TMJ, hip, wrist
3. Indications include trauma, capsular damage, meniscal tears, rupture of ligaments, arthritis
4. Joint is manipulated by hand to distribute contrast medium
a. 1, 2, 3, 4
b. All except 4
c. All except 1
d. 2, 3

25. Which of the following are true concerning myelography?
1. Injection is always made at the L3-L4 interspace
2. Oily, iodinated contrast agent is the medium of choice
3. Indications include herniated intervertebral disks, space-occupying lesions, degenerative diseases of the CNS
4. Contrast medium is distributed by manual manipulation of the subarachnoid space
5. Head must be kept hyperflexed to prevent contrast medium from entering cerebral ventricles
6. Spinal fluid may be withdrawn for laboratory analysis
a. All are true
b. None are true
c. 1, 2, 3, 5
d. 3, 6

26. An exam that uses motion and blurring to view anatomy by setting the x-ray tube and film in motion is:
a. Computed tomography
b. Autotomography
c. Conventional tomography
d. Fluoroscopy

27. The proper centering point for a PA projection of the hand is the:
    a. Third metatarsophalangeal joint
    b. Third metacarpophalangeal joint
    c. Midshaft of the third metacarpal
    d. First metacarpophalangeal joint

28. For the lateral projection of the wrist:
    a. Radius and ulna should be superimposed
    b. Radial surface must be in contact with the film
    c. Central ray is perpendicular to wrist
    d. More than one but not all of the above

29. For the lateral projection of the forearm:
    1. Ulnar surface must be in contact with the film
    2. Thumb should be in a relaxed position
    3. Humerus and forearm should be in contact with the table
    4. Elbow should be flexed 45 degrees
    5. Central ray is directed toward the injured joint
    a. All are true
    b. 1, 2, 5
    c. 1, 3
    d. 2, 4, 5

30. For the AP projection of the elbow:
    1. Forearm and humerus should be at right angles
    2. Central ray is directed perpendicular to the joint
    3. Forearm and humerus should be parallel to the table
    4. Hand must be pronated
    5. Patient may have to lean laterally to ensure AP alignment
    a. All are true
    b. 2, 3, 5
    c. 1, 4
    d. 2, 3, 4, 5

31. For the lateral projection of the humerus:
    1. Hand should be pronated
    2. Patient may be upright or supine
    3. Humeral epicondyles are placed perpendicular to cassette
    4. Arm should be slightly adducted
    5. Central ray is directed perpendicular to the midshaft
    a. 2, 3, 5
    b. 1, 4
    c. All are true
    d. 1, 2, 3, 5

32. For the PA oblique (scapular Y) projection of the shoulder:
    1. Central ray is directed to the shoulder at a 10-degree cephalad angle
    2. Anterior surface of the affected shoulder is centered to the cassette
    3. Patient is rotated so that midcoronal plane forms 60-degree angle with cassette
    4. Patient continues shallow breathing during exposure
    a. All are true
    b. 2, 3, 4
    c. 2, 3
    d. 1, 2, 3

33. For the AP projection of the AC joints:
    a. To properly demonstrate AC separation, both joints with and without weights should be demonstrated on one film if possible
    b. To properly demonstrate AC separation, separate films must be acquired—with equal weights attached to both wrists and without weights
    c. The central ray is always directed midway between the AC joints
    d. Patient should be seated upright and instructed to continue shallow breathing during the exposure

34. When the clavicle is being radiographed:
    1. PA projection must always be used
    2. Central ray angle of 25 to 30 degrees cephalad is used for the PA axial
    3. Patient's head should be turned away from the affected side
    4. AP projection may be used for patient comfort
    5. Erect position may be used for patient comfort
    6. Central ray angle of 25 to 30 degrees caudad is used for the PA axial
    a. 1, 2, 3, 4, 5
    b. 1, 3, 4, 5
    c. 2, 3, 4, 5
    d. 3, 4, 5, 6

35. For the lateral projection of the scapula:
    1. Patient should be upright to reduce pain
    2. Patient is positioned obliquely with unaffected scapula centered to the cassette
    3. Body is adjusted by palpating axillary and vertebral borders of the scapula so that the scapula is lateral
    4. Scapula must be projected free of the rib cage
    a. 1, 3, 4
    b. All are true
    c. 3, 4
    d. 2, 3, 4

Use the following list to answer questions **36-40**. Items may be used more than once.

A. Trimalleolar fracture
B. Giant cell myeloma
C. Osteoarthritis
D. Pott's fracture

36. Fracture of medial and lateral malleoli of the ankle with ankle joint dislocation _D_

37. Involves the posterior portion of the tibia and the medial and lateral malleoli _A_

38. More commonly seen in the elderly _C_

39. Tumor arising on bone with large bubble appearance; may be benign or malignant _B_

40. Characterized by the degeneration of one or several joints _C_

For the following questions, choose the single best answer.

41. For AP radiography of the foot:
1. A trough-compensating filter may be used
2. Dorsal surface rests on cassette
3. Central ray is directed 10 degrees anterior
4. Central ray is directed at the head of the third metatarsal
a. All are true
b. 1, 3, 4
c. 2, 4
d. None are true

42. When the AP axial projection is performed for the os calcis:
1. The leg should be fully extended
2. The plantar surface of the foot should be parallel to the cassette
3. The central ray is directed 40 degrees cephalad to the long axis of the foot
4. The central ray enters the foot at the head of the fifth metatarsal
5. A cylinder cone may be used for this projection
a. 1, 3, 5
b. 2, 4
c. All are true
d. 1, 3, 4, 5

43. For the medial oblique position of the ankle:
1. Leg and foot are rotated medially
2. Ankle is adjusted to a 90-degree angle
3. Medial rotation is adjusted to 45 degrees to demonstrate the mortise joint
4. Medial rotation is adjusted to 15 to 20 degrees to demonstrate the bony structure
5. Central ray is directed vertically midway between the malleoli
a. All are true
b. 1, 5
c. 1, 3, 4, 5
d. 1, 2, 3, 4

44. For the lateral lower leg projection:
1. Leg is centered to cassette
2. May be performed table top or Bucky
3. Roll patient away from affected side
4. Patella should be perpendicular to cassette
5. Include both joints
6. Tibia and fibula should be superimposed
7. Central ray is directed to midpoint of leg
a. All are true
b. 1, 2, 3, 4, 5, 7
c. 1, 4, 5, 6, 7
d. 1, 2, 4, 5, 7

45. When the lateral knee projection is performed:
1. Patient turns onto affected side
2. Knee is flexed 20 to 30 degrees
3. Patella must be parallel to film
4. Central ray is directed 5 degrees caudad
5. Central ray enters knee joint inferior to the medial condyle
a. All are true
b. 1, 2, 3, 5
c. 1, 2, 5
d. 1, 2, 4, 5

46. For the tangential projection of the patella:
1. Patient is prone
2. Affected knee is flexed so that tibia and fibula form 50- to 60-degree angle with table
3. Central ray is directed 45 degrees cephalad through patellofemoral joint
4. Tangential patella may also be performed with the patient supine
a. All are true
b. 2, 3, 4
c. 1, 2, 3
d. 1, 2, 4

47. For the AP projection of the femur:
   a. The lower leg should be rotated laterally 15 degrees
   b. The central ray is directed toward the affected joint
   c. The patient is prone
   d. The lower leg is rotated medially 15 degrees

48. The central ray for an AP projection of the hip is:
   a. Directed parallel to a point 2 inches medial to the ASIS and at the level of the superior margin of the greater trochanter
   b. Directed parallel to a point 2 inches lateral to the ASIS and at the level of the superior margin of the greater trochanter
   c. Directed parallel to a point 2 inches medial to the ASIS and at the level of the inferior margin of the greater trochanter
   d. Directed perpendicular to a point 2 inches medial to the ASIS and at the level of the superior margin of the greater trochanter

Use the following list to answer questions **49-53.** Items may be used more than once.

   A. Jefferson's fracture
   B. Hangman's fracture
   C. Spondylolysis
   D. Spina bifida

49. Commonly caused by motor vehicle accidents

50. Caused by acute hyperextension of the head on the neck; fracture of the arch of C2

51. Defect of the posterior aspect of the spinal canal caused by failure of the vertebral arch to properly form

52. Defect in pars articularis

53. Comminuted fracture of the ring of the atlas involving both anterior and posterior arches and causing displacement of the fragments

For the following questions, choose the single best answer.

54. For the lateral projection of the cervical spine:
   1. Patient may be upright, seated, or supine, depending on condition
   2. SID of 72 inches should be used because of increased object-to-image distance
   3. Shoulders should lie in the same plane
   4. Cervical collar should be removed so that it does not obstruct pertinent anatomy
   5. Chin should be in contact with chest
   a. All are true
   b. 1, 2, 3
   c. 1, 2, 3, 5
   d. 1, 2, 4, 5

55. For the lateral projection of the thoracic spine:
   1. The head and spine should be in the same plane
   2. The central ray is directed to T7, at a cephalad angle of 10 degrees
   3. Patient should continue shallow breathing during exposure
   4. Exam should not be performed in room with a falling load generator
   a. All are true
   b. 1, 3
   c. 1, 3, 4
   d. 1, 2, 3

56. For the lateral projection of L5-S1:
   1. Patient is in lateral position
   2. Hips and knees are extended
   3. Cassette is centered at the level of the transverse plane that passes midway between the iliac crests and the ASIS
   4. A cylinder cone may be used to greatly reduce the production of scatter radiation
   5. Central ray is directed to a point 1.5 inches anterior to palpated spinous process of L5
   a. All are true
   b. 1, 2
   c. 1, 2, 3, 5
   d. 1, 3, 4, 5

57. For RPO and LPO positions for sacroiliac joints:
   a. Image the joint nearest the film
   b. Require the part to be angled at 10 to 15 degrees to coincide with the angle of the joints
   c. Image the joint farthest from the film
   d. Require the central ray to be angled 25 degrees cephalad

58. For the AP projection of the coccyx:
    a. The central ray should be directed 10 degrees caudad, entering 2 inches superior to the symphysis pubis
    b. The central ray should be directed 10 degrees cephalad, entering 2 inches superior to the symphysis pubis
    c. The central ray should be directed 25 degrees caudad, entering 2 inches superior to the symphysis pubis
    d. The central ray should be directed 25 degrees caudad, entering 4 inches superior to the symphysis pubis

Use the following list to answer questions **59-64**. Items may be used more than once.

   A. Atelectasis
   B. Bronchogenic carcinoma
   C. COPD
   D. Emphysema

59. Pathology that is easy to penetrate D

60. Collapse of lung tissue; harder to penetrate A

61. Air trapped in the alveoli make this too easy to penetrate D

62. AECs should not be used to image D

63. Lung cancer arising from bronchial mucosa B

64. Progressive condition marked by diminished capabilities of inspiration and expiration C

For the following questions, choose the single best answer.

65. For the AP projection of the ribs above the diaphragm:
    1. Top of cassette placed 1 to 2 inches above shoulders
    2. Shoulders relaxed, scapulae flat against table
    3. Central ray to T7
    4. Respiration on full expiration to depress diaphragm
    a. 1, 3
    b. All are true
    c. 1, 2, 3
    d. 1, 3, 4

66. For the RAO position of the sternum:
    a. Body should be rotated 45 to 60 degrees to prevent superimposition of sternum and spine
    b. Patient is supine
    c. Breathing should be shallow during exposure; falling load generator should not be used
    d. Best image is obtained with suspended breathing

67. When radiographing the sternoclavicular articulations:
    a. PA and lateral projections are required
    b. RAO or LAO positions are used to eliminate superimposition of joints onto vertebral shadow
    c. Patient should breathe during exposure; falling load generator should be used if possible
    d. AP projection is used to reduce magnification of joints

Use the following list to answer questions **68-72**. Items may be used more than once.

   A. Hydrocephalus
   B. Paget's disease
   C. Osteoporosis
   D. Rickets

68. Soft bones resulting from deficiency of vitamin D and sunlight D

69. Bone disease causing bone destruction and unorganized bone repair; generally difficult to penetrate B

70. Abnormal demineralization of bone, seen more often in females C

71. Abnormal accumulation of CSF in the brain A

72. Most often seen in the elderly C

For the following questions, choose the single best answer.

73. For the direct PA projection of the skull, the central ray is directed:
    a. 15 degrees caudad
    b. 25 degrees caudad
    c. Perpendicular to the film
    d. Perpendicular to the film, exiting the nasion when the OML is perpendicular to the cassette

74. When the skull is radiographed in the lateral position:
    a. The MSP must be perpendicular to the cassette, the IOML must be parallel to the cassette, and the IPL must be parallel to the cassette
    b. The MSP and IOML are parallel to the cassette, and the IPL is perpendicular to the cassette
    c. The MSP is perpendicular to the cassette, and the IPL is parallel to the cassette
    d. The MSP and IOML are perpendicular to the cassette, and the IPL is parallel to the cassette

75. For the parieto-orbital (Rhese) projection of the optic foramen:
   a. The head is resting on the forehead, nose, and zygoma
   b. The MSP forms an angle of 53 degrees from the perpendicular
   c. The central ray exits the unaffected orbit
   d. The head rests on the zygoma, nose, and chin while the MSP is rotated 53 degrees from the cassette

76. When a parietoacanthial (Waters) projection is performed for the facial bones:
   a. The MSP is parallel to the cassette
   b. The MSP is perpendicular to the cassette, the head rests on the chin, and the OML forms a 53-degree angle with the plane of the film
   c. The MSP is perpendicular to the cassette, the head rests on the chin, and the OML forms a 37-degree angle with the plane of the film
   d. The MSP is perpendicular to the cassette, the head rests on the nose, and the OML forms a 37-degree angle with the plane of the film

77. For the unilateral tangential (May) projection of the zygomatic arches:
   a. The IOML is parallel to the plane of the film, the MSP is rotated 15 degrees away from the affected side, the cassette is centered 3 inches distal to the most prominent point of the zygoma, and the central ray is directed perpendicular to the IOML through the zygomatic arch 1.5 inches posterior to the outer canthus
   b. The IOML is parallel to the plane of the film, the MSP is rotated 15 degrees toward the affected side, the cassette is centered 3 inches distal to the most prominent point of the zygoma, and the central ray is directed perpendicular to the IOML through the zygomatic arch 1.5 inches posterior to the outer canthus
   c. The IOML is parallel to the plane of the film, the MSP is rotated 15 degrees away from the affected side, the cassette is centered 3 inches distal to the most prominent point of the zygoma, and the central ray is directed perpendicular to the zygomatic arch 1.5 inches posterior to the outer canthus
   d. The IOML is parallel to the plane of the film, the MSP is rotated 25 degrees away from the affected side, the cassette is centered 3 inches distal to the most prominent point of the zygoma, and the central ray is directed perpendicular to the IOML through the zygomatic arch 1.5 inches posterior to the outer canthus

78. When the mandibular body is radiographed with the patient in the SMV position:
   a. Head and neck are extended and resting on chin
   b. MSP is parallel with cassette
   c. IOML is perpendicular with plane of film, head and neck are resting on vertex, and MSP is perpendicular to the cassette
   d. IOML is parallel with plane of film, head resting on vertex, and MSP is perpendicular to the cassette

79. The best survey film of the paranasal sinuses is obtained using:
   a. Lateral
   b. Parietoacanthial (Waters)
   c. Upright lateral
   d. SMV

Use the following list to answer questions **80-84**. Items may be used more than once.

   A. Annular carcinoma
   B. Crohn's disease
   C. Hiatus hernia
   D. Ileus

80. Condition in which a portion of the stomach protrudes through the diaphragm

81. Intestinal obstruction

82. Chronic inflammation of portions of bowel

83. May be adynamic or mechanical

84. Appears in an "apple-core" pattern on barium enema

Use the following list to answer questions **85-89**. Items may be used more than once.

   A. Diverticula
   B. Ulcerative colitis
   C. Pyloric stenosis
   D. Adynamic ileus

85. Visualized by performing an upper GI series

86. Bowel obstruction caused by immobility of bowel

87. Pouchlike herniations of the colonic wall

88. Narrowing of sphincter at distal end of stomach

89. Severe inflammation of colon and rectum with loss of mucosal lining

For the following questions, choose the single best answer.

90. For the RAO position of the esophagus:
   a. Patient is rotated obliquely by elevating right side 35 to 40 degrees, esophagus is centered to film at level of T5 or T6
   b. Patient is rotated obliquely by elevating left side 35 to 40 degrees, esophagus is centered at level of T5 or T6
   c. Patient is rotated obliquely by elevating right side 55 to 60 degrees, esophagus is centered to film at level of T5 or T6
   d. Patient is rotated obliquely by elevating left side 55 to 60 degrees, esophagus is centered to film at level of T5 or T6

91. For the PA projection of the stomach:
   a. Center midway between the xiphoid process and the umbilicus
   b. Center halfway between the midline and lateral border of abdominal cavity
   c. Center midway between the manubrium and the umbilicus and halfway between the midline and lateral border of abdominal cavity
   d. Center midway between the xiphoid process and the umbilicus and halfway between the midline and lateral border of abdominal cavity

92. For the LPO or RPO positions for the colon:
   a. Patient is prone, rotated 35 to 45 degrees, central ray at level of iliac crest
   b. Patient is supine, rotated 55 to 60 degrees, central ray at level of ASIS
   c. Patient is supine, rotated 35 to 45 degrees from the AP, central ray at level of iliac crest
   d. Patient is prone, rotated 55 to 60 degrees, central ray at level of iliac crest

93. For the lateral decubitus positions of the colon:
   a. Patient lying on side, cassette centered to iliac crest, central ray horizontal to midline at level of iliac crest
   b. Patient prone, cassette centered to iliac crest, central ray horizontal to midline at level of iliac crest
   c. Patient lying on side, cassette centered 3 inches above iliac crest, central ray horizontal 3 inches above iliac crest
   d. Patient prone, cassette centered to L1, central ray horizontal to L1

94. A procedure used to evaluate biliary and pancreatic pathologies using an endoscope is:
   a. Sonography
   b. MRI
   c. ERCP
   d. IVP

Use the following list to answer questions **95-99.** Items may be used more than once.

   A. Polycystic kidney disease
   B. Renal calculus
   C. Wilms' tumor
   D. Renal cysts

95. Fluid-filled masses in kidney D

96. Malignant cancer of the kidney C

97. Enlarged kidneys containing numerous cysts A

98. Primarily seen in children C

99. Kidney stone B

For the following question, choose the single best answer.

100. For the RPO and LPO positions of the kidneys:
   a. Patient is prone, body is rotated obliquely 30 degrees, kidney farthest from film is imaged in profile and kidney nearest film is imaged in its entirety, central ray is perpendicular
   b. Patient is supine, body is rotated obliquely 45 degrees, kidney farthest from film is imaged in profile and kidney nearest film is imaged in its entirety, central ray is perpendicular
   c. Patient is supine, body is rotated obliquely 30 degrees, kidney farthest from film is imaged parallel to film and kidney nearest film is imaged perpendicular to film, central ray is perpendicular to film
   d. Patient is supine, body is rotated obliquely 30 degrees, kidney nearest the film is imaged in profile and kidney farthest from film is imaged in its entirety, central ray is perpendicular

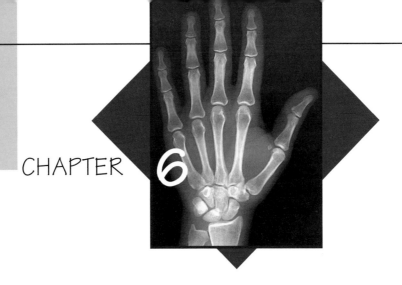

CHAPTER 6

Review of Patient Care and Management

SCHEDULING OF RADIOGRAPHIC EXAMINATIONS

A. General considerations
1. Schedule in an appropriate and timely sequence to ensure patient comfort and fiscal responsibility
2. Sequence so that exams do not interfere with one another
3. Schedule barium studies last
4. Schedule several exams in one day if the patient is able to tolerate them
5. Seriously ill or weak patients may be able to tolerate only one exam per day or must have a rest between examinations
6. If sedation is used, patient must be given time to recover from sedation before beginning fluoroscopic studies
7. Thyroid assessment must precede any examinations involving iodinated contrast media
8. Schedule radiographic examinations not requiring contrast agents first
9. Total doses of iodinated contrast media should be calculated if they are to be used in a series of examinations
10. Schedule patients who have been held NPO (nothing by mouth) first
11. Schedule pediatric and geriatric patients early
12. Schedule diabetic patients early because of their need for insulin

B. Sequencing
1. Fiberoptic (endoscopy) studies are conducted first in a series
2. Radiography of the urinary tract
3. Radiography of the biliary system
4. Computed tomography (CT) studies should be scheduled before examinations involving the use of barium sulfate
5. Lower gastrointestinal (GI) series
6. Upper GI series

PATIENT PREPARATION

A. GI system or urinary system
1. Low-residue diet
2. NPO for 8 to 12 hours before the procedure
3. Cathartics and enemas are used to cleanse the GI system
4. If scheduled as an outpatient
   a. Patient must clearly understand the routine for proper preparation
   b. Patient should be asked to explain the procedure back to the radiographer to verify understanding

B. All procedures
1. Clothing removed from area to be radiographed and replaced by patient gown when appropriate
2. All radiopaque objects removed from area of interest

PATIENT HISTORY

A. Provides information for the radiographer about the extent of the patient's injury and the range of motion the patient will tolerate

B. Assists the radiologist during interpretation of the radiographs

C. History should begin with radiographer introducing self and verifying the patient's name

D. Types of questions used to take a patient's history (depending on type and site of injury)

1. How did your injury occur?
2. When did your injury occur?
3. Where is your pain?
4. Do you have tingling or numbness?
5. Do you have any weakness?
6. Were you unconscious after your injury?
7. Why did your doctor order this exam?
8. Have you experienced shortness of breath or been coughing?
9. Have you experienced a fever or heart problems?
10. Have you experienced any nausea, vomiting, or diarrhea?

MEDICOLEGAL ASPECTS OF PRACTICE

A. Torts
1. Violations of civil law
2. Also known as *personal injury law*
3. Injured parties have a right to compensation for injury

B. Intentional misconduct
1. Assault
   a. Patient is apprehensive about being injured
   b. Imprudent conduct of radiographer that causes fear in patient is grounds for an allegation of civil assault
2. Battery
   a. Unlawful touching or touching without consent
   b. Harm resulting from physical contact with radiographer
   c. May also include radiographing the wrong patient, the wrong body part, or performing radiography against a patient's will
3. False imprisonment
   a. Unjustified restraint of a person
   b. Care must be taken when using restraint straps or having other individuals assist with holding a patient still
4. Invasion of privacy
   a. Violation of confidentiality of information
   b. Unnecessarily or improperly exposing the patient's body
   c. Unnecessarily or improperly touching a patient's body
   d. Photographing patients without their permission
5. Libel: written information that results in defamation of character or loss of reputation
6. Slander: verbally spreading false information that results in defamation of character or loss of reputation

C. Unintentional misconduct (negligence)
1. Neglect or omission of reasonable care
2. Based on doctrine of the reasonably prudent person
3. Reasonably prudent person doctrine: based on how a reasonable person with similar education and experience would perform under similar circumstances
4. Gross negligence: acts that demonstrate reckless disregard for life or limb
5. Contributory negligence: instance in which the injured person is a contributing party to the injury

D. Four conditions needed to establish malpractice
1. Establishment of standard of care
2. Demonstration that standard of care was violated by the radiographer
3. Demonstration that loss or injury was caused by radiographer who is being sued
4. Loss or injury actually occurred and is a result of the negligence

E. *Respondeat superior*
1. "Let the master answer"
2. Legal doctrine stating that an employer will be held liable for an employee's negligent act

F. Rule of personal responsibility: individuals are responsible for their own actions

G. *Res ipsa loquitur*
1. "The thing speaks for itself"
2. Legal doctrine stating that cause of the negligence is obvious (e.g., forceps left inside a patient during surgery)

H. Charting
1. Writing on the patient's chart by radiographer
2. Varies by institution
3. Radiographer's responsibilities in this regard must be carefully outlined during new employee orientation
4. Write clear statements regarding patient's condition, reaction to contrast agents, amount of contrast material injected, etc.
5. Must be clearly stated on the chart
6. Information must also include the date and time of the occurrence
7. Radiographer must sign such entries using full name and credentials

I. Radiographs
1. Radiographs are legal documents
2. Items that radiographs must include
   a. Patient identification
   b. Anatomic markings, including left and right markers
   c. Markings must be carefully placed on each radiograph using lead markers
   d. Date of exposure
   e. Other markings (using stickers, grease pencils, etc.) applied to the radiograph after processing may not be legally admissible
3. Retention of radiographs

a. Varies according to state law
b. Normally maintained for 5 to 7 years after the date of the last radiographic examination
c. Film folders on minors are normally retained for 5 to 7 years after the minor reaches age 18 or 21, depending on the state of residence

4. Careful documentation must be maintained when radiographs are checked out for use by physicians, students, or other health care practitioners

J. Patient consent
   1. Patient bill of rights provides for patient consent or refusal of any procedure
   2. Implied consent
      a. Provides for care when patient is unconscious
      b. Based on assumption that patient would approve care if conscious
   3. Valid consent
      a. Also called *informed consent*
      b. Patient must be mentally competent
      c. Consent must be offered voluntarily
      d. Patient must be adequately informed
      e. Patient must be of legal age
      f. Requires radiographer and radiologist to carefully explain all aspects of procedure and risks involved
      g. Requires that explanation be provided in lay terms that the patient understands

PATIENT TRANSFER

A. Check identification bracelet to ensure correct patient is being transferred
B. Ask patient to state name to double-check identity; ask date of birth as a backup
C. Explain transfer procedure to patient to gain cooperation and alleviate fear
D. Radiographer must always use proper body mechanics for patient transfer
   1. Keep knees slightly bent
   2. Keep back straight
   3. Perform all lifting using legs, not back

Transfer from Wheelchair to X-Ray Table

A. Wheelchair parallel to the table
B. Brakes applied with step stool nearby
C. Using face-to-face method, assist the patient to a standing position
D. Have patient place one hand on step stool handle, the other hand on your shoulder, and step up onto the stool
E. Patient pivots with back against the table into a sitting position on the edge of the table
F. Place one arm around patient's shoulder and the other arm under the knees
G. Assist patient to a supine position

Transfer from X-Ray Table to Wheelchair

A. Check to see that brakes of wheelchair have been applied
B. Assist patient to a sitting position
C. Allow patient to sit up for a short time to regain sense of balance
D. Ambulatory patient
   1. Assist to a standing position and pivot
   2. Have patient reach back with both hands and grab arms of wheelchair
   3. Assist patient to sit in the wheelchair
E. Nonambulatory patients
   1. Stand facing the patient
   2. Reach around the patient and place your hands on each scapula
   3. Lift the patient upward to a standing position
   4. Pivot so that the back of the patient's leg is touching the edge of the wheelchair
   5. Ease the patient down to a sitting position
   6. Position foot and leg rests into place
   7. Cover patient's lap with a sheet

Cart Transfer

A. Place cart near and parallel to the x-ray table
B. Do not attempt patient transfer from cart to x-ray table without assistance
C. One person supports the neck and shoulders at the head of the cart; the second individual lifts the pelvis and knees; if available, other individuals support patient at both sides
D. Transfer sheet or draw sheet should be used under the patient
E. On signal, all involved in transfer move the patient in one fluid motion to the x-ray table

PATIENT COMFORT

A. Taking into account the patient's physical condition, carefully position pillows or radiolucent sponges so that they will not interfere with the examination
B. Evaluate patient's condition
   1. Ability to breathe
   2. Presence of nausea
   3. Allow the patient to remain partially upright when possible
   4. Special care must be given to elderly patients, who may have decubitus ulcers or particularly sensitive or thin skin

INFECTION CONTROL
Routes of Transmission

A. Contact transmission

1. Direct contact: infected person touches the susceptible host, allowing the infectious organisms to come in contact with susceptible tissues
2. Indirect contact: an inanimate object containing pathogenic organisms is placed in contact with a susceptible person

B. Airborne transmission: droplets and dust

C. Droplet transmission: primarily transmitted by coughs, sneezes, or other methods of spraying onto a nearby host

D. Common vehicle transmission: primarily transmitted by contaminated items such as food, water, medications, devices, and equipment

E. Vectorborne transmission: an animal that contains and transmits an infectious organism to humans

Standard Precautions

A. The first tier of transmission-based isolation precautions

B. System that uses barriers between blood, all body fluids, nonintact skin, and mucous membranes of all individuals and susceptible persons

C. Assumes all body fluids are sources of infection

D. Assumes all patients are infected

E. Guidelines
1. Always wear gloves when any chance of being in contact with body substances exists
2. Protect clothing by wearing a protective gown or plastic apron if a chance of coming in contact with body substances exists
3. Masks and/or eye protection must be worn if a chance of body substances splashing exists
4. Handwashing is the most effective method to prevent the spread of infection
5. Uncapped needle syringe units and all sharps must be discarded in biohazard containers
6. If any contact is made with body substances, the entire area contacted must be washed completely with bleach
7. Needles should never be recapped but should be placed with the syringe in a sharps container
8. Use protective masks and/or mouthpieces when performing cardiopulmonary resuscitation (CPR)

Medical Asepsis

A. Microorganisms have been eliminated as much as possible

B. Water and chemicals are used for the disinfection

Surgical Asepsis

A. Complete removal of all organisms from equipment and the environment in which patient care is conducted

B. Includes complete sterilization of equipment and appropriate skin preparation

1. Chemical sterilization: soaking objects in germicidal solution
2. Boiling: sterilization with moist heat
3. Dry heat: placing objects in an oven at temperatures in excess of 300° F
4. Gas sterilization: items are exposed to a mixture of gases that will not harm the materials
5. Autoclaving: steam sterilization under pressure; most convenient way to sterilize materials

Sterile Technique

A. Steps to follow in opening sterile packs
1. Place pack on a clean surface
2. Break the seal and open the pack
3. Unfold first corner of the pack away from you
4. Unfold both sides
5. Pull front portion of the wrap toward you and drop it
6. Never touch the inner surface
7. If there is an inner wrap, open it using the same method
8. Separately wrapped sterile items may be added to the sterile field by opening the pack and allowing the items to drop onto the sterile field
9. Never allow the container to touch the sterile field

B. Pouring liquids into containers in a sterile field
1. Carefully determine the contents of the container
2. Pour a small amount into a waste receptacle to cleanse the lip of the bottle
3. Pour the medium into the receptacle, being careful not to touch the sterile field in the process

C. Sterile objects or fields touched by unsterile objects or persons are immediately contaminated

D. Avoid reaching across sterile fields

E. If you suspect an object is contaminated, assume that it *is* contaminated

F. Always assume damp items are contaminated

G. Do not invade the space between a physician and the sterile field

H. Never abandon a sterile field; it must be under direct observation at all times

I. Never turn your back on a sterile field

Gloving

A. Wash hands thoroughly

B. Open outer package containing gloves

C. Open inner package, exposing gloves

D. Approach glove from the open end, and touch only inner surface with opposite hand

E. Put on glove, touching only the folded cuff

F. Pick up other glove with gloved hand under the cuff

G. Place second glove on other hand and unfold cuff

H. Carefully unfold the cuff on both gloves

I. Always keep hands in front of the body without touching body covering or placing hands under arms

Isolation Precautions: Types

A. Transmission-based precautions
 1. Airborne precautions
  a. Respiratory protection required for individuals entering patient's room
  b. Gowns required to prevent contamination of clothing
  c. Use of standard precautions
 2. Droplet precautions
  a. Masks required for persons coming in close contact with the patient
  b. Use of standard precautions
 3. Contact precautions
  a. Masks, gloves, and gowns are indicated for individuals coming in contact with the patient
  b. Use of standard precautions
B. Empiric use
 1. Routine use of standard precautions
 2. Each patient condition is evaluated
 3. Appropriate isolation precaution guidelines are put in place

Isolation Technique: Mobile Radiography

A. If protective cap is indicated, it should be put on and all hair tucked inside
B. Mask should be put on next, completely covering the nose and mouth
C. Gown should be put on and tied securely at the back and neck
D. Gloves should be put on and pulled over the end of the sleeve on the gown
E. Radiographic cassette should be placed in a protective cover
F. Enter patient's room and follow all isolation guidelines that have been posted
G. When possible, have a second radiographer handle the portable x-ray machine and controls while the first radiographer touches only the patient
H. After the radiographic exposure is made
 1. Remove cassette from the vicinity of the patient
 2. Open the end of the protective covering
 3. Radiographer handling the equipment should remove cassette from the open end of the cover
I. When leaving the patient's isolation room, carefully remove attire
 1. Untie waist belt of protective gown
 2. Remove gloves
  a. Pull off one glove by grasping the cuff and inverting it as it is pulled off
  b. Remove second glove by inserting clean fingers inside the cuff and inverting it as it is removed
 3. Untie neck and back strings from gown
 4. Remove mask by using strings only
 5. Remove gown by holding it away from the body as it is removed

 6. Carefully wash hands
 7. Use paper towels to touch faucet handles
 8. After moving the portable x-ray unit safely outside the room, it should be cleaned thoroughly before it is returned to the radiology department

Isolation Technique: Patients in Radiology Departments

A. Identify isolation category and follow guidelines
B. Isolation patients should never spend time waiting in the hallway
C. Carefully cover x-ray table with a sheet
D. Work in pairs so that only one radiographer is in contact with the patient while the other manipulates the equipment
E. Carefully cover the patient with protective sheets and blankets when returning patient to the wheelchair or cart
F. All contaminated materials must be placed in an appropriate discard bag
G. Carefully clean off the x-ray table and any other equipment with which the patient came in contact
H. Remove gloves and carefully wash hands

ASSESSMENT OF CHANGING PATIENT CONDITIONS

A. Visual observation of patient
B. Changes in skin color to cyanotic or waxen pallor
C. Patient verbalizations of discomfort or dizziness
D. Cyanosis of lips or nail beds
E. Patient is cool and diaphoretic to the touch

Vital Signs

A. Temperature: normal oral temperature is 98° to 99° F
B. Pulse
 1. Taken at radial or carotid artery
 2. More than 100 beats per minute: tachycardia
 3. Fewer than 60 beats per minute: bradycardia
C. Respiration: normal rate of respiration is 12 to 16 breaths per minute
D. Blood pressure
 1. Measured using sphygmomanometer
 2. Systolic pressure: measurement of the pumping action of the heart
 3. Diastolic pressure: measures the blood pressure of the heart at rest
 4. Diastolic pressure greater than 90 mm Hg indicates increasing level of hypertension
 5. Diastolic pressure less than 50 mm Hg gives some indication of shock
 6. Always expressed as systolic pressure over diastolic pressure (e.g., 120/80 mm Hg)

Medical Emergencies

A. Oxygen administration
1. Generally administered using mask or nasal cannula
2. Usual oxygen flow rate is 3 to 5 L per minute
3. Care must be taken while radiographing patients who are on portable oxygen support; avoid pinching or kinking oxygen tubing
4. Radiographers must know how to operate oxygen tanks or wall oxygen outlets so that they can administer oxygen to a patient in the event of an emergency

B. Suction unit
1. Used to maintain patient's airway
2. Must be used any time the airway becomes obstructed by fluids
3. If you are working alone and a patient needs suctioning, call for help before beginning procedure

C. Cardiac arrest
1. Cessation of heart function
2. Specific routine for announcing cardiac arrest must be followed
3. Emergency medical assistance must be called immediately
4. CPR must commence immediately
5. Radiographer must be familiar with location and contents of "crash cart"
   a. Medications
   b. Airways
   c. Sphygmomanometers
   d. Stethoscopes
   e. Defibrillators
   f. Cardiac monitors

D. Respiratory arrest
1. Cessation of breathing
2. Possible causes of respiratory arrest
   a. Upper respiratory tract swelling
   b. Failure of the central nervous system (CNS)
   c. Choking
3. Tracheolaryngeal edema may necessitate an emergency tracheotomy
4. Tracheolaryngeal edema may follow injection of iodinated contrast material
   a. Radiographer should be aware of location of tracheotomy tray
5. Respiratory arrest secondary to CNS failure necessitates calling a respiratory arrest
6. Respiratory arrest secondary to choking necessitates the use of suction or the Heimlich maneuver

E. Shock
1. Failure of circulation in which blood pressure is inadequate to oxygenate tissues and remove byproducts of metabolism
2. Hypovolemic shock: follows the loss of a large amount of blood or plasma

3. Septic shock: occurs when toxins produced during massive infection cause a dramatic drop in blood pressure
4. Neurogenic shock: causes blood to pool in peripheral vessels
5. Cardiogenic shock: secondary to cardiac failure or other interference with heart function
6. Allergic shock (anaphylaxis)
   a. Allergic reaction to foreign proteins following injections
   b. Marked by extremely low pressure, dyspnea, and possible death
   c. May follow injection of iodinated contrast media
7. Symptoms of shock
   a. Restlessness, apprehension
   b. Accelerated pulse
   c. Pale skin
   d. Weakness
   e. Alteration in ability to think
   f. Cool, clammy skin
   g. Systolic blood pressure less than 30 mm Hg
8. Radiographer's response to shock
   a. Stop procedure
   b. Place patient in a recumbent (Trendelenburg) position
   c. Immediately obtain help, calling a code if necessary
   d. Determine blood pressure
   e. Administer oxygen
   f. Carefully document the time and occurrence of each symptom

F. Trauma
1. Serious and potentially life-threatening injuries
2. Be careful to do no additional harm to the patient
3. Be prepared to work with other health care professionals present in the radiographic room
4. Be prepared to perform a lateral crosstable cervical spine as soon as possible
5. Regardless of which area of the body is to be radiographed, assume a serious internal injury is present
6. Patient will be at one of four levels of consciousness
   a. Alert and conscious
   b. Drowsy
   c. Unconscious but reactive to stimuli
   d. Comatose
7. Carefully observe the condition of the patient when first brought to the radiographic room
8. Note any changes in patient's condition during the course of the radiographic procedures
9. Under no circumstances should trauma patients be left alone
10. Until otherwise informed by a physician, assume the presence of serious spinal injuries

11. Slight movement of patient with spinal injuries may result in paralysis or death
12. Immobilization devices such as cervical collars or splints must never be removed without the permission of a physician
13. Be prepared to alter routine positions and projections because of the inability of the anatomic part to be moved
14. Adjust radiographic technique to compensate for the presence of splints, spine boards, and other immobilization devices
15. Work carefully with patients who have wounds
16. Observe condition of wound when patient is brought for radiography, and immediately notify emergency room personnel of any changes in the wound, including fresh bleeding
17. Patients with severe burns will require protective isolation
    a. Such patients either experience no sensation at all or extreme pain
    b. Care must be exercised when working with burn patients under either condition

Patient Monitoring/Support Equipment

A. Ventilators
1. Mechanical respirators attached to tracheostomies
2. Patient with a ventilator has been intubated (a tube inserted into the trachea)
3. Care must be taken not to dislodge the tubing connected to the tracheostomy

B. Nasogastric (NG) tubes
1. Tube inserted through the nose and down the esophagus into the stomach
2. Used to feed the patient or to conduct gastric suction
3. Care must be taken by the radiographer not to pull on the NG tube while moving the patient or performing the examination

C. Chest tube
1. In place to remove fluid or air from the pleural space
2. May be connected to a suction device
3. Radiographer must be careful not to disturb the chest tube or suction devices or bottles to which the tube may be attached
4. Bottle must never be raised above chest level
5. Tubing must not be pinched

D. Venous catheters
1. May be kept in place for patients requiring long-term chemotherapy or nutrition
2. Must not be disturbed or pulled in any way

E. Urinary catheters (Foley and suprapubic)
1. Care must be taken during the transfer and radiography of patients with urinary catheters in place
2. Attention must be given to urinary catheter tubing so

that it is not bent, pinched, or caught on other equipment
3. Bag attached to urinary catheters must always be kept below the level of the bladder
4. Allowing urine to flow retrograde into the urethra and bladder can cause urinary tract infections
    a. Urinary tract infections are the number one cause of nosocomial infections (infections acquired in the hospital)

F. Oxygen
1. Oxygen should not be removed during radiographic examinations
2. Oxygen may be removed only with a physician's order
3. Care should be taken to prevent pinching the tubing

CONTRAST MEDIA

A. Negative contrast agent
1. Most commonly used is air
2. Requires fewer x rays and produces a higher density on the radiograph
3. Air may be used in combination with a positive contrast agent on double-contrast studies
4. Most common exam performed using a negative contrast agent is the routine chest radiograph

B. Positive contrast agents
1. Examples
    a. Iodine (atomic number 53)
    b. Barium (atomic number 56)
2. Relatively high atomic numbers
    a. Result in greater attenuation of x rays
    b. Provide lower density on the radiograph
    c. Provide an increase in contrast between the structure to be visualized and surrounding structures

C. Barium
1. Administered to the patient in the form of barium sulfate, an inert salt
2. For upper GI series and esophagram, the barium is most palatable when mixed with very cold water
3. For barium enema the barium powder is mixed with water at a temperature of approximately 100° F
4. For some studies of the esophagus, a barium sulfate paste, which is much thicker and more difficult to swallow, may be administered
5. Barium tends to absorb water
6. Patients must be given careful instructions regarding fluid intake following barium studies so that the barium does not cause an impaction
7. Barium sulfate escaping into the peritoneal cavity can cause peritonitis

D. Aqueous iodine compounds
1. Used for contrast studies of the GI tract

2. Used when barium could prove to be a surgical contaminant
   a. Perforated ulcers
   b. Ruptured appendix
3. Aqueous iodine compounds may also be used in patients at high risk for impactions
4. These compounds may cause significant dehydration
   E. Iodinated contrast media
   1. Ionic contrast agents
      a. Salts of organic iodine compounds
      b. Composed of positively and negatively charged ions
   2. Nonionic contrast agents
      a. Similar to ionic contrast agents
      b. Do not ionize into separate positive and negative charges, which negates their primary advantage over ionic contrast agents
      c. Provide far lower incidence of contrast agent reactions
   3. Contraindications to the use of iodinated contrast media
      a. Previous sensitivity to contrast agents
      b. Known sensitivity to iodine
   4. It should be noted that both ionic and nonionic contrast agents are iodinated (i.e., both contain various concentrations of iodine—*nonionic* does not mean *noniodinated*)

Contrast Media Reactions

A. Overdose: may occur in infants or adults with renal, cardiac, or hepatic failure
B. Anaphylactic reactions: flushing, hives, nausea
C. Cardiovascular reactions: hypotension, tachycardia, cardiac arrest
D. Psychogenic factors: may be caused by patient anxiety or suggested by the possible reactions described during the informed consent process
E. Other symptoms of contrast agent reactions
   1. Nausea and vomiting
   2. Sneezing
   3. Sensation of heat
   4. Itching
   5. Hoarseness (or change in pitch of voice during conversation)
   6. Coughing
   7. Urticaria
   8. Dyspnea
   9. Loss of consciousness
   10. Convulsions
   11. Cardiac arrest
   12. Paralysis
   13. Any change in level of orientation
F. Complications may occur at the site of injection
   1. Local irritation may occur if the contrast material extravasates

2. Phlebitis may occur in the vein in which the contrast material was injected

Patient Care Preceding Injection of Iodinated Contrast Media

A. Determine history of allergies or previous hypersensitivity to contrast media
B. Determine extent of patient's medical problems
C. Review possible reactions to the contrast medium being used
D. Know the location of all emergency equipment
E. Carefully observe and evaluate the patient, noting color of skin, tone and pitch of voice, and presence of apprehension or anxiety so that changes from these baselines may be noted after injection

Patient Care after Injection of Iodinated Contrast Media

A. Continue conversation with patient
   1. Encourage patient to speak
   2. Laryngeal swelling as a contrast agent reaction will first manifest itself as a change in the tone and pitch of the patient's voice
B. Continue to observe the patient for early signs of urticaria, profuse sweating, or extreme anxiety
C. If patient becomes overanxious, take patient's pulse and determine whether tachycardia is present
D. If patient becomes faint, immediately check respirations, pulse, and blood pressure and observe for signs of cyanosis
E. Be aware of the location of a physician in the event of an emergency
F. Remain with the patient (except when at the control panel to make exposures)
   1. Patient should never be left alone after injection or at any time during the procedure
   2. Although most contrast media reactions are noticeable and may even be violent, others are more difficult to observe
      a. A patient who appears to be resting comfortably or sleeping may have experienced cardiac arrest
   3. Summon help immediately upon observing the onset of a contrast agent reaction
      a. Although a calm response is required to avoid alarming the patient, urgency is important because a mild contrast agent reaction may quickly accelerate into a more serious reaction

VENIPUNCTURE

A. Use of hypodermic needle
   1. May be used for small injections

2. Described by gauge
    a. Unit of measurement that indicates diameter
    b. The larger the gauge, the smaller the diameter of the needle opening
    c. Higher-gauge needles are useful for intravenous (IV) injection of contrast agents because they make a smaller hole and limit bleeding at the site
    d. Higher-gauge needles limit the rate at which contrast material may be injected and consequently limit the size of the bolus that may be injected
3. If a hypodermic needle is used, the contrast medium must fill the needle before venipuncture so that air is not injected

B. Butterfly set
1. Smaller and sometimes easier to handle
2. Plastic projections make the needle easier to hold during venipuncture and injection
3. Radiographer must remember to fill plastic tubing and needle with contrast medium before venipuncture so that air is not injected
4. Butterfly may also be taped to the patient's arm so that the radiographer's hands are free to hold syringe and plunger

C. IV catheter
1. Combination unit with a needle inside a flexible plastic catheter
2. Combined unit is inserted into the vein, needle first
3. Once in place, the catheter is pushed in over the needle
4. Afterward, the needle is withdrawn
5. Catheter may then be connected to the syringe containing contrast medium
6. Entire system is more flexible than a hypodermic needle or butterfly
7. Also allows for attachment to IV tubing leading to bag or bottle that can be used in the event of a serious contrast agent reaction

D. Procedure for performing venipuncture
1. Wash hands
2. Always wear gloves
3. Secure tourniquet in place
4. Select vein
5. Thoroughly cleanse the skin using departmental protocol
6. Insert needle into vein
7. Observe blood return into catheter, plastic tubing, or syringe depending on equipment used; remove tourniquet
8. Tape catheter or butterfly in place and begin injection
9. If using hypodermic needle, begin injection immediately
10. If using hypodermic needle, remove needle at conclusion of injection
    a. Place small piece of gauze or alcohol wipe on puncture site and bend patient's arm
11. If using catheter or butterfly, continue until all contrast medium has been injected, then disconnect syringe and observe site for swelling

HAZARDOUS MATERIALS

Handling and Disposal of Biohazardous Materials (Figure 6-1)

A. General chemicals
1. Chemicals may cause harm if taken into the body by any route
2. Possible routes of entry
    a. Inhalation
    b. Swallowing
    c. Absorption through the skin or mucous membranes
3. Material Safety Data Sheets (MSDS) must be available, and radiographers should be familiar with their content and warnings
4. MSDS provide direction for the following
    a. Handling precautions
    b. Safe use of the product
    c. Clean-up and disposal
5. Guidelines for handling chemicals
    a. Use only if container is clearly labeled
    b. Read container label several times before actually using the contents to be certain of what is being handled
    c. Handle carefully to prevent contact with skin, eyes, and mucous membranes
    d. Wear personal protective equipment (PPE)
    e. Use chemicals only as directed
    f. Never mix chemicals unless compatibility can be verified

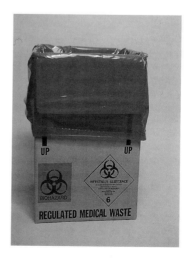

Figure 6-1 Biohazardous waste container and symbol.

g. Store chemicals only as directed on the label

h. Never pour toxic chemicals down the drain; this includes irritating or flammable materials

i. Clean up spills immediately according to written procedures

j. Following contact with the skin, rinse immediately with cool water for at least 5 minutes

k. Following contact with eyes, rinse for at least 15 minutes

l. Always notify the supervisor on duty and follow guidelines for medical follow-up and incident reports

B. Processing chemistry

1. MSDS must be displayed

2. Always use eye protection, such as full-face or non-vented goggles when working with processing chemistry

3. An eyewash station should be used immediately should contact occur

4. The Environmental Protection Agency (EPA) regulates processing chemistry as follows

   a. Amount of chemistry used

   b. Dilution of liquid waste

   c. Shipping requirements

5. The Occupational Safety and Health Administration (OSHA) requires eye and skin protection because of the corrosive properties of processing chemicals

6. Eye protection, protective apron, and rubber gloves should always be used when mixing chemistry

7. Silver is a toxic heavy metal and requires recovery and the same careful handling as processing chemistry

8. Silver contained in fixer and wash solutions is regulated by the EPA

C. Infectious waste

1. Anything that has the potential to transmit disease

2. Handle using Centers for Disease Control and Prevention (CDC) guidelines for standard precautions

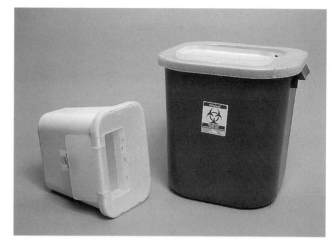

Figure 6-2 Puncture-proof containers for needle and syringe disposal.

3. Place in containers or bags properly labeled as to the type of waste therein

4. Be familiar with the facility's procedures for handling, containment, and disposal of all infectious waste

5. Exposure to infectious waste must be reported for medical follow-up and incident reports

6. Gloves must always be worn when

   a. Handling used needles and syringes

   b. Handling bandages and dressing

   c. Assisting patients with urinals or bedpans

7. Needles and syringes must be disposed of in special sharps containers (Figure 6-2)

8. Needles should not be recapped

9. Used bandages and dressings must be placed into waterproof bags and sealed

10. Bedpans and urinals must be emptied immediately and rinsed

REVIEW QUESTIONS

Read the following paragraph. Determine the accuracy of each underlined word or phrase. Then refer to questions **1-6** following the paragraph, and choose the answer that best corrects and completes the corresponding underlined item.

When scheduling radiography examinations, it is important to (1) schedule barium studies first, because these are the most difficult for the patient to tolerate. Several (2) nonconflicting exams should be scheduled the same day, if possible. (3) Elderly patients should be scheduled later in the day to give them time to get up their strength for the exam(s). (4) Patients who have been held NPO should be scheduled first so that they may eat or drink as allowed once the exam is over. It is important for (5) patients with diabetes to be scheduled later in the morning so that they may take their insulin and have a higher energy level for the exam. (6) Endoscopic procedures should be scheduled after ingestion of barium for increased contrast.

1. a. The underlined word or phrase is accurate as written
   b. True; barium hardens quickly and must be used first thing in the morning
   c. True; fluoroscopy must be done first so that the radiologists have time to dictate reports
   d. False; barium may interfere with the visibility of anatomic structures; nonbarium studies should be performed first

2. a. The underlined word or phrase is accurate as written
   b. False; exams should be spread out so that patients and staff are under less stress
   c. True; it is generally easier, more convenient, and possibly less costly for the patient to make one trip to radiology either as an inpatient or outpatient
   d. True; discounts are given when all exams can be combined, and films on the same patient can be interpreted all at once; in addition, it aids in the determination of a diagnosis if the radiologist can see the images from all the exams on one view box

3. a. The underlined word or phrase is accurate as written
   b. True; radiography exams can be exhausting to the elderly
   c. False; radiography exams must be scheduled at the convenience of the radiology department
   d. False; elderly patients should be scheduled early when they are the strongest, especially if they have been held NPO

4. a. The underlined word or phrase is accurate as written
   b. False; trauma cases should be scheduled first
   c. False; it is important that the GI system be as empty as possible; scheduling these cases last ensures the GI system will be totally empty
   d. True; NPO all night is sufficient time; in addition, patients are extremely hungry and may be weak if the exam is postponed

5. a. The underlined word or phrase is accurate as written
   b. False; patients with diabetes should be scheduled first because of their need for insulin
   c. False; patients with diabetes may experience hyperglycemia if they have taken their insulin but have not eaten
   d. True; the need for insulin is great, and the diabetic patient needs the extra sugar from the insulin to be alert and cooperative

6. a. The underlined word or phrase is accurate as written
   b. False; barium will interfere with most endoscopic procedures
   c. True; barium is an excellent contrast medium
   d. False; barium may harden and damage the fiber optics

For the following questions, choose the single best answer.

7. Torts:
   a. Are violations of civil law
   b. Are considered part of personal injury law
   c. Provide for compensation for injury
   d. All of the above

8. Which of the following may be considered an example of battery?
   a. Touching the patient without consent
   b. Threatening the patient
   c. Radiographing the wrong patient
   d. All of the above

9. Assault means:
   a. Threatening the patient or causing the patient to be apprehensive
   b. Striking the patient
   c. Touching the patient without consent
   d. Performing radiography against the patient's will

10. Which of the following is not an example of invasion of privacy?
   a. Violation of confidentiality, such as discussing the patient's case in public
   b. Unjustified restraint of patient
   c. Improperly exposing the patient's body
   d. Improperly touching the patient's body

11. Unintentional misconduct is also called:
   a. Negligence
   b. An accident
   c. Libel
   d. Slander

12. The concept of the reasonably prudent person is interpreted as:
   a. How a reasonable jury member would perform the act
   b. How a professional with similar education, training, and experience would perform the act
   c. How a prudent attorney would interpret the act
   d. How a reasonable and prudent judge will rule on the act

13. *Respondeat superior* means:
   a. "The thing speaks for itself"
   b. A radiographer has no need to carry malpractice insurance
   c. The reasonable and prudent person should make the decision
   d. "Let the master answer"

14. Gross negligence is:
   a. A case that includes the injured person as a contributing party to the injury
   b. Loss of life or limb
   c. An act that shows reckless disregard for life or limb
   d. Found in criminal cases only

15. Which of the following conditions must be met to prove malpractice?
   a. The injury actually occurred and is a result of negligence
   b. The standard of care was violated
   c. The injury was caused by the person being sued
   d. All of the above

16. A case involving obvious negligence would be defined by the doctrine of:
   a. *Respondeat superior*
   b. Slander
   c. Libel
   d. *Res ipsa loquitur*

17. Which of the following is (are) true concerning valid (informed) consent?
   1. Patient must be of legal age
   2. Patient must be given a brochure describing the procedure's risks in lay terms
   3. Consent must be offered voluntarily
   4. Patient must be mentally competent
   5. Patient must completely understand all aspects of the procedure
   a. 1, 3, 4
   b. All are true
   c. 1, 2, 3, 4
   d. 1, 2, 3, 5

18. Patient transfers from cart to x-ray table and back to cart should be performed:
   a. By the radiographer alone if the patient is ambulatory
   b. By two or more radiographers to ensure patient and radiographer safety
   c. By the radiographer alone if the department is short-staffed
   d. By the radiographer alone so as not to frighten the patient

19. A history on the patient should be taken by the radiographer:
   a. To assist the radiologist with interpretation of the radiographs
   b. To verify patient name and condition
   c. To assist the radiographer in understanding the patient's injury and range of motion
   d. All of the above

Read the following paragraph. Determine the accuracy of each underlined word or phrase. Then refer to questions **20-26** following the paragraph, and choose the one statement that best completes and corrects the corresponding underlined item.

The most obvious route of infection transmission is direct contact. (20) <u>Direct contact allows the infectious organism to move from the susceptible host directly to the infected person.</u> The other route of transmission is called (21) <u>*indirect contact.*</u> There are several routes of indirect contact. (22) <u>Fomiteborne transmission involves an animal that contains and transmits an infectious organism to a human.</u> (23) <u>Vectors may be animals such as rabid dogs and bats.</u> (24) <u>Common vehicle transmission is the spreading of infection in crowded forms of public transportation such as jet aircrafts, subways, and trains.</u> (25) <u>Airborne transmission of infection may occur as a result of contact with bird droppings, acid rain, air pollution, etc.</u> In addition, (26) <u>droplets such as those resulting from coughs or sneezes also spread infections.</u>

20. a. The underlined word or phrase is accurate as written
   b. False; infectious organisms do not move easily
   c. False; the organism moves from the infected person to the susceptible host
   d. False; this type of transmission is called *indirect contact*

21. a. The underlined word or phrase is accurate as written
   b. False; the other route is called *direct contact*
   c. Droplet transmission
   d. Infectious transmission

22. a. The underlined word or phrase is accurate as written
   b. False; vectorborne transmission involves an animal that develops an infectious disease and transmits it to humans
   c. False; a fomite is another term for an infected person
   d. False; a bacterium is an animal that contains an infectious organism and that transmits the infection to a human

23. a. The underlined word or phrase is accurate as written
   b. False; vectors are only microscopic
   c. False; vectors live only on the scalp of humans
   d. False; vectors are objects containing pathogenic organisms

24. a. The underlined word or phrase is accurate as written
   b. False; actually very little transmission of infections occurs in crowded places
   c. False; common vehicle transmission involves contaminated items (e.g., food, water, equipment)
   d. False; a human cannot become infected just by touching an object

25. a. The underlined word or phrase is accurate as written
   b. False; none are part of this category
   c. False; airborne infections are contracted only on long airplane trips
   d. False; only acid rain has been shown to transmit infection

26. a. The underlined word or phrase is accurate as written
   b. False; no scientific evidence exists to support this concept
   c. Partially false; infections can only be spread in this manner during cold and flu season
   d. False; such infection can be spread only if the exposed person has low resistance to droplet infections

Read the following paragraph. Determine the accuracy of each underlined word or phrase. Then refer to questions **27-34** following the paragraph, and choose the one statement that best corrects and completes the corresponding underlined item.

Standard precautions (27) comprise a system that emphasizes the placement of barriers between the health care worker and the patient. This system assumes that (28) all patients are infected with the human immunodeficiency virus (HIV) and that most body fluids are sources of infection. Because the system of standard precautions emphasizes barriers, (29) gloves are the most effective method used to prevent the spread of infection. Given that barium enemas increase the possibility of contact between body substances and clothing, (30) disposable gowns or surgical scrubs should be worn by the radiographer in these cases. Because blood needs to enter the body to cause infection, (31) there is no need to wear eye protection for any radiologic procedures. In the interest of safety, (32) needles should be carefully recapped following injections for intravenous pyelograms (IVPs) so that no one else is stuck by the needle. (33) Any area that is touched by body fluids must be washed completely. Finally, (34) hands should be washed at least five times during each shift to help stop the spread of infections.

27. a. The underlined word or phrase is accurate as written
   b. False; in the interest of compassionate patient care, barriers should not come between patient and health care worker
   c. False; barriers have been shown to be quite ineffective
   d. False; standard precautions do not comprise a system; they are the law

28. a. The underlined word or phrase is accurate as written
   b. False; this system assumes that all patients younger than 50 years of age are infected with HIV
   c. False; standard precautions apply only to patients with HIV and hepatitis
   d. False; the system of standard precautions assumes that all patients are infectious, regardless of diagnosis

29. a. The underlined word or phrase is accurate as written
   b. False; gloves are permeable
   c. False; handwashing is the most effective method
   d. False; as with radiation, the most effective method is distance

30. a. The underlined word or phrase is accurate as written
   b. False; the use of disposable gowns or surgical scrubs is against the dress code
   c. False; the use of disposable gowns or surgical scrubs is too expensive
   d. False; there is little chance of disease transmission during barium enemas because most patients are not infected

31. a. The underlined word or phrase is accurate as written
   b. False; any radiologic procedure (e.g., angiography) that may involve blood splashing requires eye protection
   c. False; eye protection should be worn for all exams requiring venous injection
   d. False; eye protection should be worn for all radiologic exams

32. a. The underlined word or phrase is accurate as written
   b. False; needles should be recapped after all injections
   c. False; all sharps should be disposed of in appropriate containers and never recapped
   d. False; after injection for an IVP, the needle should be kept nearby in the event of a contrast medium reaction

33. a. The underlined word or phrase is accurate as written
   b. False; the radiographer does not have time to perform housekeeping duties
   c. False; not all body fluids are infectious
   d. False; this is an expensive process and it is not justified by scientific research

34. a. The underlined word or phrase is accurate as written
   b. False; hands should be washed after contact with each patient and before touching equipment and other patients
   c. False; the CDC determined that handwashing has little effect on the spread of infection
   d. False; handwashing should be done only at the start and end of the shift

For the following questions, choose the single best answer.

35. The process of eliminating as many organisms as possible by the use of water and chemical disinfectants is called:
a. Surgical asepsis
b. Sterilization
c. Medical asepsis
d. Boiling

36. The process of eliminating all organisms from the environment by gas sterilization, use of germicides, or use of dry heat is called:
a. Surgical asepsis
b. Sterilization
c. Medical asepsis
d. Autoclaving

37. When putting on gloves for a procedure, which of the following should take place first?
a. Carefully open glove package, and avoid touching outside of gloves
b. Wash hands
c. Place glove package in center of sterile field in preparation for the procedure
d. Put on one glove immediately so that one hand is protected and the other is free

38. Once gowned and gloved for a procedure, hands may *not* be placed:
a. Anywhere on the body because the gown and gloves are sterile
b. Anywhere on the front or sides of the gown
c. Anywhere on the table containing the sterile field
d. Under the arms or on the sides or back of the gown

39. A radiographer who is assisting with a sterile procedure but is not gloved and gowned:
a. Should never step between the physician and the sterile field
b. Should carefully place all utensils needed in the center of the sterile field by dropping them from above out of their packages
c. Should not come in contact with the sterile field under any circumstances
d. All of the above

40. What route of transmission involves touching a susceptible person with a contaminated object (e.g., a radiographic cassette)?
a. Droplet transmission
b. Indirect contact
c. Direct contact
d. Airborne transmission

41. Which of the following transmission-based precautions also require the use of standard precautions?
a. Airborne precautions
b. Droplet precautions
c. Contact precautions
d. All of the above

42. Which of the following rules must always be followed regardless of the route of transmission of infection?
a. Gloves must be worn
b. Gowns must be worn
c. Patient must not have any direct contact with the health care worker
d. Handwashing must be performed

Use the list that follows to answer questions **43-50**. Items may be used more than once.

A. Strict isolation
B. Respiratory isolation
C. Enteric isolation
D. Body substance precautions
E. Reverse isolation

43. Does not require the use of gloves

44. All equipment and personnel must be carefully covered

45. Used to totally protect the health care worker from every method of transmission possible in the work setting

46. Used if there is any chance of coming in contact primarily with products of GI system of infected person

47. Gowns and gloves not required

48. Masks not required; needlestick injuries must be avoided

49. Used to protect the worker from airborne droplets

50. Used with patients who are not infectious

For the following questions, choose the single best answer.

51. Assessment of changing patient conditions includes observing for:
a. Skin that becomes cool and diaphoretic
b. Patient expressions of discomfort or dizziness
c. Lips or nail beds that become cyanotic
d. All of the above indicate changing patient conditions

52. The normal adult body temperature taken orally is:
a. 98.6° C
b. 98° to 99° C
c. 99.6° F
d. 98° to 99° F

53. Which of the following are true concerning the pulse?
a. All of these are true
b. Normally taken at the radial artery
c. Normal range of values is 60 to 72 beats per minute
d. May be counted at the carotid artery

54. Normal respiration is:
a. 30 breaths per minute
b. 12 to 16 breaths per minute
c. 10 to 12 breaths per minute
d. 60 to 72 breaths per minute

55. A sphygmomanometer is used to:
a. Hear the heartbeat
b. Hear the blood pressure
c. Measure blood pressure
d. Measure body temperature

56. A blood pressure of 120/80 mm Hg reveals that:
a. The pressure is 120 mm Hg when the heart is at rest
b. The diastolic pressure is 120 mm Hg
c. The systolic pressure is 80 mm Hg
d. The pressure is 80 mm Hg when the heart is at rest

57. When administering oxygen the usual rate is:
a. 3 to 5 lb per minute
b. 3 to 5 L per hour
c. 3 to 5 L per minute
d. 5 to 7 L per minute

58. A mechanical method used to clear the patient's airway is called:
a. The Heimlich maneuver
b. CPR
c. Suctioning
d. NG tube insertion

59. The device that contains all the instruments and medications necessary for dealing with cardiac or respiratory arrest is called the:
a. Crash cart
b. Tackle box
c. IVP cabinet
d. Code blue cabinet

Use the list that follows to answer questions **60-65**. Items may be used more than once.

A. Anaphylaxis
B. Cardiogenic shock
C. Hypovolemic shock
D. Septic shock
E. Neurogenic shock

60. Caused by loss of a large amount of blood or plasma

61. Causes blood to pool in peripheral vessels

62. Allergic reaction to foreign proteins

63. Caused by infection that results in extremely low blood pressure

64. Occurs secondary to heart failure or interference with heart function

65. May occur after injection of iodinated contrast agent

For each of the following questions, choose the single best answer.

66. Which of the following is a symptom of shock?
a. Accelerated pulse
b. Cool, clammy, pale skin
c. Systolic pressure less than 30 mm Hg
d. All of the above

67. Which of the following should the radiographer perform first when a patient is suspected of going into shock?
a. Call for assistance
b. Place patient in Trendelenburg position
c. Take patient's blood pressure to confirm shock status
d. Administer oxygen

68. Which of the following are true when radiographing trauma patients?
1. Work quickly and efficiently
2. Patient may be left alone if unconscious
3. Spinal injury may be ruled out if patient is not on spine board or wearing a cervical collar
4. Observe for changes in wound dressing while performing radiography
5. Document, in writing, changes in patient condition
a. 1, 3, 4
b. 1, 2, 3
c. 1, 4, 5
d. All are true

Use the list that follows to answer questions **69-73**. Items may be used more than once.

- **A.** Urinary catheter
- **B.** Chest tube
- **C.** Ventilator
- **D.** Nasogastric tube
- **E.** Venous catheter

69. Used to feed patient or conduct gastric suction

70. Used to administer nutrition or long-term chemotherapy

71. Site of most nosocomial infections

72. Helps remove fluid or air from pleural space

73. Mechanical respirator

For the following questions, choose the single best answer.

74. The most frequently performed exam using a contrast medium is a(n):
a. Small bowel study
b. IVP
c. Barium enema
d. Chest x-ray study

75. Which of the following are true concerning positive contrast media?
1. Air is the most commonly used
2. Aqueous iodine compounds may be used if perforations are suspected
3. Barium should be mixed with cold water for retrograde administration
4. Nonionic contrast media are ideal for injection because they do not contain iodine, reducing the risk of reactions
5. Barium is an inert substance
6. Aqueous iodine compounds may cause serious dehydration
7. Barium is a surgical contaminant
a. 2, 5, 6, 7
b. All are true
c. 1, 2, 3, 4, 7
d. 1, 2, 4, 5, 6, 7

76. Which of the following are legitimate contraindications to the use of iodinated contrast media?
a. Allergy to seafood
b. Known sensitivity to iodine
c. Previous sensitivity to contrast agents
d. b and c

77. Reaction at the site of injection of iodinated contrast media may be caused by:
a. b and d
b. Extravasation of contrast agent
c. Anaphylaxis
d. Phlebitis

78. Which of the following is *not* a symptom of a contrast agent reaction?
a. Hoarseness
b. Sneezing
c. Urticaria
d. All are symptoms

79. Following injection of iodinated contrast media, the radiographer should:
a. b and d
b. Remain with the patient
c. Tell the patient about his or her previous weekend as a means of allaying anxiety about the procedure
d. Have a conversation with the patient, listening for signs of laryngeal swelling

80. At the first indication of a contrast agent reaction, the radiographer should:
a. Immediately shout for help
b. Stop the exam and obtain help so as not to alarm the patient
c. Continue with exam because most reactions turn out to be minor
d. Call a code blue

81. Hypodermic needles are described by their gauge, which is a:
a. List of the uses of the needle
b. Measure of the length of the needle
c. Measure of the diameter of the needle
d. Measure of the diameter of the needle opening; the larger the gauge, the smaller the diameter

82. Air must not be injected when performing venipuncture because:
a. An air embolus will form that may be fatal to the patient
b. Most exams requiring injection are not air contrast studies
c. It will interfere with the iodine
d. It will prevent the iodine from visualizing

83. A smaller, easier to handle injection set that includes plastic projections on both sides of the needle and may be used for venipuncture is called a:
a. Venous catheter
b. Butterfly
c. Hypodermic needle
d. Single-injection needle

84. A venous catheter:
a. Consists of a long plastic tube that is inserted into the artery during angiography
b. Is more flexible and easier to use than a needle or butterfly
c. Is a combination unit with a needle inside a flexible plastic catheter; both the needle and the catheter are inserted into the vein, after which the needle is withdrawn
d. b and c

85. Place the following steps for performing venipuncture in the proper order.
1. Secure tourniquet in place
2. Thoroughly cleanse the skin
3. Wash hands
4. Select vein
5. Put on gloves
6. Perform puncture
7. Cover wound and compress site
8. Inject contrast agent
9. Check wound for swelling
10. Observe blood return
a. 5, 4, 1, 6, 8, 7
b. 3, 1, 4, 5, 2, 6, 10, 8, 7, 9
c. 3, 5, 1, 4, 2, 6, 10, 8, 7, 9
d. 4, 1, 3, 5, 2, 6, 8, 9, 10, 7

86. Venipuncture:
a. May be performed only where allowed by state law
b. May be performed by a nurse only
c. May be performed by a radiology supervisor only
d. a and c

87. A contrast medium overdose:
a. Cannot occur because it is not a drug
b. May occur in infants
c. May occur if contrast material was injected during the week before the exam
d. May occur in infants or adults with renal, cardiac, or hepatic failure

88. Barium and iodine are excellent contrast media because:
a. They are inert substances
b. Both are high atomic number elements, resulting in low attenuation of x-ray photons
c. Both are high atomic number elements, resulting in high attenuation of x-ray photons
d. Both are negative contrast media (the most commonly used)

89. When performing patient care after the injection of an iodinated contrast medium, the radiographer must make full use of which senses?
a. Vision
b. Hearing
c. Touch
d. All of the above

Use the list that follows to answer questions **90-100**. Items may be used more than once.

A. Mild to moderate reaction to contrast agent
B. Severe reaction to contrast agent
C. Not considered a reaction to contrast agent

90. Intermittent sneezing

91. Vomiting

92. Constipation

93. Dyspnea

94. Sensation of heat

95. Cardiac arrest

96. Loss of consciousness

97. Nausea

98. Disorientation

99. Hoarseness

100. Convulsions

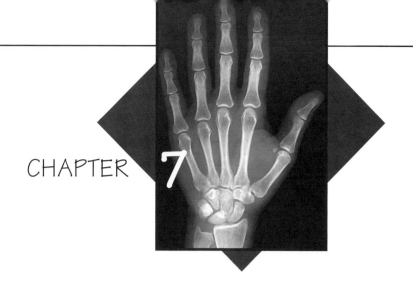

CHAPTER 7

Review Activities
and Challenge Tests

NOTE TO READER

It is very important to read the following paragraphs before you begin to work through this chapter.

The review activities and challenge tests in this chapter constitute a system of self-assessment. Simply answering hundreds or even thousands of multiple-choice questions will not help you assess what you know or do not know regarding this material. However, interacting with the information and recalling it in different formats will help you reach your goal of mastering the material. In this way, you will be more fully prepared to take the certification exam.

The first two challenge tests are not written in Registry exam format and are not meant to be representative of the actual ARRT exam. Rather, these first two tests will push your critical thinking and mental abilities to the limit and will help you assess how much you really know in each of the subject areas. This will be of great value when you finally take the certification exam. If you were in training to run a marathon, you would practice by regularly pushing your body to its limits. The race itself would then not seem so grueling.

Special Note: It is important to wait until you are finished with a test to correct it. When you do correct a test, be sure to read the rationales for the answers in the back of the book. Understand why the correct answer is the one best answer. Review the subject matter again by going to the appropriate chapter in this book.

Challenge Test #1

Challenge Test #1 includes different types of activities, not just multiple-choice questions and answers. This variety of

activities will help you better assess your areas of strength and weakness in each of the five major subject areas. These activities do not cover every detail of each subject area. However, they do cover major points and key items in which you need to be proficient, and to round out your review, Challenge Test #2 covers other aspects of the subject areas.

After you complete Challenge Test #1, correct your test using the answer key in the back of the book. Then, fill in the scoring table that follows the test to identify areas in which you are strong and those in which you may need additional review.

Challenge Test #2

Next, take Challenge Test #2. It will assess your knowledge in even greater depth. This test uses story problems and multilayered multiple-choice questions to help you interact more closely with the information. After you are done, correct your test and calculate your score in the table at the end of the test.

Challenge Test #3

For practice taking traditional multiple-choice questions, use Challenge Test #3, which is written in a format similar to the ARRT exam. After you are done, correct your test and calculate your score in the table at the end of the test.

Book Companion CD-ROM

After you complete your review work and take the challenge tests, you are ready to move on to the CD-ROM provided with this book. There you will find hundreds of traditional, multiple-choice questions presented randomly in 200-question blocks, sectioned to simulate the actual ARRT exam. This will ultimately be your best practice and preparation. You will be answering questions on a computer at random, just as you will when you take the ARRT exam.

There are enough questions to give you many different exams with countless combinations of questions, always according to ARRT test specifications. By drilling yourself using this test bank, you will be as prepared as possible for test day.

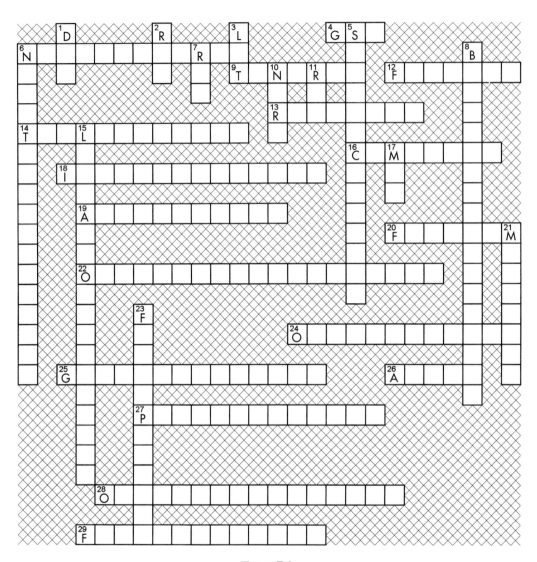

Figure 7-1

Challenge Test #1
Self-Assessment Activities and Questions

Topic: Radiation Protection (30 Crossword Entries, Figure 7-1)

Note: Answers with more than one word do *not* contain spaces.

Across

4. Average gonadal dose to the childbearing population
6. Angle from the patient where there is the least amount of scatter
9. Lowest dose recorded by a film badge
12. Quality of radiation is measured by this part of a film badge
13. Unit of radiation exposure in air
14. Minimum source-to-skin distance for portable radiography and fluoroscopy
16. Photon-tissue interaction that is the source of scatter radiation
18. Effect on cell in which the radiation strikes the cytoplasm, creating free radicals and hydrogen peroxide
19. Changes in the x-ray beam as it traverses an object
20. Annual effective absorbed dose equivalent limit for radiographers
22. Thickness preferred for lead aprons, thyroid shields, protective curtains, and Bucky slot shields
24. Amount of radiation leakage allowed per hour at a distance of 1 m from the tube housing
25. Radiation effects that manifest themselves in offspring of those exposed
26. Concept that encourages radiation workers to keep the dose as low as reasonably achievable
27. Photon-tissue interaction that results in the photon being completely absorbed; responsible for producing contrast on the radiograph
28. Intensity of the scattered beam compared with the primary beam at a 90-degree angle from the patient at a distance of 1 m
29. Minimum source-to-tabletop distance for fixed fluoroscopes

Down

1. Part of the cell that is struck by radiation, resulting in direct effect
2. Unit of dose equivalency; a product of rads times a quality factor
3. Amount of radiation deposited per unit length of tissue irradiated
5. Effects of exposure to ionizing radiation that are manifested in the individual being exposed
6. Gonadal shielding of males may reduce exposure by this percentage
7. Unit of absorbed dose
8. Law described by these two scientists that states cells are most sensitive to radiation when they are immature, undifferentiated, and rapidly dividing
10. Organization that publishes scientific research and recommendations regarding radiation exposure limits
11. The ability of radiation to produce biologic damage, which varies with LET
15. Dose-response relationship stating there is no level of radiation that may be considered completely safe and that the degree of response is directly proportional to the amount of radiation received
17. Average dose to active bone marrow
21. Annual effective absorbed dose equivalent for the general public is 500 of this unit
23. Percentage of reduction to female gonads when using gonadal shielding

```
O N E M I L L I S E C O N D J O P W I F I B J A H M
U A U T O T R A N S F O R M E R N H M V O Y I Y O E
T L R H N C H A R A C T E R I S T I C N E D W J L X
P S E E I I A R L P U C G N I S U C O F F E M F P T
U A O R Z R N T E I N P U T P H O S P H O R V M U R
T N I M A C O V H E N Z I C A T O M I C N U M B E R
P O D I T U D T W O P E R C E N T O F S I D R C R V
H D Y O I I E D Y L D H A C I W I V K B B K T K L R
O E R N O T B U L J C E A R R E M G V Y I I U B V E
S C T I N J E X J F U Q G S I Q J L V F F Y B Z C P
P O V C C G Y B G P N L X K E T U A N I Y K E P U R
H O R E H C K R W F G B A C G I Y I E V J D R H P O
O L C M A L T E R N A T I N G C U R R E N T A O N D
R I H I M S K M T K A E K F U X Z U D U B L T T V U
U N P S B D H S M W V S Y C N E U Q E R F W I O P C
F G S S E L X S K D O P Y F C Z Y S M V A H N C B I
W C U I R W O T K K X D T U V U I D A V L M G A J B
H U K O M I V R R V R T K I V Q E L E N L R C T R I
L R M N J X F A E V O N U I M V U L L V I D H H E L
V V H I E G W H B P K H T B L E E I C V N Y A O B I
L E S V H J C L O F W Y R N L N S C F S G H R D C T
O D X A M K G U R U V C Y A G V E M W U L X T E M Y
R I P S K I U N A C R S Y T O V M G A M O R B M J T
H P K R O W M G M F F E H D H Y I O U S A J Y N L D
V U I S T E P U P T R A N S F O R M E R D I U K D J
```

Figure 7-2

Topic: Equipment Operation and Maintenance (Questions 31-60)

Use the blanks to fill in the answers to the following questions. Then find your answers in the word search (Figure 7-2).

31. Current produced by generators and required for operation of transformers _____

32. Site of bremsstrahlung radiation production; the positive electrode in the x-ray tube _____

33. Chart used to determine the safety of a series of exposures, taking into account heat units and the number of exposures to be made _____

34. Represented by the letter Z; indicates the number of protons in the atomic nucleus _____

35. Variable transformer _____

36. Process that produces x rays as a result of the braking action between the atomic nucleus and an incident electron _____

37. Site of thermionic emission; the negative electrode in the x-ray tube _____

38. Type of x rays produced when energy is released by electrons falling from an outer shell to an inner shell _____

39. Path electrons take, usually over copper wire
_____

40. Type of x-ray generator that uses the maximum heat storage capacity of the x-ray tube at each mA station, dropping the mA each fraction of a second during the exposure _____

41. Surrounds the filaments on three sides; carries a negative charge during the exposure _____

42. For quality control testing, accuracy of kVp must be plus or minus this amount _____

43. Number of sine waves passing a certain point per unit time _____

44. Measure of the quality of the x-ray beam; the amount of absorbing material that reduces the intensity of the x-ray beam by half _____

45. Most of the energy produced at the anode is in this form _____

46. The portion of the image intensifier that converts x-ray energy to light energy _____

47. Automatic exposure control most commonly used; composed of a wafer-thin device placed between the patient and the film _____

48. Equation multiplied by a constant; used to calculate heat units _____

49. Tested to verify that adjacent mA stations are within 10% of one another _____

50. Shortest exposure time available with electronic timers _____

51. The portion of the image intensifier that converts electron energy to light energy _____

52. The portion of the image intensifier that converts light energy to electron energy _____

53. Changes alternating current to direct current just before passing through the x-ray tube _____

54. Tested to verify successive exposures, indicating that variation in radiation intensity is no more than 5% _____

55. Operates on principle of mutual induction, increases voltage to kilovoltage levels _____

56. Process that produces electron cloud surrounding the filament _____

57. Type of current used in x-ray production wherein the current never falls to zero _____

58. Chart used to determine the safety of a single exposure _____

59. Required accuracy of a collimator _____

60. Distance from one crest of a sine wave to the next crest _____

Topic: Image Production and Evaluation (Questions 61-110)

Matching: Match the following items with their answers (A-XX, see p. 171). Each answer is only used once.

_____ **61.** Logarithm of opacity

_____ **62.** Primary controlling factor of density

_____ **63.** Reciprocity law

_____ **64.** kVp

_____ **65.** 15% rule

_____ **66.** Increased kVp

_____ **67.** Inverse square law

_____ **68.** Anode heel effect

_____ **69.** Reduces number of soft, long wavelengths reaching the patient

_____ **70.** Photoelectric effect

_____ **71.** Contrast produced by the anatomy and pathology of the body

_____ **72.** Recorded detail

_____ **73.** Causes magnification of the image

_____ **74.** Algae in wash water

_____ **75.** Distortion causing image to appear longer than it really is

_____ **76.** Foreshortening

_____ **77.** Serve as centers of development in the film emulsion's silver halide crystals

_____ **78.** Reasons blue tint is added to film's base

_____ **79.** Graphs used to illustrate film's response to exposure

_____ **80.** Portion of H & D curve that illustrates base plus fog

_____ **81.** Portion of H & D curve that illustrates usable densities

_____ **82.** Temperature range in which film should be stored

_____ **83.** Caused by static electricity discharge on a film

_____ **84.** Caused by bending film over the fingernail

_____ **85.** Contained in the active layer of intensifying screens

_____ **86.** High-speed film-screen system

_____ **87.** Slow-speed film-screen system

_____ **88.** Unit of measurement of resolution

_____ **89.** Relative speed numbers

_____ **90.** Spectral matching

_____ **91.** Used to evaluate film-screen contact

_____ **92.** Height of lead strips divided by the space between the lead strips

_____ **93.** Absorbs the product of Compton's interaction

_____ **94.** Number of lead strips per centimeter

_____ **95.** Grid type with lead strips parallel to one another

_____ **96.** Grid type with lead strips angled to coincide with divergence of the x-ray beam

_____ **97.** Decreased density on film resulting from absorption of image-forming rays by the grid

_____ **98.** Converts exposed silver halide crystals to black metallic silver

_____ **99.** Clears and removes unexposed silver halide crystals from the film

_____ **100.** Agitates chemistry and moves film in the processor

_____ **101.** Adds fresh developer and fixer as film is fed into processor

_____ **102.** Agitates solution, stabilizes temperatures, filters developer solution

_____ **103.** 90 to 102 degrees

_____ **104.** Straight-line scratches on the film running in direction of film travel

_____ **105.** Produces odor of ammonia in the processor

_____ **106.** May produce films with a greasy appearance

_____ **107.** May produce films with a milky appearance

_____ **108.** Should be cleaned daily

_____ **109.** Should be cleaned weekly

_____ **110.** Should be cleaned monthly

A. mAs = mAs
B. Crinkle or half-moon artifact
C. Subject contrast
D. Density
E. Filtration
F. Produces differential absorption of the x-ray beam by the body
G. Body or slope
H. Produces x-ray beam with shorter wavelengths
I. Static artifact
J. $\dfrac{\text{Old mAs}}{\text{New mAs}} = \dfrac{\text{New distance squared}}{\text{Old distance squared}}$
K. Used to double or halve density using kVp
L. Intensity of x-ray beam varies along the longitudinal axis of the beam
M. Reduce glare, enhance contrast
N. 68 to 70 degrees
O. Sharpness, definition, image resolution
P. Toe
Q. H & D curves, characteristic curves, sensitometric curves
R. Primary controlling factor of contrast
S. Distortion causing image to appear shorter than it really is
T. Phosphors
U. Sensitivity specks
V. Increased OID
W. mAs
X. Elongation
Y. Line pairs per millimeter
Z. Crossover rollers

AA. Focused
BB. Produces images with high contrast, narrow latitude, and less recorded detail
CC. Grid frequency
DD. Linear
EE. Contamination of developer by fixer
FF. Wire mesh test
GG. Poor fixer replenishment
HH. Grid ratio
II. Wavelength of light emitted by screens is compatible with wavelengths to which the film is most sensitive
JJ. Grids
KK. Recirculation system
LL. Inadequate washing
MM. Cut-off
NN. Guide shoe scratches
OO. Usual range for developer temperature in a 90-second processor
PP. Allow for exposure calculations when moving from one speed of screens to another
QQ. Transport system
RR. Deep racks
SS. Replenishment system
TT. Developer
UU. Produces images with lower contrast, wider latitude, greater recorded detail
VV. Fixer
WW. Entire processor
XX. Dark flakes on processed film

Topic: Radiographic Procedures (Questions 111-170)

Using Figure 7-3, identify the radiographic anatomy of the urinary system:

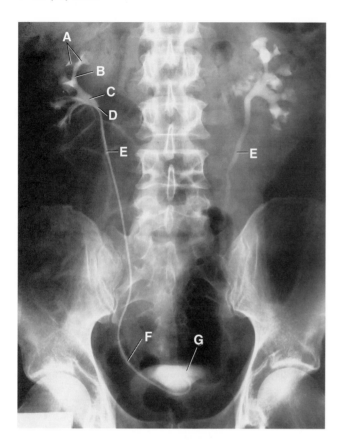

Figure 7-3 Retrograde pyelogram.

111. A is the _____.

112. B is the _____.

113. C is the _____.

Using Figure 7-4, identify the radiographic anatomy of the colon:

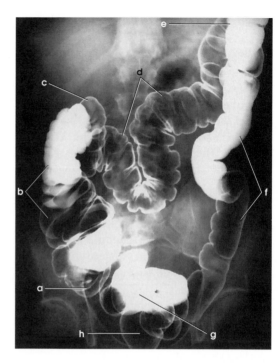

Figure 7-4 Anteroposterior projection, barium enema (double-contrast enema).

114. B is the _____.

115. C is the _____.

116. D is the _____.

117. F is the _____.

Using Figure 7-5, identify the radiographic anatomy visualized during an upper gastrointestinal series:

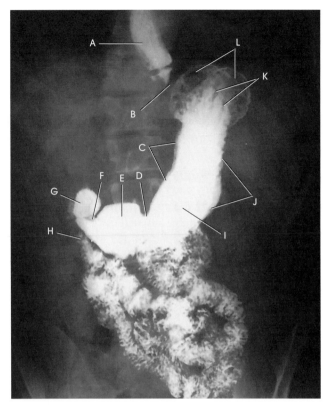

Figure 7-5 Posteroanterior projection of the stomach.

118. D is the _____.

119. E is the _____.

120. K is the _____.

121. L is the _____.

Using Figure 7-6, identify the anatomy of a lumbar vertebra:

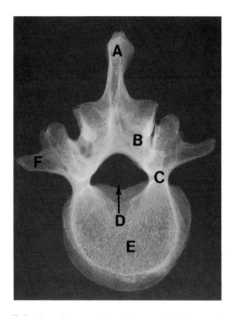

Figure 7-6 Lumbar vertebra (superoinferior projection).

122. A is the _____.

123. B is the _____.

124. C is the _____.

125. F is the _____.

Using Figure 7-7, identify the radiographic anatomy of the cervical spine:

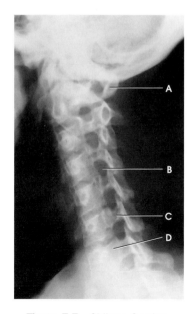

Figure 7-7 Oblique C-spine.

126. B is the _____.

127. C is the _____.

Using Figure 7-8, identify the radiographic anatomy of the hip:

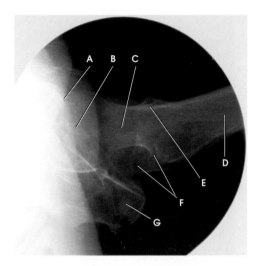

Figure 7-8   Lateral hip, inferosuperior projection.

128. E is the _____.

129. F is the _____.

130. G is the _____.

Using Figure 7-9, identify the radiographic anatomy of the knee:

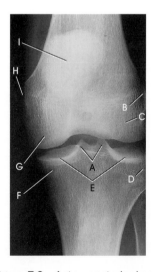

Figure 7-9   Anteroposterior knee.

131. B is the _____.

132. D is the _____.

133. E is the _____.

134. G is the _____.

Using Figure 7-10, identify the radiographic anatomy of the hand:

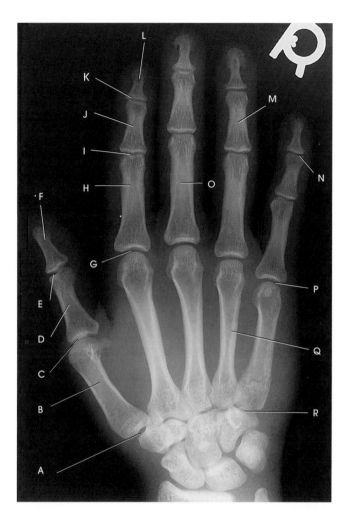

Figure 7-10   Posteroanterior radiograph of right hand.

135. A is the _____.

136. G is the _____.

137. I is the _____.

138. K is the _____.

Using Figure 7-11, identify the radiographic anatomy of the wrist:

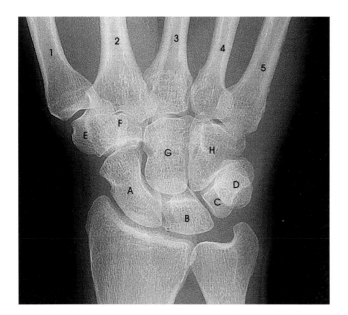

Figure 7-11 Posteroanterior wrist.

Using Figure 7-12, identify the radiographic anatomy of the shoulder:

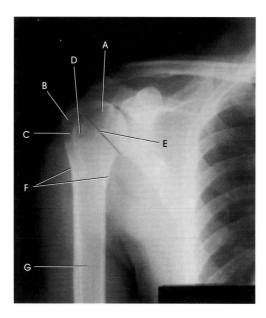

Figure 7-12 Anteroposterior shoulder in external rotation.

139. A is the _____.

140. B is the _____.

141. C is the _____.

142. D is the _____.

143. E is the _____.

144. F is the _____.

145. G is the _____.

146. H is the _____.

147. B is the _____.

148. D is the _____.

149. E is the _____.

150. F is the _____.

Using Figure 7-13, identify the radiographic anatomy of the foot:

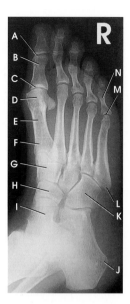

Figure 7-13 Oblique right foot.

Using Figure 7-14, identify the radiographic anatomy of the elbow:

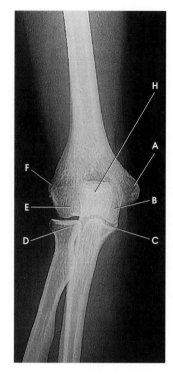

Figure 7-14 Anteroposterior elbow.

151. G is the _____.

152. H is the _____.

153. I is the _____.

154. J is the _____.

155. K is the _____.

156. M is the _____.

157. A is the _____.

158. D is the _____.

159. E is the _____.

160. H is the _____.

Using Figure 7-15, identify the radiographic anatomy of the skull:

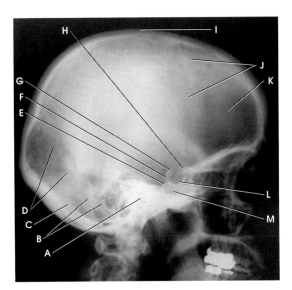

Figure 7-15 Lateral projection of skull.

Using Figure 7-16, identify the radiographic anatomy of the facial bones:

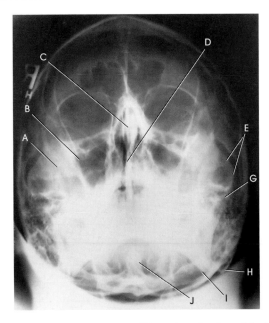

Figure 7-16 Parietoacanthial (Waters) projection of facial bones.

161. C is the _____.

162. F is the _____.

163. H is the _____.

164. M is the _____.

165. B is the _____.

166. C is the _____.

167. D is the _____.

168. E is the _____.

169. I is the _____.

170. J is the _____.

Topic: Patient Care (Questions 171-200, Figure 7-17)

Note: Answers with more than one word do *not* contain spaces.

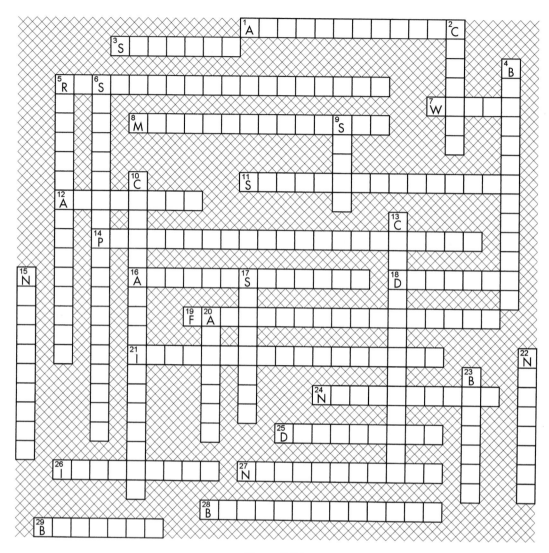

Figure 7-17

Across

1. Type of contrast agent reaction characterized by flushing, hives, or nausea
3. Type of technique used when handling supplies used in interventional procedures
5. Legal concept meaning the employer is responsible for the actions of the employee
7. Absorbed by barium as it moves through the alimentary canal
8. Use of water and chemical disinfectants to eliminate as many microorganisms as possible
11. Complete removal of all organisms
12. Type of transmission-based precaution requiring respiratory protection
14. Must precede all initiation of patient care
16. Contrast agent used when barium is contraindicated
18. Type of transmission-based precaution used when infection could be spread by droplets
19. Unjustified restraint of a patient
21. Violation of confidentiality
24. Hospital-acquired infection
25. Blood pressure of the heart at rest
26. Contrast agents containing organic iodine compounds
27. Tube inserted into patient for feeding or to suction the stomach
28. Measured using a sphygmomanometer
29. The bag attached to a urinary catheter must not be placed above this level to prevent retrograde flow

Down

2. Type of transmission-based precaution requiring masks, gloves, and gowns
4. Contrast medium administered to patient in the form of an inert salt
5. Legal concept meaning "the thing speaks for itself"
6. Actions that make use of barriers to prevent the spread of infection
9. Medical emergency caused by failure of circulation in which blood pressure is inadequate to oxygenate tissues and remove byproducts of metabolism
10. Reasons why medical procedures may not be performed on a given patient
13. Type of contrast agent reaction characterized by hypotension, tachycardia, or cardiac arrest
15. Unintentional misconduct
17. Blood pressure that measures the pumping action of the heart
20. Imprudent conduct that causes patient to fear injury
22. Type of iodinated contrast media that have lower incidence of reactions
23. Unlawful touching of the patient, radiographing the wrong patient, radiographing the wrong part, performing radiography against the patient's will

Scoring

Traditionally you have probably focused on how many questions you miss on an exam. As you prepare for the certification exam, I am encouraging you to focus on how many you answer correctly. Use Table 7-1 to calculate the percentage of questions you answered correctly in each category and on the test as a whole. Remember, a score below 75% on any topic or on an entire test is an indication that more review is needed on that topic. Now, go back and concentrate on the items that were missed and figure out the reason why. Then, go on to Challenge Test #2.

TABLE 7-1	Calculating Your Score for Challenge Test #1	
Topic	**Percentage calculation**	**Your score**
Radiation protection	Number correct _____ times 100, ÷ 30 =	
Equipment operation and maintenance	Number correct _____ times 100, ÷ 30 =	
Image production and evaluation	Number correct _____ times 100, ÷ 50 =	
Radiographic procedures	Number correct _____ times 100, ÷ 60 =	
Patient care	Number correct _____ times 100, ÷ 30 =	
TOTAL	Number correct _____ times 100, ÷ 200 =	

Challenge Test #2
Higher-Level Questions Requiring Analysis and Critical Thinking

Note to Reader: The questions on this test are written to challenge your critical thinking skills and specific knowledge of the subject matter. *This is a difficult test; do not be surprised if you score lower than usual.* Use the results of this test to assess your strengths and weaknesses.

Read each question and the answer choices carefully. For some questions, more than one answer may be correct. However, you must choose the one best, most complete answer for each item. Do not look up any of the answers until you have completed the entire test. Correct the test using the answer key in the back of the book. Then use Table 7-2 to calculate the percentage of questions you answered correctly in each category and on the test as a whole. Your scores will let you see where you are strong and where you may need additional review. Refer to the appropriate chapter in this book for review of questions you miss.

Topic: Radiation Protection
(Questions 1-30)

Questions **1-14** are based on the following real-life drama at a major metropolitan medical center. Choose the answer that best completes the sentence.

Scenario

You have been chosen as the student representative for the advisory committee that is planning to establish a new radiology department at your place of employment. It is your task to assist in developing the radiation protection policies in the new department. Your conversation with the department head and the chief of radiology, Dr. Raydee Ologist, goes something like this:

"I think it is very important for each room to be constructed properly right from the start. First, we must consider several factors that determine selection of protective barriers: (1). As you both know, we need a primary protective barrier of (2). The secondary protective barrier must be installed to extend from the primary barrier to the (3)."

"Very good," says Dr. Ologist. "I'm glad you learned your structural requirements so well. It's time to move on to the equipment in the room. Can you help us out on this too?"

"I sure can!" you begin happily. "Let's talk about fluoroscopic facilities first." The department head and Dr. Ologist nod in agreement.

"As you know, each x-ray tube must have total filtration of at least (4). The fluoroscopic source-to-tabletop distance must be (5). The x-ray intensity during fluoroscopy may not exceed (6) at the tabletop. We must install two protective devices for Dr. Ologist and her colleagues. The Bucky slot cover and the protective curtain each must be at least (7)."

"Golly, these second-year students are sure on the ball. I'm glad we have them around!" Dr. Ologist says excitedly.

"You're right," says the department head. "I hope they can help us with personnel radiation protection policies also."

"I sure can," you begin. "I have a list here of some things we will need to consider."

"Go right ahead!" (Isn't it nice to see everyone working so well together?)

"We want to be sure we have the right lead aprons available. Different thicknesses of lead provide different levels of protection, but we must ensure that the minimum thickness available is (8). If the staff will combine the use of the lead apron with the inverse square law, their total dose will remain very, very low."

"Just a minute," interrupts Dr. Ologist. "I think you will need to refresh my memory of the inverse square law."

"Gladly," you begin. "My instructor taught me well! Let's say the exposure measured is 10 R per minute at a distance of 2 feet from the x-ray table. If the radiographer will step back to a distance of 4 feet, the new exposure measured will be only (9). It's really quite simple and shows how effective distance can be. Also, remember that the x-ray tube may put out some leakage radiation, which should (10)."

"Now, about mobile units," you continue. "The minimum distances are as follows: (11)."

"Finally, we need to review our personnel monitoring policies. Traditionally, we have used film badges. Among the advantages and disadvantages are (12). Also available are thermoluminescent dosimeters that the nuclear medicine technologists wear on their fingers but which can be worn as badges. Their advantages and disadvantages are (13). Of course, we could always issue everyone a pocket ionization chamber."

"Wait a minute," declared the department head. "Those are expensive; besides, a reading of 200 mR concerns me because (14)."

"Well, this has been a very productive committee meeting. I am happy to be able to help," you finish. "I'm sure we all agree that it is important to keep the dose to the patients and staff ALARA!"

1. a. Distance, occupancy, workload, use factor
   b. Fluoroscopy, radiography, computed tomography, tomography
   c. Inverse square law, lead thickness, total fluoroscopy time, number of patients
   d. Distance, occupancy (divided between controlled and uncontrolled area), workload (measure in mA minutes per week), use (amount of time beam is on and directed at a barrier)

2. a. ¹⁄₁₆-inch aluminum equivalent
b. 0.25-mm lead equivalent
c. ¹⁄₃₂-inch lead equivalent
d. ¹⁄₃₂-inch aluminum equivalent

3. a. Ceiling, ¹⁄₃₂-inch lead equivalent, with a ½-inch overlap
b. Ceiling, ¹⁄₃₂-inch aluminum equivalent, with a 1-inch overlap
c. Ceiling, ¹⁄₁₆-inch lead equivalent, with a ½-inch overlap
d. Ceiling, ¹⁄₁₆-inch aluminum equivalent, with a 2-inch overlap

4. a. 2.5-mm lead equivalent
b. 2.5-mm aluminum equivalent
c. 1.5-mm lead equivalent
d. 1.5-mm aluminum equivalent

5. a. No less than 5 inches
b. No less than 12 inches
c. No less than 12 inches, should be 15 inches
d. No less than 15 inches, should be 20 inches

6. a. 10 roentgens per minute
b. 10 rads per minute
c. 10 roentgens per hour of fluoroscopy
d. 10 rem per minute

7. a. 0.5-mm aluminum equivalent
b. 2.5-mm aluminum equivalent
c. 0.25-mm lead equivalent
d. 0.5-mm lead equivalent

8. a. 0.25-mm lead equivalent
b. 0.5-mm lead equivalent, but 0.25-mm lead equivalent preferred
c. 0.5-mm lead equivalent preferred
d. 1-mm lead equivalent preferred

9. a. 5 R per minute
b. 2 R per minute
c. 2.5 R per minute
d. 2.5 rem per minute

10. a. Not exceed 100 R per hour, 1 m from the housing
b. Not exceed 100 mR per hour, 1 m from the housing
c. Not exceed 100 mR per hour
d. Not exceed 100 R per hour

11. a. Radiography (minimum source-to-skin distance = 12 inches); fluoroscopy (minimum source-to-skin distance = not less than 12 inches, 15 inches preferred)
b. Radiography (minimum source-to-skin distance = 15 inches); fluoroscopy (minimum source-to-skin distance = not less than 15 inches)
c. Radiography (minimum source-to-skin distance = 12 inches); fluoroscopy (minimum source-to-skin distance = not less than 12 inches)
d. Radiography (minimum source-to-skin distance = 10 inches); fluoroscopy (minimum source-to-skin distance = not less than 10 inches, 15 inches preferred)

12. a. Advantages: accurate as low as 5 mrem; disadvantages: costly, sensitive to temperature extremes
b. Advantages: accurate as low as 10 mrem; disadvantages: may not be used longer than 1 month
c. Advantages: inexpensive, accurate as low as 10 mrem, simple to use; disadvantages: sensitive to temperature and humidity extremes, not accurate at extremely low doses
d. Advantages: inexpensive; disadvantages: none

13. a. Advantages: accurate as low as 5 mrem, dilithium crystals may be reused, may be worn up to 3 months; disadvantages: expensive
b. Advantages: accurate as low as 5 mrem, lithium fluoride chips may be reused, may be worn up to 3 months; disadvantages: expensive
c. Advantages: accurate as low as 1 mrem, lithium fluoride chips may be reused, may be worn up to 6 months; disadvantages: expensive
d. Advantages: accurate as low as 10 mrem, dilithium crystals may be reused, may be worn up to 3 months; disadvantages: expensive

14. a. It is the maximum dose
b. 200 mR is beyond the monthly absorbed dose equivalent limit
c. Work must stop at that reading while the unit is charged
d. Maximum reading is 200 mR; one does not know how much over that amount the dose is

For the following questions, choose the single best answer.

15. The amount of radiation deposited per unit length of tissue traversed by incoming photons is called:
a. Tissue exposure
b. Linear deposition of energy
c. Linear energy transfer
d. Absorbed dose equivalent limit

16. Cataractogenesis, life span shortening, embryologic effects, and carcinogenesis are examples of:
   a. Short-term somatic effects
   b. Genetic effects
   c. Acute radiation syndrome
   d. Long-term somatic effects

17. Compton's interaction:
   a. Produces contrast in the radiographic image
   b. Results in scattering of the incident photon
   c. May produce a fog on the radiograph
   d. More than one but not all of the above

18. Rem multiplied by a quality factor equals:
   a. Rads
   b. Roentgens
   c. Grays
   d. No such equation is used

19. Effective absorbed dose equivalent limit:
   a. Is the level of radiation that an organism can receive and probably sustain no appreciable damage
   b. Is a safe level of radiation that can be received with no effects
   c. Should be absorbed annually to maintain proper immunity to radiation
   d. Is 5000 mrem per year for the general public

20. Radiation with a high LET:
   a. Has low ionization
   b. Is highly ionizing
   c. Carries a low quality factor
   d. Equates with a low RBE

21. Radiation protection is based on which dose-response relationship?
   a. Linear-threshold
   b. Nonlinear-nonthreshold
   c. Linear-nonthreshold
   d. Nonlinear-threshold

22. Which of the following states that the radiosensitivity of cells is directly proportional to their reproductive activity and inversely proportional to their degree of differentiation?
   a. Inverse square law
   b. Law of Bergonié and Tribondeau
   c. Reciprocity law
   d. Ohm's law

23. Which of the following causes about 95% of the cellular response to radiation?
   a. Direct effect
   b. Law of Bergonié and Tribondeau
   c. Target theory
   d. Indirect effect

24. When radiation strikes DNA, which of the following will occur?
   a. Direct effect
   b. Law of Bergonié and Tribondeau
   c. Target theory
   d. Indirect effect

25. The amount of radiation that causes the number of genetic mutations in a population to double is called the:
   a. Threshold dose
   b. Doubling dose
   c. Mutagenic dose
   d. Genetic dose

26. The units of dose equivalency, activity, in-air exposure, and absorbed dose are (respectively):
   a. Roentgen, rad, rem, curie
   b. Rad, coulomb per kilogram, curie, becquerel
   c. Rem, curie, roentgen, rad
   d. Sievert, becquerel, gray, coulomb per kilogram

27. Medical x rays are an example of:
   a. Natural background radiation
   b. Artificial radiation
   c. Nonionizing radiation
   d. Ionizing, natural background radiation

28. The absorbed dose equivalent limit for the embryo-fetus is:
   a. 500 mrem during gestation
   b. 5 rem per year
   c. 0.5 rem per month
   d. 50 mrem per year

29. The photoelectric effect:
   a. Results in absorption of the incident photon
   b. Results in absorption of the incident electron
   c. Produces contrast fog on the radiographic image
   d. Is the same as brems radiation

30. The effective absorbed dose equivalent limit for radiographers is:
   a. 3 rem per quarter
   b. 500 mrem per year
   c. 5000 mrem per year
   d. 100 mrem per month

Topic: Equipment Operation and Maintenance (Questions 31-60)

31. Voltage ripple of 100% is characteristic of:
a. Single-phase power
b. Three-phase, six-pulse power
c. Three-phase, twelve-pulse power
d. High-frequency power

32. Which of the following is true regarding frequency and wavelength of electromagnetic radiation?
a. Frequency and wavelength are directly proportional
b. Frequency and wavelength are unrelated
c. Wavelength and frequency are inversely proportional to the square of the distance between wave crests
d. Wavelength and frequency are inversely proportional

33. The smallest particle of a compound that retains the characteristics of the compound is a(n)
a. Element
b. Atom
c. Molecule
d. Neutron

34. Which of the following does not belong in the definition of matter?
a. Travels at the speed of light
b. Has shape
c. Has form
d. Occupies space

35. A step-up transformer:
a. Has more turns in the primary coil than in the secondary coil
b. Has more turns in the secondary coil than in the primary coil
c. Steps down voltage
d. Steps up current

36. An ionization chamber circuit places:
a. A photomultiplier tube between the film and the patient
b. An ionization chamber beneath or behind the film
c. An ionization chamber between the patient and the x-ray tube
d. An ionization chamber between the film and the patient

37. Full-wave rectification uses:
a. A single semiconductor
b. Four silicone-based semiconductors
c. The x-ray tube as a semiconductor
d. Four silicon-based semiconductors

38. Which of the following is (are) false?
a. The octet rule states that no more than eight electrons may occupy the *K* shell at any time
b. Falling load generators are extremely efficient and should be used when breathing techniques are required, such as during radiography involving a lateral view of the thoracic spine and an oblique view of the sternum
c. The nucleus of an atom contains protons and electrons
d. All are false

39. A full-wave rectified, three-phase, twelve-pulse x-ray machine produces approximately _____% more average photon energy than a full-wave rectified, single-phase x-ray machine.
a. 35
b. 50
c. 41
d. 100

40. According to the anode heel effect, the intensity of radiation is greater at the _____ side of the x-ray tube.
a. Anode
b. Central x-ray
c. Neither side; the beam is of uniform intensity
d. Cathode

41. The amount of time needed for an AEC to terminate the exposure is called:
a. Exposure latitude
b. Minimum reaction time
c. Chamber response time
d. Electronic time

42. A tube rating chart is used to determine:
a. The safety of a single exposure
b. The safety of a series of exposures such as those performed in tomography
c. Patient dose per mAs
d. The number of exposures made on the anode

Use the list that follows to answer questions **43-48**. Items may be used more than once.

A. Characteristic radiation
B. Photoelectric effect
C. Pair production
D. Bremsstrahlung
E. Compton's interaction

43. Occurs when an incident electron interacts with the force field of an atomic nucleus

44. Occurs when an incident photon interacts with an outer-shell electron, producing a scatter photon and a recoil electron

45. Occurs when an incident electron dislodges a *K*-shell electron

46. Produces contrast in the radiographic image

47. Occurs when an incident photon interacts with an atomic nucleus above 1.02 MeV

48. Primary source of diagnostic x rays

Using Figure 7-18, answer questions **49-52**.

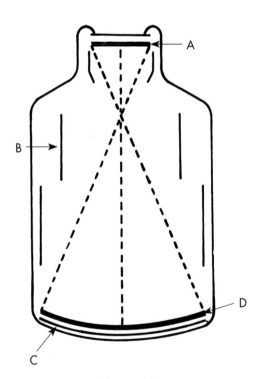

Figure 7-18

49. Electron beam is focused here

50. Electronic image is produced here

51. Visible image is distributed to viewing and/or recording media from here

52. X-ray energy is converted to visible light here

For the following questions, choose the single best answer.

53. A particular x-ray room is "shooting dark." The problem arises when changing from 200 to 300 mA using fixed kVp techniques at 0.16 seconds. Which of the following would lead to an accurate diagnosis of the problem?
a. Wire mesh test
b. Pinhole camera test
c. Use of a digital dosimeter to determine HVL
d. Use of digital dosimeter to determine exposure linearity

54. An outpatient radiographic room is used primarily for tabletop radiography of the extremities. On a particularly busy afternoon, the radiographers find that similar exposure techniques on successive patients result in substantially different radiographs. Which of the following would lead to an accurate diagnosis of the problem?
a. Wire mesh test
b. Pinhole camera test
c. Use of a digital dosimeter to determine HVL
d. Use of a digital dosimeter to determine exposure reproducibility

55. Localized lack of sharpness on a radiograph may be diagnosed using which of the following tests?
a. Wire mesh test
b. Pinhole camera test
c. Use of a digital dosimeter to determine HVL
d. Use of a digital dosimeter to determine exposure linearity

56. X-ray beam quality is expressed in terms of:
a. Half-value layer
b. Exposure linearity
c. Exposure reproducibility
d. mAs

57. The accuracy of collimation at a 40-inch SID must be:
a. ±4 inches
b. ±8/10 inch
c. ±1 inch
d. ±1/10 inch

58. The accuracy of kVp at 80 kVp must be:
   a. No lower than 75 kVp and no higher than 85 kVp
   b. No lower than 79kVP and no higher than 81 kVp
   c. No lower than 76 kVp and no higher than 84 kVp
   d. No lower than 78 kVp and no higher than 82 kVp

59. The apparent size of the focal spot as viewed by the image receptor is called the:
   a. Actual focal spot
   b. Target angle spot
   c. Anode heel effect
   d. Effective focal spot

60. As the angle of the anode decreases, the:
   a. Actual focal spot decreases
   b. Effective focal spot increases
   c. Actual focal spot increases
   d. Effective focal spot decreases

Topic: Image Production and Evaluation (Questions 61-110)

For questions **61** and **62,** indicate which set of exposure factors would produce the greatest density.

61. a. 100 mAs, 70 kVp, 0.5-mm focal spot, 60-inch SID
   b. 200 mAs, 60 kVp, 1.2-mm focal spot, 60-inch SID
   c. 100 mAs, 70 kVp, 1.2-mm focal spot, 60-inch SID
   d. 50 mAs, 90 kVp, 0.5-mm focal spot, 60-inch SID

62. a. 80 mAs, 85 kVp, 40-inch SID, 1.2-mm focal spot
   b. 40 mAs, 80 kVp, 40-inch SID, 0.5-mm focal spot
   c. 160 mAs, 70 kVp, 40-inch SID, 1.2-mm focal spot
   d. 160 mAs, 60 kVp, 40-inch SID, 0.5-mm focal spot

For questions **63-68,** choose the best answer.

63. The components of a grid are:
   a. Pb strips and Pb interspacers
   b. Al strips and Pb interspacers
   c. Pb strips and Al interspacers
   d. Pb strips and cardboard interspacers

64. What is the purpose of a grid?
   a. To remove scatter radiation from the exit beam
   b. To increase radiographic contrast
   c. To decrease dose to the patient
   d. More than one but not all of the above

65. Of the following substances that make up the human body, which list places them in increasing order of density?
   a. Air, fat, water, muscle, bone
   b. Bone, muscle, water, fat, air
   c. Air, fat, muscle, water, bone
   d. Air, fat, water, muscle, bone, tooth enamel

66. The solution filtered through the Ag recovery unit is:
   a. Developer
   b. Fixer
   c. Water
   d. Replenishment solution

67. The action of the developer solution on the film is controlled by:
   a. Chemical activity
   b. Solution temperature
   c. Film immersion time
   d. All of the above

68. If it is necessary to reduce radiographic density by half, and it is not possible to do so by changing mAs, the radiographer may:
   a. Reduce SID by half
   b. Double SID
   c. Decrease kVp by 15%
   d. Reduce time a "step"

Use the list that follows to answer questions **69-74.** Items may be used more than once.

   A. Replenishment system
   B. Transport system
   C. Recirculation system
   D. Dryer system
   E. Starter solution

69. Controls immersion time

70. Seals the film's emulsion

71. Moves film through the processor

72. "Seasons" fresh developer solution

73. Replaces developer and fixer

74. Filters reaction particles from developer

For questions **75-84,** indicate what effect the change has on the item in parentheses. Answer *A* if it increases, *B* if it decreases, *C* if it has no effect.

75. Increase phosphor size (speed)

76. Increase active layer thickness (resolution)

77. Decrease phosphor layer thickness (IF)

78. Decrease film-screen contact (resolution)

79. Decrease phosphor size (resolution)

80. Increase kVp (speed)

81. Decrease phosphor size (speed)

82. Decrease active layer thickness (resolution)

83. Increase active layer thickness (speed)

84. Increase light-absorbing dye in active layer (speed)

Using Figure 7-19, answer questions **85-92.**

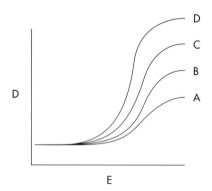

Figure 7-19

Which film:

85. Has the largest AgBr crystals?

86. Demonstrates the least number of gray tones?

87. Results in the patient being exposed to the least amount of radiation?

88. Has the ability to image the greatest number of LP/MM?

89. Is the least sensitive to x rays and light?

90. Has the lowest number of sensitivity specks?

91. Demonstrates the narrowest range of OD numbers?

92. Has the ability to cause radiographers the most trouble?

For questions **93-110,** indicate what effect the change has on the item in parentheses. Answer *A* if it increases, *B* if it decreases, *C* if it has no effect.

93. Decrease anode angle (recorded detail)

94. Increase mAs (contrast)

95. Increase SID (density)

96. Decrease OID (recorded detail)

97. Decrease developer temperature (density)

98. Increase kVp (contrast)

99. Decrease film-screen system speed (recorded detail)

100. Conversion from nongrid to 12:1 grid (contrast)

101. Decrease SID from 60 to 30 inches (magnification)

102. Decrease kVp (recorded detail)

103. Move film from tabletop to Bucky (recorded detail)

104. Decrease source-to-object distance (recorded detail)

105. Increase film immersion time (recorded detail)

106. Increase added filtration (contrast)

107. Tighten collimation (density)

108. Use cylinder cone (contrast)

109. Switch large focal spot to small focal spot (density)

110. Change kVp when using AEC (density)

Topic: Radiographic Procedures (Questions 111-170)

For the following questions, choose the single best answer.

111. The carpal bones are arranged in two rows as follows:
   a. Proximal row (scaphoid, lunate, triquetral, pisiform) and distal row (trapezium, trapezoid, capitate, hamate)
   b. Distal row (scaphoid, lunate, triquetral, pisiform) and proximal row (trapezium, trapezoid, capitate, hamate)
   c. Proximal row (scaphoid, triquetral, capitate, pisiform) and distal row (trapezium, trapezoid, lunate, hamate)
   d. The carpals are not arranged in rows

112. The prominent point of the elbow is called the:
   a. Olecranon, part of the radius
   b. Semilunar notch
   c. Trochlea
   d. Olecranon, part of the ulna

Use the following list to answer questions **113-117.** Items may be used more than once or not at all.

   A. Talipes
   B. Colles' fracture
   C. Boxer's fracture
   D. Jefferson's fracture
   E. Ankylosing spondylitis

113. Imaging of this pathologic condition would require radiography of the cervical spine

114. Imaging of this pathologic condition would require radiography of the hand

115. Imaging of this pathologic condition would require radiography of the distal forearm

116. Imaging of this pathologic condition would require radiography of the feet

117. Imaging of this pathologic condition would require radiography of the entire spine

Using Figure 7-20, answer questions **118-123.**

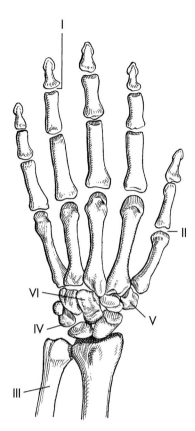

Figure 7-20

118. The structure designated as *I* is the:
   a. Carpometacarpal joint
   b. Interphalangeal joint
   c. Proximal phalanx
   d. Distal interphalangeal joint

119. The structure designated as *II* is the:
   a. Carpometacarpal joint
   b. Interphalangeal joint
   c. Proximal phalanx
   d. Metacarpophalangeal joint

120. The structure designated as *III* is the:
   a. Ulna
   b. Metacarpal
   c. Radius
   d. Humerus

121. The structure designated as *IV* is the:
   a. Lunate
   b. Triquetral
   c. Capitate
   d. Pisiform

122. The structure designated as *V* is the:
   a. Lunate
   b. Scaphoid
   c. Trapezium
   d. Trapezoid

123. The structure designated as *VI* is the:
   a. Lunate
   b. Triquetrum
   c. Capitate
   d. Scaphoid

Using Figure 7-21, answer questions **124-128.**

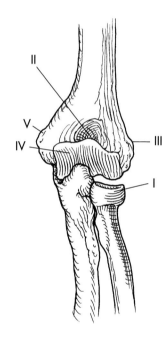

Figure 7-21

124. The structure designated as *I* is the:
   a. Head of ulna
   b. Radial head
   c. Medial epicondyle
   d. Lateral epicondyle

125. The structure designated as *II* is the:
   a. Coronoid fossa
   b. Olecranon
   c. Semilunar notch
   d. Radial head

126. The structure designated as *III* is the:
   a. Head of the ulna
   b. Radial head
   c. Medial epicondyle
   d. Lateral epicondyle

127. The structure designated as *IV* is the:
   a. Medial epicondyle
   b. Trochlea
   c. Lateral epicondyle
   d. Ulnar head

128. The structure designated as *V* is the:
   a. Medial epicondyle
   b. Trochlea
   c. Lateral epicondyle
   d. Ulnar head

Using Figure 7-22, answer questions **129-133.**

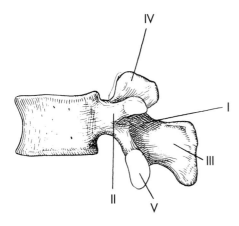

Figure 7-22

129. The structure designated as *I* is the:
   a. Pedicle
   b. Superior vertebral notch
   c. Interior vertebral notch
   d. Lamina

130. The structure designated as *II* is the:
   a. Pedicle
   b. Superior vertebral notch
   c. Interior vertebral notch
   d. Spinous process

131. The structure designated as *III* is the:
   a. Lamina
   b. Spinous process
   c. Superior articular process
   d. Pedicle

132. The structure designated as *IV* is the:
   a. Superior vertebral notch
   b. Superior articular process
   c. Transverse process
   d. Spinous process

133. The structure designated as *V* is the:
   a. Lamina
   b. Spinous process
   c. Inferior vertebral notch
   d. Inferior articular process

Using Figure 7-23, answer questions **134-137.**

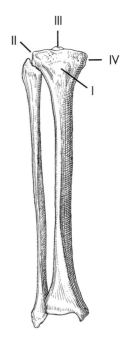

Figure 7-23

134. The structure designated as *I* is the:
   a. Head of the fibula
   b. Head of the tibia
   c. Tuberosity
   d. Styloid process

135. The structure designated as *II* is the:
   a. Medial condyle
   b. Lateral condyle
   c. Intercondylar eminence
   d. Head of the fibula

136. The structure designated as *III* is the:
   a. Tubercle
   b. Lateral condyle
   c. Medial condyle
   d. Intercondylar eminence

137. The structure designated as *IV* is the:
   a. Tubercle
   b. Lateral condyle
   c. Medial condyle
   d. Intercondylar eminence

Using Figure 7-24, answer questions **138-143**.

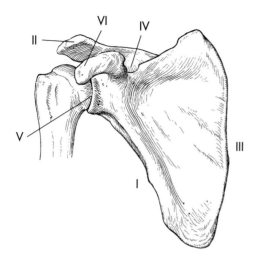

Figure 7-24

138. The structure designated as *I* is the:
    a. Vertebral border
    b. Scapular notch
    c. Body
    d. Axillary border

139. The structure designated as *II* is the:
    a. Humeral head
    b. Acromion
    c. Coracoid process
    d. Coronoid process

140. The structure designated as *III* is the:
    a. Vertebral border
    b. Scapular notch
    c. Body
    d. Subscapular fossa

141. The structure designated as *IV* is the:
    a. Coracoid process
    b. Coronoid process
    c. Scapular notch
    d. Glenoid fossa

142. The structure designated as *V* is the:
    a. Glenoid fossa
    b. Acromion
    c. Coronoid process
    d. Coracoid process

143. The structure designated as *VI* is the:
    a. Glenoid fossa
    b. Acromion
    c. Coronoid process
    d. Coracoid process

Using Figure 7-25, answer question **144.**

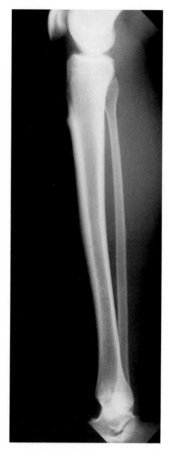

Figure 7-25

144. Critique the radiograph:
    a. Radiograph is not acceptable; radius and ulna should be superimposed
    b. Radiograph is not acceptable; tibia and fibula should be superimposed
    c. Radiograph is acceptable, but only one joint is needed
    d. Radiograph is acceptable

Using Figure 7-26, answer question **145.**

Using Figure 7-27, answer question **146.**

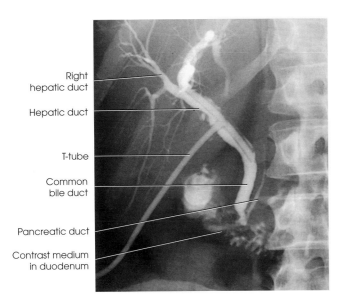

Right
hepatic duct

Hepatic duct

T-tube

Common
bile duct

Pancreatic duct

Contrast medium
in duodenum

Figure 7-26

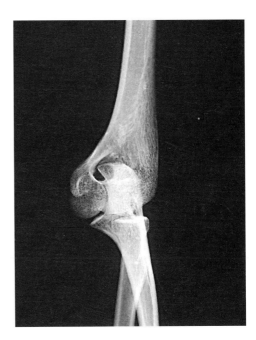

Figure 7-27

145. Critique the radiograph:
   a. Radiograph taken during surgery; acceptable
   b. Radiograph taken during surgery; unacceptable
   c. Radiograph taken postoperatively; unacceptable
   d. Radiograph taken postoperatively; acceptable

146. Critique the radiograph:
   a. Radiograph unacceptable; arm rotated
   b. Radiograph acceptable for medial oblique
   c. Radiograph acceptable for lateral oblique
   d. Radiograph unacceptable; humerus and forearm
      must be in same plane

Using Figure 7-28, answer question **147.**

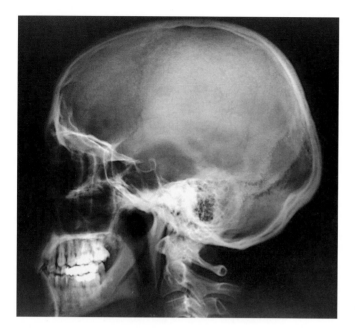

Figure 7-28

147. Critique the radiograph:
   a. Radiograph was taken with interpupillary line parallel to film
   b. Radiograph was taken with MSP perpendicular to film
   c. Radiograph was taken with interpupillary line perpendicular to film
   d. Radiograph was taken with MSP parallel to central ray

Using Figure 7-29, answer question **148.**

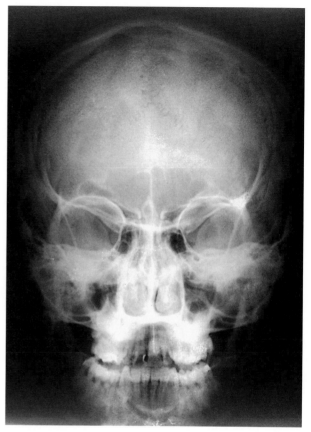

Figure 7-29

148. Critique the radiograph:
   a. Radiograph was taken with central ray angled 15 degrees caudad
   b. Radiograph was taken with central ray angled 0 degrees
   c. Radiograph was taken with central ray angled 15 degrees cephalad
   d. Radiograph was taken with MSP perpendicular to central ray

Using Figure 7-30, answer questions **149-153**.

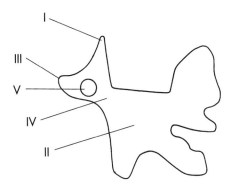

Figure 7-30

149. The structure designated as *I* is the:
    a. Pars interarticularis
    b. Superior articular process
    c. Pedicle
    d. Lamina

150. The structure designated as *II* is the:
    a. Pars interarticularis
    b. Superior articular process
    c. Pedicle
    d. Lamina

151. The structure designated as *III* is the:
    a. Spinous process
    b. Transverse process
    c. Pedicle
    d. Inferior articular process

152. The structure designated as *IV* is the:
    a. Spinous process
    b. Transverse process
    c. Pedicle
    d. Pars interarticularis

153. The structure designated as *V* is the:
    a. Spinous process
    b. Transverse process
    c. Pedicle
    d. Inferior articular process

For the following questions, choose the single best answer.

154. The lateral transthoracic humerus, oblique sternum, and lateral thoracic spine may be imaged best by using a technique called:
    a. Tomography
    b. Zonography
    c. Autotomography
    d. Computed tomography

155. A patient unable to supinate the hand for an AP projection of the forearm:
    a. Should be made to do so to provide a diagnostic radiograph
    b. Probably has a fracture of the radial head and must be handled carefully
    c. Probably has a low pain tolerance and must be handled carefully
    d. May require radiographs with and without weights

156. When a PA axial projection of the clavicle is performed, the central ray should be angled:
    a. 15 degrees cephalad
    b. 15 degrees caudad
    c. 25 to 30 degrees cephalad
    d. 25 to 30 degrees caudad

157. When a lateral projection of the knee is performed, the knee should be:
    a. Extended 20 to 30 degrees
    b. Flexed to a 90-degree angle
    c. Flexed 20 to 30 degrees
    d. Fully extended

158. When a tangential projection of the patella is performed with the patient prone, the central ray should be angled:
    a. 15 degrees cephalad
    b. 15 degrees caudad
    c. 25 degrees cephalad
    d. 45 degrees cephalad

159. Use of which of the following would provide an improved image of the femur?
    a. Trough filter
    b. Anode heel effect
    c. Short SID
    d. Long OID

160. When an AP projection of the hip is performed, the central ray is directed:
   a. Perpendicular to a point 2 inches medial to the ASIS at the level of the superior margin of the greater trochanter
   b. Parallel to a point 2 inches medial to the ASIS at the level of the superior margin of the greater trochanter
   c. At a 15-degree cephalad angle
   d. To the level of the ASIS

161. When the AP oblique projection is performed for the cervical vertebrae, the central ray is directed:
   a. 25 to 30 degrees cephalad
   b. 15 to 20 degrees caudad
   c. 5 to 10 degrees cephalad
   d. 15 to 20 degrees cephalad

162. When the AP oblique projection is performed for the lumbar vertebrae, the side of interest is:
   a. Farthest from the film
   b. Closest to the film
   c. Rotated 30 degrees
   d. Rotated 20 degrees

163. When the PA oblique projection for the sacroiliac joints is performed, the side of interest is:
   a. Farthest from the film
   b. Closest to the film
   c. Rotated 10 degrees
   d. Rotated 45 degrees

164. Routine chest radiography is performed:
   a. At the end of full inspiration
   b. At the end of full expiration
   c. At the end of the second full inspiration
   d. With the patient supine or upright

165. The primary purpose of performing the oblique projections of the ribs is:
   a. To image the axillary portion of the ribs
   b. To image the ribs above the diaphragm
   c. To image the ribs below the diaphragm
   d. To determine the extent of the patient's pain tolerance

166. When the PA projection of the skull is performed to image the frontal bone:
   1. The central ray is directed perpendicular to the cassette
   2. The OML is perpendicular to the cassette
   3. The central ray exits at the glabella
   4. MSP is parallel to cassette
   a. All are true
   b. 1, 2
   c. 1, 3, 4
   d. 1, 3

167. When the AP axial projection of the skull is performed:
   1. The OML is parallel to cassette
   2. The central ray is directed through the foramen magnum 37 degrees to the OML
   3. The central ray is directed through the foramen magnum 30 degrees to the IOML
   4. The MSP is parallel to the plane of the film
   a. All are true
   b. 1, 2
   c. 1, 3, 4
   d. None are true

168. When performing the SMV projection of the skull, the IOML:
   a. Is placed perpendicular to the plane of the cassette
   b. Is not used in positioning for the SMV
   c. Is placed parallel to the plane of the cassette
   d. Is placed parallel to the central ray

169. When the parieto-orbital oblique projection of the optic foramen is performed, the MSP is placed:
   a. 53 degrees from the central ray
   b. 37 degrees from the cassette
   c. 37 degrees from the perpendicular
   d. 12 degrees cephalad

170. For the parietoacanthial projection of the facial bones, the OML:
   a. Forms a 37-degree angle with the plane of the film
   b. Forms a 53-degree angle with the plane of the film
   c. Forms a 37-degree angle with the central ray
   d. Is not used, but the IOML forms a 37-degree angle with the plane of the film

Topic: Patient Care (Questions 171-200)

171. The radiographer must be proficient in the use of which medical instruments?
 a. Angiography catheter
 b. Sphygmomanometer
 c. Thermometer
 d. Oxygen administration equipment

172. A tube used to feed the patient or to perform gastric suction is called a:
 a. Tracheostomy tube
 b. Tracheotomy tube
 c. Nasogastric tube
 d. Ventilator tube

173. Nosocomial infections are acquired:
 a. In radiology
 b. Through the nose
 c. During cold and flu season
 d. In the hospital

174. During movement and transfer of patients, urinary catheter bags should be:
 a. Safely placed on the patient's abdomen
 b. Kept below the level of the urinary bladder
 c. Kept below the level of the x-ray table
 d. Kept on the cart or wheelchair

175. The first task that must be performed when beginning a radiographic examination on a patient is to:
 a. Verify patient identity
 b. Determine accuracy of physician's orders
 c. Verify exam to be performed
 d. Remove radiopaque objects from area of interest

176. Which of the following is *not* required for valid consent?
 a. Patient must be of legal age
 b. Patient must be adequately informed and sign consent form
 c. Patient must be mentally competent
 d. Consent must be offered voluntarily

177. The most common site injured by radiographers while caring for patients is the:
 a. Head
 b. Arms and shoulders
 c. Lumbosacral spine
 d. Lower leg

178. When taking a patient's history, which of the following questions is inappropriate?
 a. Why did your doctor order this exam?
 b. Have you experienced any difficulty breathing or shortness of breath?
 c. Have you experienced nausea or vomiting?
 d. How long ago was your cancer diagnosed?

179. A system that uses barriers between individuals and assumes all patients are infectious is called:
 a. Standard precautions
 b. Whole body isolation
 c. Sterile technique
 d. Surgical asepsis

180. When you are performing patient care in radiology:
 a. Hands should be washed after each procedure
 b. Gowns and gloves should always be worn
 c. Hands should be washed only after caring for obviously infectious patients
 d. Gloves should be worn only when performing gastrointestinal procedures or performing venipuncture

181. Patient transfer from cart to x-ray table should be performed:
 a. Alone when working evenings or nights
 b. By radiographers working in pairs at all times
 c. Alone when the department is busy or has a staff shortage
 d. In pairs only when other radiographers are available to assist

182. When seeking the latest information regarding universal precautions, the best source is the:
 a. Radiology administrator
 b. Radiology purchasing manager
 c. Infection control department
 d. Radiologist

183. Following all radiographic or fluoroscopic procedures, the radiographer should clean surfaces with which the patient was in contact using:
 a. Alcohol
 b. Surgical asepsis
 c. Soap and water
 d. Medical asepsis

184. When sterile fields are prepared, damp packages:
 a. Are always considered contaminated
 b. Are always considered sterile because the dampness confirms they were cleaned
 c. Should be unwrapped first and placed in the center of the sterile field
 d. Are always considered sterile; the dampness is only a remnant of the gassing process

185. When mobile radiography is performed, the mobile unit:
   a. Does not have to be cleaned because it is never in contact with sterile fields
   b. Must be cleaned before and after each use
   c. Must be cleaned before entering surgical areas or reverse isolation units
   d. Must be cleaned before entering surgical areas or reverse isolation units and after leaving most isolation units

186. When radiography is performed on patients in isolation, the cassette:
   a. Needs to be placed in a protective covering only if the patient is in reverse isolation
   b. Must always be placed in a protective covering
   c. Needs to be placed in a protective covering to keep it free of microbes
   d. Needs to be placed in a protective covering so that no microbes leave the room

187. A radiographer should be prepared to assist with which of the following procedures at any time?
   a. CPR
   b. Intubation
   c. Suctioning
   d. All of the above

188. In addition to performing radiography on a trauma victim, the radiographer should be:
   1. Continually assessing the patient's condition
   2. Interpreting the radiographs for the emergency room physician
   3. Taking additional projections as indicated by the patient's condition or preliminary radiographs
   4. Keeping all other health care workers out of the room because of radiation protection standards
   5. Providing comfort and communicating quietly with the patient, whether the patient is conscious or unconscious
   a. 1, 3
   b. All are true
   c. 1, 3, 5
   d. 1, 3, 4, 5

189. For a barium enema the contrast agent should be mixed with:
   a. Cold water
   b. Water at or below body temperature
   c. Water at approximately 120° F
   d. Water at approximately 100° F

190. All iodinated contrast media used today contain:
   a. Iodine and free ions
   b. Free ions
   c. Only iodine
   d. Salts of organic iodine compounds

191. The highest incidence of contrast agent reactions occurs when using:
   a. Negative contrast media
   b. Ionic iodinated contrast media
   c. Nonionic iodinated contrast media
   d. Barium sulfate

192. It is important for the radiographer to obtain the recent history of radiographic examinations performed on a patient so that:
   a. An overdose of iodinated contrast media does not occur from exams performed in the past week
   b. An overdose of radiation is not administered
   c. A pattern of unnecessary exams may be established
   d. None of the above

193. For patients with a history of intravenous urography and no contrast agent reactions:
   a. The radiographer may assume there will be no reaction on subsequent intravenous urograms
   b. The radiographer must assume there is a chance of a reaction on other contrast examinations
   c. The radiographer must assume there is a chance of a reaction on subsequent intravenous urograms
   d. There is no chance of reactions on subsequent intravenous urograms

194. When venipuncture is performed:
   a. The radiographer is not responsible for obtaining patient history because the exam was ordered by a physician
   b. The contrast agent should be flushed through the syringe, any tubing used, and the needle before injection
   c. The contrast agent must be cooled to make it easier to inject
   d. The contrast agent must always be flushed through the syringe, any tubing used, and needle before injection

195. After cleansing the injection site, before performing venipuncture, the radiographer should:
   a. Immediately perform the puncture
   b. Palpate the vein once more just before the puncture to make certain of the site
   c. Apply a tourniquet
   d. If using a butterfly, tape the tubing to the patient's arm

196. Factors that contribute to contrast media reactions caused by patient anxiety or suggestibility (e.g., resulting from the informed consent process) are called:
a. Psychosomatic factors
b. Psychogenic factors
c. Psychologic factors
d. Anxiety factors

197. Contrast agent reactions such as flushing, hives, and nausea are called:
a. Psychosomatic
b. Cardiovascular
c. Anaphylactic
d. Nonsystemic

198. Aqueous iodine compounds are used as contrast media when radiographing the:
a. Urinary system
b. Gastrointestinal system
c. Reproductive system
d. Central nervous system

199. When entering data on a patient's chart, the radiographer must:
a. Sign and date the entry
b. Date the entry and sign with name and credentials—RT(R), which means radiologic technologist (radiography)
c. Date the entry and sign with name and credentials—RT(R), which means registered technician (radiography)
d. Date the entry and sign with name and credentials—RT(R), which means registered technologist (radiography)

200. In an attempt to maintain the quality of patient care at the highest level possible over time, proof of continuing education is mandatory for renewal of certification with the:
a. State licensing board in all 50 states
b. American Society of Radiologic Technologists
c. Joint Commission on Accreditation of Healthcare Organizations
d. American Registry of Radiologic Technologists

Scoring

Traditionally you have probably focused on how many questions you miss on an exam. As you prepare for the certification exam, I encourage you to focus on how many you answer correctly. Use Table 7-2 to calculate the percentage of questions you answered correctly in each category and on the test as a whole. Remember, a score below 75% on any topic or the entire test is an indication that more review is needed on that topic. Now, go back and concentrate on which items were missed and the reason why. When you are done reviewing, go on to Challenge Test #3.

TABLE 7-2	Calculating Your Score for Challenge Test #2	
Topic	**Percentage calculation**	**Your score**
Radiation protection	Number correct _____ times 100, ÷ 30 =	
Equipment operation and maintenance	Number correct _____ times 100, ÷ 30 =	
Image production and evaluation	Number correct _____ times 100, ÷ 50 =	
Radiographic procedures	Number correct _____ times 100, ÷ 60 =	
Patient care	Number correct _____ times 100, ÷ 30 =	
Total	Number correct _____ times 100, ÷ 200 =	

Challenge Test #3
Practice for Taking Traditional Multiple-Choice Exams

Read each question and the answer choices carefully. For some questions, more than one answer may be correct. However, you must choose the one best, most complete answer for each item. Use the results of this test to assess your strengths and weaknesses. Do not look up any of the answers until you have completed the entire test. Correct the test using the answer key in the back of the book. Then compute your scores using Table 7-3 to see where you are strong and where you need additional review. Refer to the appropriate chapter in this book for review of the questions you miss.

Topic: Radiation Protection
(Questions 1-30)

For the following questions, choose the single best answer.

1. Radiation that exits the x-ray tube from the anode is called:
   a. Remnant radiation
   b. Gamma radiation
   c. Nonionizing radiation
   d. Primary radiation

2. The photon-tissue interaction in diagnostic radiography that results in the total absorption of an x-ray photon and the production of contrast in the radiographic image is:
   a. Compton's
   b. Coherent
   c. Photoelectric
   d. Pair production

3. Which photon-tissue interaction produces a recoil electron and a scattered photon in diagnostic radiography?
   a. Compton's
   b. Coherent
   c. Photoelectric
   d. Pair production

4. The traditional unit of in-air exposure is the:
   a. Coulombs/kilogram
   b. Rem
   c. Becquerel
   d. Roentgen

5. The SI unit of absorbed dose is the:
   a. Coulombs/kilogram
   b. Gray
   c. Curie
   d. LET

6. The traditional unit of dose equivalency is the:
   a. Rem
   b. Gray
   c. Quality factor
   d. LET

7. The SI unit of dose equivalency is the:
   a. Rem
   b. Gray
   c. Quality factor
   d. Sievert

8. The traditional unit of activity is the:
   a. Becquerel
   b. Gray
   c. Quality factor
   d. Curie

9. One hundred ergs of energy deposited per gram of tissue defines the:
   a. Becquerel
   b. Gray
   c. Quality factor
   d. Rad

10. The amount of radiation deposited per unit length of tissue traversed by incoming photons is called:
    a. Tissue exposure
    b. Linear deposition of energy
    c. Linear energy transfer
    d. Absorbed dose equivalent limit

11. Rem multiplied by a quality factor equals:
    a. Rads
    b. Roentgens
    c. Grays
    d. No such equation is used

12. Compton's interaction:
    a. Produces contrast in the radiographic image
    b. Results in scattering of the incident photon
    c. May produce a fog on the radiograph
    d. More than one but not all of the above

13. The quality factor for x rays is:
    a. 10
    b. 1
    c. 20
    d. 5

14. Cataractogenesis, life span shortening, embryologic effects, and carcinogenesis are examples of:
    a. Short-term somatic effects
    b. Genetic effects
    c. Acute radiation syndrome
    d. Long-term somatic effects

15. Effective absorbed dose equivalent limit:
    a. Is the level of radiation that an organism can receive and probably sustain no appreciable damage
    b. Is a safe level of radiation that can be received with no effects
    c. Should be absorbed annually to maintain proper immunity to radiation
    d. Is 5000 mrem per year for the general public

16. What agency publishes radiation protection recommendations?
    a. ICRP
    b. NCRP
    c. NRC
    d. ASRT

17. Radiation protection is based on which dose-response relationship?
    a. Linear-threshold
    b. Nonlinear-nonthreshold
    c. Linear-nonthreshold
    d. Nonlinear-threshold

18. Which of the following states that the radiosensitivity of cells is directly proportional to their reproductive activity and inversely proportional to their degree of differentiation?
    a. Inverse square law
    b. Law of Bergonié and Tribondeau
    c. Reciprocity law
    d. Ohm's law

19. Which of the following causes about 95% of the cellular response to radiation?
    a. Direct effect
    b. Law of Bergonié and Tribondeau
    c. Target theory
    d. Indirect effect

20. When radiation strikes DNA which of the following will occur?
    a. Direct effect
    b. Law of Bergonié and Tribondeau
    c. Target theory
    d. Indirect effect

21. The absorbed dose equivalent limit for the embryo-fetus is:
    a. 500 mrem per year
    b. 5 rem per year
    c. 0.5 rem per month
    d. 500 mrem during gestation

22. The effective absorbed dose equivalent limit for radiographers is:
    a. 3 rem per quarter
    b. 500 mrem per year
    c. 5000 mrem per year
    d. 100 mrem per month

23. The cumulative occupational exposure for a 29-year-old radiographer is:
    a. 29 mrem
    b. 55 rem
    c. 11 mrem
    d. 29 rem

24. The annual effective absorbed dose equivalent for the general public, assuming infrequent exposure, is:
    a. 0.5 mrem
    b. 500 rem
    c. 0.5 rem
    d. 50 mrem

25. The upper boundary dose that can be absorbed that carries a negligible risk of somatic or genetic damage to the individual defines:
    a. Maximum permissible dose
    b. ALARA
    c. The Law of Bergonié and Tribondeau
    d. Effective absorbed dose equivalent limit

26. Film badges are generally accurate down to the level of:
    a. 10 rem
    b. 5 rem
    c. 0.1 mrem

27. The exposure switch on a portable x-ray machine must be attached to a cord that is at least _____ feet long?
    a. 3
    b. 6
    c. 12
    d. 2

28. Under what conditions may the radiographer be exposed to the primary beam?
   a. When performing mobile radiography, as long as the exposure is low
   b. Never, under any conditions
   c. When performing crosstable projections, if needed to hold the cassette in place
   d. When assisting with fluoroscopy

29. For purposes of radiation protection, the x-ray beam is filtered. X-ray tubes operating above 70 kVp must have total filtration of:
   a. At least 0.25-mm aluminum equivalent
   b. At least 0.25-mm lead equivalent
   c. No more than 2.5-mm aluminum equivalent
   d. At least 2.5-mm aluminum equivalent

30. Gonadal shielding should be used:
   a. On every exam performed
   b. Whenever it will not obstruct the area of clinical interest
   c. Only on children and women of childbearing age
   d. Only during pregnancy

Topic: Equipment Operation and Maintenance (Questions 31-60)

31. The smallest particle of a compound that retains the characteristics of the compound is a(n):
   a. Element
   b. Atom
   c. Molecule
   d. Neutron

32. Atomic number refers to:
   a. The number of protons plus the number of neutrons
   b. The number of electrons
   c. The number of electron shells
   d. The number of protons

33. Atoms with the same number of protons but with a different number of neutrons are called:
   a. Electrons
   b. Isotopes
   c. Ions
   d. Particulate radiation

34. The force that holds electrons in orbit around a nucleus is called:
   a. Gravity
   b. Atomic force
   c. Electron binding energy
   d. Ionization energy

35. X rays travel as bundles of energy called:
   a. Protons
   b. Phasers
   c. Particles
   d. Quanta

36. The distance between the peaks of a sine wave of x rays is called:
   a. Wavelength
   b. Altitude
   c. Amplitude
   d. Frequency

37. The transformer with a single coil of wire serving as both the primary and secondary coils is the:
   a. Step-up transformer
   b. Step-down transformer
   c. Induction transformer
   d. Autotransformer

38. The transformer that makes the use of variable kVp possible is the:
   a. Step-up transformer
   b. Step-down transformer
   c. Induction transformer
   d. Autotransformer

39. When an ionization chamber is used, where is the chamber located?
   a. Between the patient and the film
   b. Between the x-ray tube the patient
   c. Between the film and the detector
   d. Behind the film

40. What safety feature is set when using an automatic exposure control?
   a. The minimum response time
   b. The falling load generator
   c. The backup timer
   d. The ionization chamber

41. An x-ray machine that cannot provide long exposure times such as those required for autotomography uses a(n):
   a. Ionization chamber
   b. Phototimer
   c. AEC
   d. Falling load generator

42. Devices in the x-ray circuit that increase or decrease voltage are called:
   a. Rectifiers
   b. Generators
   c. Timers
   d. Transformers

43. The filament circuit makes use of what type of transformer?
a. Step-up
b. Autotransformer
c. Step-down
d. Falling load

44. Because the x-ray tube requires DC to operate properly, what device is required in the x-ray circuit?
a. Autotransformer
b. Step-up transformer
c. Rectifier
d. Falling load generator

45. Where is the rectifier located in the x-ray circuit?
a. Between the timer and the step-up transformer
b. Between the step-up transformer and the step-down transformer
c. Between the primary and secondary coils of the step-up transformer
d. Between the step-up transformer and the x-ray tube

46. Thermionic emission occurs at the:
a. Anode
b. Control panel
c. Rectifier
d. Cathode

47. At the time of exposure, the charge on the focusing cup is:
a. Irrelevant
b. Positive
c. Negative
d. Alternating

48. An interaction that primarily produces heat at the anode but that also produces x rays is called:
a. Characteristic
b. Photoelectric
c. Compton's
d. Bremsstrahlung

49. Examples of video tubes that may be used in fluoroscopy are:
a. Brems and characteristic
b. Vidicon and Plumbicon
c. Digital and analog
d. Anode and cathode

50. When a quality control test for exposure linearity is performed, adjacent mA stations must be within this amount of one another:
a. 2% of SID
b. 4%
c. 10%
d. 5%

51. When a quality control test for exposure reproducibility is performed, successive exposures must be within this amount of one another:
a. 2% of SID
b. 4%
c. 10%
d. 5%

52. When a quality control test for collimator accuracy is performed, the result must be within this amount:
a. 2% of SID
b. 4%
c. 10%
d. 5%

53. When a quality control test for accuracy of kVp is performed, the result must be within this amount of the control panel setting:
a. 2% of SID
b. 4%
c. 10%
d. 4

54. When a spinning top test is performed on single-phase equipment, a radiograph exhibiting six dots would indicate:
a. An accurate timer, if set on $\frac{1}{20}$ second
b. A malfunctioning timer, if set on $\frac{1}{20}$ second
c. A malfunctioning autotransformer, if set on $\frac{1}{20}$ second
d. An accurate timer, if set on $\frac{1}{6}$ second

55. When a spinning top test is performed on three-phase equipment, a timer setting of 0.5 second should indicate the following on the resultant radiograph:
a. 180 dots
b. 90 dots
c. A 180-degree arc
d. A 90-degree arc

56. The accuracy of collimation at a 72-inch SID must be:
a. ±1.44 inches
b. ±7.2 inches
c. ±3.6 inches
d. ±0.02 inch

57. The accuracy of kVp at 90 kVp must be:
a. No lower than 85 kVp and no higher than 95 kVp
b. No lower than 89kVP and no higher than 91 kVp
c. No lower than 86 kVp and no higher than 94 kVp
d. No lower than 88 kVp and no higher than 92 kVp

58. The feature of the image intensifier that ensures the radiation dose striking the input phosphor is constant is the:
a. Photocathode
b. Electron focusing lens
c. Automatic brightness control
d. Vidicon tube

59. Instead of vidicon or Plumbicon tubes, what device may be used in the television system?
a. Charge-coupled device (CCD)
b. C-arm
c. Automatic brightness control
d. Output phosphor

60. The electronic device that may be used for many quality control tests on x-ray equipment is the:
a. Automatic exposure control
b. Digital dosimeter
c. Penetrometer
d. Densitometer

Topic: Image Production and Evaluation (Questions 61-110)

For the following questions, choose the single best answer.

61. The amount of darkness on a radiograph is best described as:
a. Contrast
b. Detail
c. Density
d. mAs

62. The image in the emulsion of a film, before processing, is called:
a. Manifest image
b. Image-in-waiting
c. Preprocessed image
d. Latent image

63. mAs = mAs is the equation that describes which of the following?
a. Inverse square law
b. mAs-density law
c. Reciprocity law
d. 15% law

64. Given an original technique of 20 mAs and 80 kVp, which of the following will produce a radiograph with double the density?
a. 40 mAs, 90 kVp
b. 30 mAs, 92 kVp
c. 40 mAs, 80 kVp
d. 15 mAs, 92 kVp

65. Distance and density are governed by what law or rule?
a. Reciprocity law
b. 15% rule
c. Inverse square law
d. Density maintenance rule

66. Unwanted markings on a radiograph are called:
a. Processing irregularities
b. Processing artifacts
c. Artifacts
d. Plus-density markings

67. Small marks on a radiograph approximately 3.1416 inches apart are called:
a. Guide shoe scratches
b. Plus-density markings
c. Pi lines
d. Chemical scratches

68. The entire processor should be cleaned every:
a. Day
b. Week
c. Month
d. 6 months

69. The wash tank should be drained every:
a. Day
b. Week
c. Month
d. 6 months

70. The developer filter should be changed every:
a. Day
b. Week
c. Month
d. 6 months

71. Sensitometric testing should be performed every:
a. Day
b. Week
c. Month
d. 6 months

72. Speed and contrast values measured during sensitometric testing should not vary more than how much from the baseline?
   a. 5%
   b. 1%
   c. 15%
   d. 10%

73. Speed step used during sensitometric testing is the step closest to what density value?
   a. 0.25
   b. 1.0
   c. 1.5
   d. 2.0

74. A malfunction in which the developer temperature runs too high will cause:
   a. Dark films
   b. Light films
   c. Milky films
   d. Greasy films

75. A malfunction in which the developer replenishment runs too high will cause:
   a. Dark films
   b. Light films
   c. Milky films
   d. Greasy films

76. A malfunction in which there is a white light leak into the processing room will cause:
   a. Dark films
   b. Light films
   c. Milky films
   d. Fogged films

77. Poor fixer replenishment will cause:
   a. Dark films
   b. Light films
   c. Milky films
   d. Greasy films

78. A malfunction in which there are dark flakes in the wash water is caused by:
   a. Dirty developer
   b. Dirty fixer
   c. Dryer temperature set too high
   d. Algae in the wash water

79. Use of outdated film will cause:
   a. Dark films
   b. Light films
   c. Milky films
   d. Fogged films

80. A malfunction in which fixer solution has entered the developer tank will cause:
   a. Dark films
   b. Light films
   c. Milky films
   d. Fogged films

81. In which section of the processor are unexposed silver halide crystals washed out of the emulsion?
   a. Wash
   b. Fixer
   c. Developer
   d. Dryer

82. In which section of the processor is the emulsion sealed?
   a. Wash
   b. Fixer
   c. Developer
   d. Dryer

83. In which section of the processor is the temperature set from 90° to 95° F?
   a. Wash
   b. Fixer
   c. Developer
   d. Dryer

84. Which of the following systems moves the film and agitates the chemistry?
   a. Transport
   b. Replenishment
   c. Recirculation
   d. Dryer

85. Which of the following systems provides fresh chemistry to process each film?
   a. Transport
   b. Replenishment
   c. Recirculation
   d. Dryer

86. Which of the following systems removes reaction particles from the developer solution by sending it through a filter?
   a. Transport
   b. Replenishment
   c. Recirculation
   d. Dryer

87. The settings on which of the following systems is determined by the average number of 14- × 17-inch films fed through the processor in a typical workday?
    a. Transport
    b. Replenishment
    c. Recirculation
    d. Dryer

88. Which of the following grid errors will result in an image that shows normal density in the middle but decreased density on the sides, assuming the correct side of the grid faces the x-ray tube?
    a. Upside down
    b. Off-level
    c. Lateral decentering
    d. Grid-focus decentering

89. Which of the following grid errors will result in an image that shows decreased density more to one side than the other?
    a. Upside down
    b. Off-level
    c. Lateral decentering
    d. Grid-focus decentering

90. Grid ratio is described by which of the following?
    a. H & D
    b. H / D
    c. mAs = mAs
    d. 15% rule

91. Grid radius is described as:
    a. The height of the lead strips divided by the distance between the lead strips
    b. The distance between the lead strips divided by the height of the lead strips
    c. The number of lead strips per inch or centimeter
    d. The SID at which the grid may be used

92. The aspect of a film-screen system that may be examined by conducting a wire mesh test is the:
    a. Phosphor layer
    b. Reflective layer
    c. Protective layer
    d. Film-screen contact

93. The portion of an intensifying screen that helps prevent damage from scratching is the:
    a. Active layer
    b. Reflective layer
    c. Protective layer
    d. Base

94. The portion of an intensifying screen that is made of polyester is the:
    a. Active layer
    b. Reflective layer
    c. Protective layer
    d. Base

95. A faster film-screen system will exhibit:
    a. Higher contrast
    b. Wider latitude
    c. Better recorded detail
    d. Decreased density

96. A slower film-screen system will exhibit:
    a. Lower contrast
    b. Narrower latitude
    c. Poorer recorded detail
    d. Increased density

97. A faster film-screen system will exhibit:
    a. Lower contrast
    b. Narrower latitude
    c. Better recorded detail
    d. Decreased density

98. The section of an H & D curve that represents base plus fog is the:
    a. Shoulder
    b. Toe
    c. Body
    d. x-axis

99. The section of an H & D curve that represents D-max is the:
    a. Shoulder
    b. Toe
    c. Body
    d. x-axis

100. The section of an H & D curve on which exposure is plotted is the:
    a. Shoulder
    b. Toe
    c. Body
    d. x-axis

101. The function of the blue tint added to the film's base is to:
    a. Increase speed
    b. Reduce glare
    c. Increase recorded detail
    d. Decrease latitude

102. As kVp is increased:
a. Density decreases
b. Contrast increases
c. Recorded detail increases
d. Contrast decreases

103. As kVp is decreased:
a. Density increases
b. Contrast decreases
c. Recorded detail decreases
d. Scale of contrast shortens

104. Which of the following sets of exposure factors will produce the radiograph with the best recorded detail?
a. 60 mAs, 80 kVp, 40-inch SID, 4-inch OID
b. 30 mAs, 92 kVp, 40-inch SID, 4-inch OID
c. 120 mAs, 92 kVp, 40-inch SID, 4-inch OID
d. All would produce equal recorded detail

105. Which of the following sets of exposure factors will produce the radiograph with the highest contrast?
a. 60 mAs, 80 kVp, 40-inch SID, 4-inch OID
b. 30 mAs, 92 kVp, 40-inch SID, 4-inch OID
c. 120 mAs, 92 kVp, 40-inch SID, 4-inch OID
d. 15 mAs, 100 kVp, 40-inch SID, 4-inch OID

106. Which of the following sets of exposure factors will produce the radiograph with the most magnification?
a. 60 mAs, 80 kVp, 40-inch SID, 4-inch OID
b. 30 mAs, 92 kVp, 40-inch SID, 4-inch OID
c. 120 mAs, 92 kVp, 20-inch SID, 4-inch OID
d. 15 mAs, 100 kVp, 40-inch SID, 4-inch OID

107. Which of the following statements is true?
a. High kVp = low contrast = long-scale contrast = many gray tones
b. Low kVp = low contrast = long-scale contrast = many gray tones
c. When kVp is increased, there is an increase in the number of photoelectric interactions that occur
d. When kVp is decreased, there is an increase in the number of Compton's interactions that occur

108. Which of the following statements is true?
a. High kVp = high contrast = short-scale contrast = few gray tones
b. Low kVp = low contrast = long-scale contrast = many gray tones
c. When kVp is increased, there is an increase in the number of photoelectric interactions that occur
d. When kVp is decreased, there is an increase in the number of photoelectric interactions that occur

109. Differential absorption of the x-ray beam produces:
a. Density
b. Subject contrast
c. Recorded detail
d. Characteristic radiation

110. Beam restriction has the following effect on contrast:
a. Decreases contrast
b. Increases contrast
c. Longer scale of contrast
d. No effect on contrast

Topic: Radiographic Procedures (Questions 111-170)

For the following questions, choose the single best answer.

111. An enlargement at the end of a bone is called a:
a. Prominence
b. Sharp prominence
c. Tubercle
d. Head

112. A rounded projection of moderate size is called a:
a. Prominence
b. Sharp prominence
c. Tubercle
d. Tuberosity

113. A spine describes a:
a. Prominence
b. Sharp prominence
c. Tubercle
d. Tuberosity

114. A pit is described as a:
a. Fossa
b. Groove
c. Sulcus
d. Sinus

115. A furrow is described as a:
a. Fossa
b. Groove
c. Sulcus
d. Sinus

116. A "typical" skull would be described as:
a. Synarthroses
b. Amphiarthroses
c. Diarthroses
d. Mesocephalic

117. Synovial joints are called:
   a. Synarthroses
   b. Amphiarthroses
   c. Diarthroses
   d. Mesocephalic

118. Fibrous joints are called:
   a. Synarthroses
   b. Amphiarthroses
   c. Diarthroses
   d. Mesocephalic

119. The radiocarpal joint has what type of movement?
   a. Hinge
   b. Pivot
   c. Saddle
   d. Condyloid

120. The proximal radioulnar articulation has what type of movement?
   a. Hinge
   b. Pivot
   c. Saddle
   d. Gliding

121. Which of the following bones has a temporal process?
   a. Sphenoid bone
   b. Ethmoid bone
   c. Mandible
   d. Zygomatic bone

122. Which of the following bones has an alveolar process?
   a. Sphenoid bone
   b. Ethmoid bone
   c. Mandible
   d. Maxilla

123. Which of the following bones has wings?
   a. Sphenoid bone
   b. Ethmoid bone
   c. Mandible
   d. Maxilla

124. Which of the following bones has a coronal suture?
   a. Frontal bone
   b. Temporal bone
   c. Occipital bone
   d. Parietal bone

125. Which of the following bones has an external protuberance?
   a. Frontal bone
   b. Temporal bone
   c. Occipital bone
   d. Mandible

126. Which of the following bones consists of five fused segments?
   a. Sacrum
   b. Axis
   c. Thoracic vertebra
   d. Lumbar vertebra

127. Which of the following bones has a dens?
   a. Atlas
   b. Axis
   c. Thoracic vertebra
   d. Lumbar vertebra

128. Which of the following individual vertebrae are larger and heavier than other individual vertebrae?
   a. Atlas
   b. Axis
   c. Thoracic vertebra
   d. Lumbar vertebra

129. The eleventh and twelfth pairs of ribs are called:
   a. Manubrium
   b. Floating
   c. Xiphoid
   d. Jugular notch

130. The blunt cartilaginous tip of the sternum is the:
   a. Manubrium
   b. Floating
   c. Xiphoid
   d. Jugular notch

131. Between the greater and lesser tubercles of the humerus is (are) located the:
   a. Greater and lesser tubercles
   b. Bicipital groove
   c. Capitulum
   d. Trochlea

132. Below the tubercles of the humerus is (are) the:
   a. Greater and lesser tubercles
   b. Bicipital groove
   c. Capitulum
   d. Surgical neck

133. Which of the following part(s) of the humerus articulate(s) with the ulna?
   a. Greater and lesser tubercles
   b. Bicipital groove
   c. Capitulum
   d. Trochlea

134. This bone is located in the wrist, between the trapezoid and the hamate:
a. Scaphoid
b. Hamate
c. Pisiform
d. Capitate

135. This bone is located in the wrist, between the lunate and the pisiform:
a. Scaphoid
b. Hamate
c. Pisiform
d. Triquetrum

136. This bone distributes body weight from the tibia to the other tarsal bones:
a. Navicular
b. Calcaneus
c. Talus
d. Cuboid

137. This bone lies along the lateral border of the navicular bone:
a. Navicular
b. Calcaneus
c. Talus
d. Cuboid

138. Which of the following articulate(s) with the first, second, and third metatarsal bones?
a. Navicular
b. Calcaneus
c. Talus
d. Cuneiforms

139. This structure has superior, middle, and inferior lobes:
a. Trachea
b. Left lung
c. Right lung
d. Hilus

140. This structure is approximately 12 cm long and is located in front of the esophagus:
a. Trachea
b. Left lung
c. Right lung
d. Hilus

141. The narrow distal end of the stomach that connects with the small intestine is called the:
a. Rugae
b. Pylorus
c. Fundus
d. Greater curvature

142. The section of the stomach where the esophagus enters is called the:
a. Rugae
b. Pylorus
c. Fundus
d. Cardiac portion

143. The lateral surface of the stomach is called the:
a. Rugae
b. Pylorus
c. Fundus
d. Greater curvature

144. The portion of the colon located between the splenic flexure and the sigmoid portion is called the:
a. Duodenum
b. Descending
c. Ileum
d. Ascending

145. The portion of the small bowel that connects with the cecum is called the:
a. Duodenum
b. Jejunum
c. Ileum
d. Ascending

146. The portion of the small bowel that connects with the stomach is called the:
a. Duodenum
b. Jejunum
c. Ileum
d. Ascending

147. The outer part of the kidney is called:
a. Cortex
b. Medulla
c. Nephron
d. Glomeruli

148. The part of the kidney through which blood is first filtered is called the:
a. Cortex
b. Medulla
c. Nephron
d. Glomeruli

149. For radiography of the fingers, the central ray enters:
a. Perpendicular to the distal interphalangeal joint
b. Parallel to the distal interphalangeal joint
c. Parallel to the proximal interphalangeal joint
d. Perpendicular to the proximal interphalangeal joint

150. For a PA projection of the hand, the central ray is centered:
    a. Perpendicular to the first metacarpophalangeal joint
    b. Perpendicular to the third metatarsophalangeal joint
    c. Parallel to the third metacarpophalangeal joint
    d. Perpendicular to the third metacarpophalangeal joint

151. For a lateral projection of the wrist, the elbow must be flexed:
    a. 45 degrees
    b. 90 degrees
    c. Only slightly
    d. Approximately 25 degrees

152. For the PA axial projection of the clavicle, the central ray is angled:
    a. 25 to 30 degrees caudad
    b. 25 to 30 degrees cephalad
    c. 20 degrees caudad
    d. 20 degrees cephalad

153. For an AP projection of the toes, the central ray enters at the:
    a. Third metatarsophalangeal joint
    b. Second metacarpophalangeal joint
    c. First metatarsophalangeal joint
    d. Second metatarsophalangeal joint

154. For an AP projection of the foot, the central ray enters at the:
    a. Head of the third metatarsal
    b. Head of the second metatarsal
    c. Base of the first metatarsal
    d. Base of the third metatarsal

155. For an axial projection of the calcaneus, the central ray is angled how many degrees to the long axis of the foot?
    a. 25
    b. 15
    c. 10
    d. 40

156. For an AP projection of the ankle, the central ray is directed perpendicular to the:
    a. Lateral malleolus
    b. Ankle joint midway between malleoli
    c. Medial malleolus
    d. Tibia

157. For an AP projection of the knee, the central ray is angled:
    a. 5 to 7 degrees cephalad
    b. 5 to 7 degrees caudad
    c. 10 degrees cephalad
    d. 10 degrees caudad

158. For an AP projection of the cervical spine, the central ray is directed:
    a. 10 degrees cephalad
    b. Parallel to C4
    c. 15 to 20 degrees caudad
    d. 15 to 20 degree cephalad

159. For a lateral projection of the cervical spine, the central ray is directed:
    a. Perpendicular to C4
    b. Parallel to C4
    c. 15 to 20 degrees caudad
    d. 20 to 25 degree cephalad

160. For an AP projection of the thoracic spine, the central ray is directed:
    a. 5 degrees cephalad
    b. Parallel to T7
    c. 3 to 4 degrees caudad
    d. Perpendicular to T7

161. For an AP projection of the lumbar spine, the central ray is directed:
    a. Parallel to the midline, entering at the level of the iliac crests
    b. Perpendicular to L2
    c. Perpendicular to the midline, entering at the level of the iliac crests
    d. Perpendicular to L4

162. For the AP oblique projections of the sacroiliac joints, the central ray is directed:
    a. 1 inch lateral to the elevated ASIS
    b. 1 inch medial to the elevated ASIS
    c. 1 inch lateral to the dependent ASIS
    d. 1 inch medial to the dependent ASIS

163. For the PA projection of the chest, the central ray is directed:
    a. Perpendicular to T10
    b. Parallel to the thoracic spine
    c. Perpendicular to T7
    d. Perpendicular to the posterior ribs

164. For the AP projection of the lower ribs, the central ray is directed:
a. Perpendicular to T10
b. Perpendicular to T5
c. Perpendicular to T7
d. Perpendicular to T12

165. For the AP axial (Towne) projection for the skull, the central ray is directed:
a. 30 degrees to the IOML
b. 37 degrees to the OML
c. 25 degrees to the IOML
d. 30 degrees to the OML

166. For the lateral projection for the facial bones, the central ray enters at the:
a. Glabella
b. Medial surface of the zygomatic bone
c. Medial surface of the nasal bone
d. Lateral surface of the zygomatic bone

167. For the parietoacanthial projection (Waters) for the sinuses, the OML forms an angle of how many degrees with the cassette?
a. 53
b. 45
c. 25
d. 37

168. For the PA axial projection for the colon, the central ray is angled caudad how many degrees?
a. 10 to 20
b. 20 to 30
c. 30 to 40
d. 25 to 45

169. The pelvocalyceal system will reach greatest visualization approximately how many minutes after injection?
a. 1 to 2
b. 2 to 5
c. 2 to 8
d. 15 to 20

170. For the RPO and LPO projections for the kidneys, how many degrees is the patient's body rotated?
a. 15
b. 25
c. 30
d. 45

Topic: Patient Care (Questions 171-200)

171. Violations of civil law are known as:
a. Assault
b. Battery
c. False imprisonment
d. Torts

172. Unjustified restraint of a patient defines:
a. Assault
b. Battery
c. False imprisonment
d. Invasion of privacy

173. Unlawful touching of the patient without consent is called:
a. Assault
b. Battery
c. False imprisonment
d. Invasion of privacy

174. Verbally spreading false information that defames another's character could lead to a charge of:
a. *Respondeat superior*
b. *Res ipsa loquitur*
c. Gross negligence
d. Slander

175. A legal doctrine that states that the cause of the negligence is obvious is known as:
a. *Respondeat superior*
b. *Res ipsa loquitur*
c. Gross negligence
d. Slander

176. Tachycardia indicates a pulse of:
a. More than 100 beats per minute
b. Fewer than 60 beats per minute
c. Greater than 90 beats per minute
d. Less than 50 beats per minute

177. Some level of hypertension is indicated when diastolic pressure is:
a. More than 100 beats per minute
b. Fewer than 60 beats per minute
c. Greater than 90 beats per minute
d. Less than 50 beats per minute

178. When oxygen is administered to the patient, the usual flow rate is:
a. 3 to 5 L per second
b. 5 L per hour
c. 1 to 3 L per minute
d. 3 to 5 L per minute

179. This item is used to clear an obstructed airway:
   a. Crash cart
   b. Suction unit
   c. Defibrillator
   d. Sphygmomanometer

180. This item is used to restore the heart to normal rhythm:
   a. Crash cart
   b. Suction unit
   c. Defibrillator
   d. Sphygmomanometer

181. The type of shock that is caused by a severe allergic reaction is called:
   a. Hypovolemic shock
   b. Septic shock
   c. Neurogenic shock
   d. Anaphylactic shock

182. The item that is used to feed the patient or to suction gastric contents is the:
   a. Ventilator
   b. Nasogastric tube
   c. Chest tube
   d. Venous catheter

183. The item that must never be placed above the level of the bladder is the:
   a. Ventilator
   b. Nasogastric tube
   c. Chest tube
   d. Urinary catheter

184. A mechanical respirator is called a:
   a. Ventilator
   b. Nasogastric tube
   c. Chest tube
   d. Venous catheter
   e. Urinary catheter

185. Barium sulfate should be mixed with water at what temperature for a barium enema?
   a. 100° C
   b. 75° F
   c. 85° C
   d. 100° F

186. A positive contrast agent administered to the patient in the form of an inert salt is:
   a. Barium sulfate
   b. Iodine
   c. Perforated ulcers or ruptured appendix
   d. Air

187. Indications for using aqueous iodine as a contrast agent include:
   a. Barium sulfate
   b. Iodine
   c. Perforated ulcers or ruptured appendix
   d. Air

188. A positive contrast agent usually used in nonionic form is:
   a. Barium sulfate
   b. Iodine
   c. Perforated ulcers or ruptured appendix
   d. Air

189. Factors that may cause the patient to react to a contrast agent simply as a result of anxiety are termed:
   a. Local irritation
   b. Cardiovascular
   c. Anaphylactic
   d. Psychogenic

190. A reaction that may occur in the vein in which the injection occurred is:
   a. Local irritation
   b. Cardiovascular
   c. Anaphylactic
   d. Phlebitis

191. This type of infection transmission occurs when an animal contains and transmits an infectious organism to humans:
   a. Contact transmission
   b. Airborne transmission
   c. Droplet transmission
   d. Vectorborne transmission

192. This type of infection transmission occurs as a result of coughing or sneezing:
   a. Contact transmission
   b. Airborne transmission
   c. Droplet transmission
   d. Common vehicle transmission

193. This type of infection transmission occurs when an infected person or contaminated object touches a host:
   a. Contact transmission
   b. Airborne transmission
   c. Droplet transmission
   d. Common vehicle transmission

194. The complete removal of all organisms from equipment and the environment in which patient care is conducted is called:
a. Medical asepsis
b. Surgical asepsis
c. Standard precautions
d. Gas sterilization

195. The system that uses barriers between blood, all body fluids, nonintact skin, and mucous membranes of all individuals and susceptible persons is called:
a. Medical asepsis
b. Surgical asepsis
c. Standard precautions
d. Gas sterilization

196. Soaking objects in germicidal solution causes:
a. Medical asepsis
b. Surgical asepsis
c. Standard precautions
d. Chemical sterilization

197. The abbreviation that means "biopsy" is:
a. hx
b. bx
c. CVA
d. MI

198. The abbreviation that means "nothing by mouth" is:
a. hx
b. bx
c. CVA
d. NPO

199. The word part that means "organ" is:
a. viscer
b. megal
c. trans
d. emia

200. The word part that means "kidney" is:
a. viscer
b. megal
c. trans
d. nephr

Scoring

Traditionally you have probably focused on how many questions you miss on an exam. As you prepare for the certification exam, I encourage you to focus on how many you answer correctly. Use Table 7-3 to calculate the percentage of questions you answered correctly in each category and on the test as a whole. Remember, a score below 75% on any topic or the entire test is an indication that more review is needed on that topic. Now, go back and concentrate on which items were missed and the reason why. When you are done reviewing, go on to the tutorials and tests found on the companion CD-ROM included with this book.

TABLE 7-3	**Calculating Your Score for Challenge Test #3**	
Topic	**Percentage calculation**	**Your score**
Radiation protection	Number correct _____ times 100, ÷ 30 =	
Equipment operation and maintenance	Number correct _____ times 100, ÷ 30 =	
Image production and evaluation	Number correct _____ times 100, ÷ 50 =	
Radiographic procedures	Number correct _____ times 100, ÷ 60 =	
Patient care	Number correct _____ times 100, ÷ 30 =	
TOTAL	Number correct _____ times 100, ÷ 200 =	

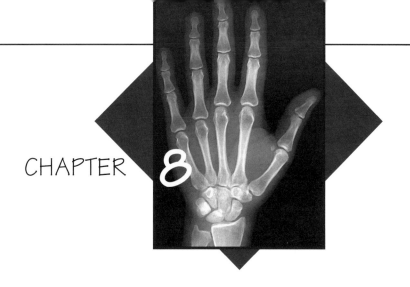

CHAPTER *8*

Examination Procedure

APPLICATION PROCESS

At the appropriate point in your educational program, your program director will provide you with a booklet published by the American Registry of Radiologic Technologists titled *Examinee Handbook*. Read everything in the handbook that pertains to the radiography examination. You should also pay close attention to the ARRT Rules and Regulations as well as the Standards of Ethics. Although your program director may highlight certain portions of the booklet, it remains your responsibility to understand everything it contains. This is probably the most important exam you have taken thus far in your life, so be sure to read the materials provided.

After reading the entire booklet, it is important to fill out the application, providing all of the information requested. Be sure to fill in all information and dates accurately and print legibly. Be sure to observe the rule that requires you to attach a photograph to the application. You should submit the application up to 3 months before your anticipated graduation date.

Once you have signed the application, attach the check or money order for the application fee and insert these documents into the envelope provided in the *Examinee Handbook*. It is important that you mail the envelope yourself. Do not include it in a large envelope with applications from other members of your class, and do not trust anyone else to mail the application for you. When you mail your application, be sure to send it as certified mail and to request a return receipt. Although this will cost more than regular mail, it will ensure that you receive verification of the delivery of your application.

Some time after your application is received, your program director will receive a form on which to verify your status, and he or she will sign the form and return it to the ARRT to verify that you have in fact completed the educational program and are eligible to take the examination. This also includes verification that you have completed all required clinical and didactic competencies.

You will receive an application status report and admission ticket from the ARRT. This can be expected to arrive up to 6 weeks after receipt of your application. When you receive the admission ticket, you should immediately check it to verify the examination window dates, the examination to be taken, and the personal identification on the form. If any of this information is incorrect or has changed, or if you fail to receive an admission ticket within this time period, it is your responsibility to immediately contact the ARRT office at (651) 687-0048. Once you have received the admission ticket, put it in a safe place until the day of the exam.

You must have completed all of the educational requirements of your program to take the exam. This may be particularly significant if your program requires you to make up missed time after graduation. If missed time must be made up as a condition of program completion, you must fulfill this requirement before taking the exam.

MATERIALS NEEDED FOR THE EXAMINATION

You should take very few items with you to the exam center. No papers, books, calculators, purses, pagers, telephones, or food or drink of any kind may be taken into the testing room. The items that you should bring include your admission ticket with your picture attached and a photo ID (e.g., a driver's license). If you wish to use a calculator during the examination, it will be provided, upon request, by the test center personnel.

EXAMINATION APPOINTMENTS

The radiography examination is administered by appointment at designated Sylvan Technology Centers in cities listed in *Examinee Handbook*. Appointments may be made after receiving the application status report and admission ticket using a provided toll-free number. The appointment may be during the examination window that extends for 90 days beginning on the Wednesday after the application is processed by the ARRT. The test centers are usually open from 8 AM to 6 PM Monday through Friday.

It is important to note that environmental conditions can vary. As a result, the exam room may be warmer or cooler than you would prefer. If being too cool is a concern for you, consider taking a sweater into the exam room. A good way to prepare for a less-than-ideal situation is to study and take practice examinations under different conditions. By doing so, you will be able to adapt more easily to the variations in temperature and to the room arrangements that you may face when you take the real exam.

Careful reading of *Examinee Handbook* will ensure that you have everything you need for the examination. Addressing these issues well ahead of time will free your mind for the more important task—passing the examination.

WAITING FOR EXAMINATION RESULTS

Many graduates have commented that the most difficult period in this entire process is waiting for the results. You should plan on receiving your results about 4 weeks after taking the exam, although many receive theirs in far less time. You should call the ARRT office if you do not receive your score by then.

Problems outside the control of the ARRT may delay your receipt of the exam results. Weather or labor problems may cause delays in the delivery of the mail from the ARRT office to your address. Energy or weather problems may delay the printing of results. Unforeseen computer glitches may cause additional delays. Be aware that neither exam results nor explanations for delay are given over the telephone. The ARRT insists on quality control at all stages of the process to ensure that you receive excellent service and accurate results and credentials.

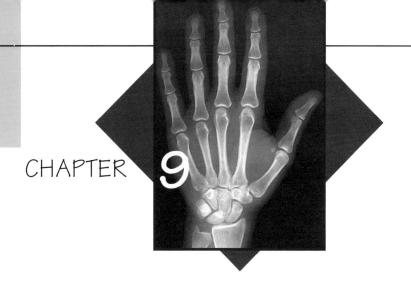

> *Do not fear the winds of adversity. Remember, a kite rises against the wind rather than with it.*

CHAPTER 9

Test-Taking Skills

PHYSICALLY AND MENTALLY PREPARING FOR EXAMINATION DAY

Although most of your preparation for the exam centers on reviewing your course work, the physical and mental preparation must be taken into account as well. The question of when, in relation to the exam date, to discontinue your review has no definite answer. It is a very individual decision based on how lengthy and thorough a review you have done and how comfortable you are with the material. Consulting your instructors to clarify your specific needs will prove most helpful in answering this question. A brief discussion of the points involved may assist you in deciding how long to study.

If you are the type of student who conducts a well-thought-out, carefully planned review of all of the material, as suggested in Chapter 1, it is reasonable to expect that studying will taper off within 2 to 3 weeks before the examination. If you use this review book effectively and cover all of the content areas over a period of at least 6 months, you should be well prepared for the examination and can draw your review to a close several weeks before the exam.

On the other hand, if you have not allowed yourself sufficient time to review and are attempting to compress your studying into a few weeks, you may wish to stop reviewing at a date that is closer to the exam. Be aware that anxiety, which will tend to increase as the exam approaches, may interfere with learning and recalling even the most basic information as you continue to review. It may also be true that if you have not learned the material over a period of time, there is little that you can learn in the last few weeks. Trying to cram for the exam is futile. If you have waited too long to begin studying, limit your review to the key points in all of the major subject areas.

As you prepare mentally for the day of the test, realize that apprehension about the exam may surface in unex-pected ways; it is not unusual for students to report having strange dreams about the exam. The content of these dreams involves driving for hours but never reaching the test center or starting the exam, falling asleep, and waking up with only 5 minutes left and nearly 200 questions to answer. These are all normal responses to your anticipation of a major event. They may also serve as a motivation to continue reviewing and preparing for the exam. You may wish to share your dream experiences with other students in your class. You will come to realize that most of them are having this response and that it is perfectly normal.

Another important aspect of preparation for the exam involves your physical readiness, which means having gathered all the materials you will need for the test and having prepared your body physically to take an exam of this type. Having the appropriate materials ready well in advance of the test has been discussed previously. Again, do not wait until the day before or the day of the exam to get your paperwork in order. Allowing several days to accomplish these tasks will ensure that you are prepared for any emergency that arises.

In preparing your body to take the exam, the basic rule of thumb is to treat exam day much as you would any other day. This phase of your preparation should actually begin the evening before the test. Intake of alcohol or large amounts of food should be avoided. You should get approximately the same amount of sleep as usual, waking at your normally scheduled time.

On the day of the exam, depending on the time of your appointment, use the time before the test to enhance your mental and physical readiness. Start the day by eating a substantial and healthy breakfast. Although you should do this every day, it is particularly important on test day. As the hour of the exam nears, you may feel less like eating. Having a light snack is a good idea; however, avoid high-sugar snacks so that you do not experience a blood sugar drop as you go in to take the exam.

If you have an exercise regimen that you follow daily, follow it on test day as well. For many, exercise helps relieve stress and anxiety. You will likely find that trips to the rest room will increase in number on test day. This is a normal physiologic response to the stress associated with the anticipation of a major event.

Is such physical preparation really necessary? Why should you be attentive to this aspect of test taking? With all of the time and effort expended during your 2 years of education in medical radiography and during the review process, you want to be certain that fatigue and physical stress do not impede your ability to take the examination.

Your instructors probably gave you a series of review examinations in the last few months of the program and you probably will have used the computer exams that accompany this text. This was to help assess your strengths and weaknesses in the various subject areas. Another reason was to help you become accustomed to sitting for 3 or 4 hours while taking an examination. It is important not to let the physical aspect of test taking hamper your ability to pass the exam.

The writing of this book is grounded in many years of experience preparing students to take the ARRT exam. Attention to the details in this section will help relieve your anxiety about the exam and allow you to focus on the more important aspects of reviewing and writing the exam.

STRATEGIES FOR TAKING THE EXAMINATION

Everyone tends to have a preferred system for taking a lengthy, multiple-choice format examination. If you have a method that has worked well in the past, then continue to use it. However, if you seem to lose focus when taking such a test, consider the following suggestions for structuring your approach to this exam.

Just getting started may be difficult for some individuals and cause them to experience discomfort. Many graduates have reported that upon beginning the test they were very uneasy. This is usually the result of the apprehension and stress surrounding this important event. Such an initial response should not be viewed as abnormal, and you can be assured that several of your peers are experiencing that same discomfort. Should this occur, close your eyes, breathe deeply several times, and start again. Unless you have severe exam anxiety or failed to review and prepare carefully ahead of time, you will be ready to begin answering the questions.

There are 200 test items on the exam, plus up to 20% additional pilot questions. You will have 3.5 hours to answer all of the questions. Additional time is allotted to complete a tutorial before beginning the exam and a survey after the exam. Questions are asked randomly, not by category. A test item includes the stem, or question, and the set of possible answers. The stem will ask a question or make an incomplete statement. Of the possible answers, one will be correct. The others are called distracters. Distracters are choices designed to make you think they are the correct answer. They will usually consist of the most common incorrect response or will include all but a small portion of the correct answer. There can be only one correct answer to the question.

Those who construct the exam attempt to include only those items for which there is a broad consensus regarding the correct response. Questions about specific departmental routines and information drawn from only one textbook are not used. Several sources are consulted when screening questions for the exam, and only the information common to most sources is used. There are no textbooks officially endorsed by the ARRT to screen or write test items, so you may be assured that you will not be penalized on the exam because you did not use a certain textbook as a student.

As you begin taking the exam, be sure to read each question carefully. It is extremely important to comprehend what is being asked. Do not attempt to read more into the question than is printed. Do not assume that it is a "trick" question. The exam is a carefully written, well-constructed document. There should be nothing on the test that you have not seen before in your studies and during your review. Be careful not to read the question the way you want it to be asked. Take the question at face value. Beware of words such as *none, every, always, never,* and *all.* These are qualifiers that often indicate a statement is false. In addition, be aware of the different types of items that may be asked. One type, called a *completion* or *open-ended question,* will simply give you a statement to complete, as in the following example:

1. The negative electrode in the x-ray tube is called the:
   a. Cathode
   b. Rotor
   c. Anode
   d. Focusing cup

Another type of item that may be used is the question. Here a complete question will be asked and you will need to choose the answer. An example of such an item follows:

2. Which interaction results in complete absorption of the energy of the incoming photon?
   a. Compton's
   b. Pair production
   c. Coherent scattering
   d. Photoelectric effect

The third form of test question—called a *negative-type item*—causes problems for many students. This item will measure your knowledge of exceptions to the data you have learned. Following is an example of a negative-type item:

3. Which of the following is not part of an image intensifier tube?
   a. Rotor
   b. Photocathode
   c. Input phosphor
   d. Cesium iodide

Becoming familiar with the types of items that may be used will help you anticipate what the exam will be like and will assist you in studying and preparing. A wide variety of question types are used in this book. Some will be found on the exam, whereas others are included only to encourage use of your critical thinking skills. Being aware of all of the types of questions will aid in your exam preparation.

After determining the type of item and reading the stem of the item, read each answer choice. Be certain to read all of the answers! Although choice *a* may appear to be correct, choice *d* may be a more complete answer:

4. An example of natural background radiation is:
   a. Radon gas
   b. The sun
   c. Radioactive elements in the earth
   d. All of the above

Reading the question and the first answer, *radon gas*, might lead you to answer *a* and move to the next question. After all, you learned that radon gas is a type of natural background radiation. However, taking the time to read all of the answers leads you to choices *b* and *c*. You remember that they are all types of natural background radiation, making choice *d* the correct answer. This is not a trick question; it is assessing whether you know the different sources of natural background radiation.

Be particularly careful of answer choices that may include several correct answers, such as *more than one but not all of the above, a and c,* or *b and d*. In such cases, take your time. Read each possible choice, and determine whether it is a correct answer on its own. One method used is to reread the question, complete it with each possible answer, and determine whether the resulting statement is true or false. A previous question has been rewritten below to provide an example:

5. An example of natural background radiation is:
   1. Cosmic radiation
   2. Medical and dental x rays
   3. Radon gas
   4. Radioactive elements in the earth
   5. Radioactive substances in food, water, and air
   6. Nuclear weapons testing
   a. 1, 2, 3
   b. 4, 5, 6
   c. 1, 3, 5, 6
   d. 1, 3, 4, 5

Take your time with this type of question. You will have plenty of time to complete the exam, even if you spend extra time on these items. Read the question, then look at choice *a*. Check to see whether every item in this choice makes a true statement when it is used to complete the test question. Ask yourself, "An example of natural background radiation is cosmic radiation, true or false?" The answer is true. Next, "An example of natural background radiation is medical and dental x rays, true or false?" The answer is false. You know that medical and dental x rays are a source of artificial or human-made radiation. This single false statement rules out choice *a* as a possible answer. Continue in this fashion until you have found a choice in which all of the possible statements are true. Using this example, that would be choice *d*.

Not all such questions will require you to take as much time to answer. However, having a specific method to use will reduce your anxiety when you are presented with a multiple-choice question that has several correct answers. Remember that after reading the question and all of the choices, the first answer you choose will usually be correct. Be careful not to begin second-guessing your choice of an answer. In addition, do not watch for patterns of answers. For example, resist choosing *a* because you haven't used it in a while, and do not be surprised if a certain answer choice is used for several consecutive questions.

There is no guessing penalty on the exam, so if you have no idea what the answer is, guess. However, have a strategy even when guessing. Do not choose an answer with terms that are unfamiliar to you. Students sometimes reason that such a choice must be the answer because they have never heard of it before. Most often, this is not the case. Make an educated guess by ruling out answers you are sure are wrong. Then choose from among those containing familiar terminology.

The certification exam is nothing to fear if you review and prepare properly. Be sure to consider the suggestions and strategies presented here and those identified by your instructors. If you have practiced and studied and have your strategy ready, the exam will be just another quiz.

PART II

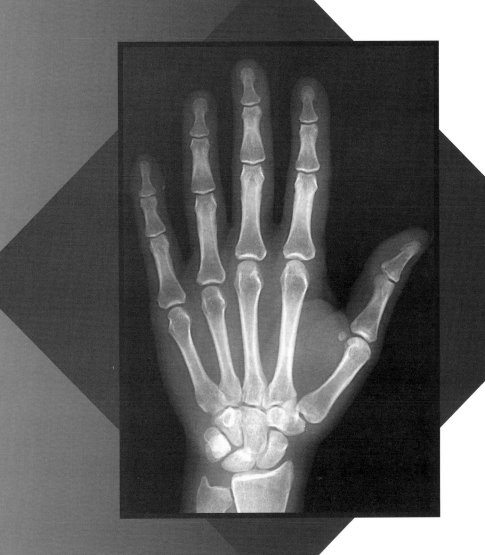

Preparation for Employment

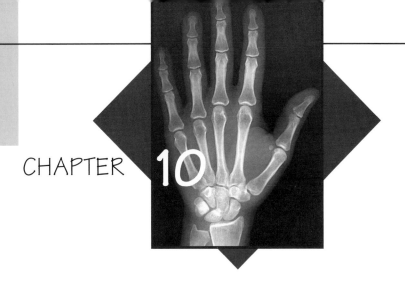

CHAPTER **10**

Career Planning

MOTIVATION

Individuals pursue chosen careers for a variety of reasons. Their sources of motivation for enrolling in an educational program and satisfying all of the graduation requirements may include the need for a stable income, the desire to become established in a career, or an interest in expanding their horizons. Incentives to undertake such a process are unique to each individual and may clearly distinguish a 45-year-old from an 18-year-old. It is also true that incentives can change as you move toward a goal, so that the circumstances that led you to select this educational program may differ considerably from those influencing you to establish a career in this field.

As the requirements for graduation from the educational program are met, it would be wise to examine your motivation for seeking employment and actually establishing a career in radiologic technology. You should reexamine your motivation and adjust your goals regularly—perhaps annually. The questions that follow will help with that process and assist you in establishing career goals.

1. Based on my studies and clinical education so far, what aspects of this profession am I really excited about?
2. Which aspects of patient care have I found the most satisfying?

Rationale: Questions 1 and 2 attempt to help you focus on what has brought you true satisfaction so far in the educational program. Being excited about what you do is critical to your longevity in the field. It is a daily reinforcement to your motivation. It helps you bring a positive attitude to class and to the clinical environment. Many individuals have certain aspects of patient care that they find particularly satisfying. Identifying yours will help you set goals for job placement or for continuing your education.

For example, if you find great satisfaction working with children, pediatric radiography may be an excellent choice for a career. You could consider job possibilities at children's hospitals. Perhaps trauma radiography is particularly challenging and satisfying for you. Pursuing employment at an institution with a trauma center and a shift with a high level of trauma cases would be a wise choice. Maybe teaching and working with students appeals to you. If so, your goals may include completing advanced academic degrees and finding a clinical job in a teaching institution.

Take time now to answer questions 1 and 2 in the space provided. Remember, you are examining situations you find motivating and exciting. You will have an opportunity to set your goals later in this chapter.

I am really excited about:

_____

_____

_____

The aspects of patient care that have been most satisfying are:

_____

_____

_____

3. Of the people with whom I have worked in clinical education, who has been most helpful?
4. Which characteristics do I want to emulate most?

Rationale: As a radiography student, you may be profoundly influenced by the personnel in the clinical department. It is important to identify people who have been particularly helpful to you as you have acquired your clinical skills. All too often, it is tempting to think about, talk about, and remember only those who have been hindrances to your education or who simply did not enjoy working with students. Concentrate instead on the positive people, and prepare a list of their names. Describe the personal and professional characteristics they possess. Explain why you enjoy working with them. Everyone benefits from role models. Describe why you wish to emulate, or pattern your professional attitudes and demeanor after, certain people with whom you have worked.

The most helpful individuals in clinical education have been:

_____

_____

_____

They have been great to work with because:

_____

_____

_____

I will emulate these positive behaviors (also explain why):

_____

_____

_____

5. When during the educational process have I been happiest?
6. When during the educational process have I been least happy?

Rationale: An awareness of events, people, or situations that have caused you to feel happy or unhappy will be helpful in setting goals for employment. Although it is not possible to be happy on the job all of the time or to always avoid unpleasant situations, being aware of such times can help you decide where you may or may not wish to work. In addition, addressing these issues now will help you gain an understanding of how you respond to positive and negative situations and how to alter your responses if necessary. You may also wish to consider ways in which you can retain a positive outlook when dealing with unpleasant situations or individuals by recalling successful self-motivating strategies

from the past. The mark of a true professional is the ability to summon the highest level of performance from yourself and those around you even during difficult times.

I have been happiest during my education when:

_____

_____

_____

I have been most dissatisfied during my education when:

_____

_____

_____

7. What employment needs will I have after graduation?
8. What financial needs will I have after graduation?
9. What housing needs and living conditions will I seek to meet after graduation?
10. Do I want or need to stay in this geographic area, or do I want or need to relocate?

Rationale: Unfortunately, individuals too often do little or no planning for their employment, financial needs, or living conditions and are consequently buffeted about by the winds of change and quirks of chance.

Consider what your needs will be for employment when you graduate. Decide whether you will need to begin work immediately and have to accept the first job offer you receive or whether you can wait a short time to scout the job market more thoroughly. It is crucial to have some idea of what your financial needs will be. Be aware of the cost of setting up your own living arrangements, paying back school loans, or providing for your family. If you are not currently responsible for your own housing, decide how it will be arranged. With a fluctuating job market, you must consider whether you will remain rooted where you are or relocate to find the type of position you desire. Perhaps relocating is something you have wanted to do all along. Or maybe relocating is simply not possible at this point in your life.

Answer each question in the space that follows. Describe what your needs and wants will be after graduation.

Employment:

_____

_____

_____

Financial:

_____

_____

_____

Housing:

_____

_____

_____

Location:

_____

_____

_____

Use the financial planning worksheet shown in Figure 10-1 to determine what your actual salary needs are. Be sure to base your salary needs on your income alone, even if you are or will be married.

11. Am I more excited about working with the high-touch (people-oriented) aspects of this profession or the high-tech (equipment) aspects of the field?

Annual Living Expenses

These are for the *entire year;* be sure to calculate *annual* figures.

Federal income tax (annual salary × 15%)	$ _____
Social Security tax (annual salary × 7.65%)	_____
State income tax (annual salary × ___%)	_____
Savings	_____
Health insurance	_____
Rent or house payment	_____
Child care	_____
College loan repayment	_____
Phone (monthly and long-distance)	_____
Electricity	_____
Water	_____
Gas	_____
Cable	_____
Cellular phone service	_____
Pager service	_____
Internet service provider	_____
Food (excluding eating out)	_____
Car payment	_____
Car insurance	_____
Car operation (gasoline, oil changes, etc.)	_____
Clothing	_____
Entertainment (night out, movie rentals, music, etc.)	_____
Gifts (for birthdays, holidays, weddings, anniversaries, etc.)	_____
Donations (place of worship, United Way, etc.)	_____
Debt, credit card payments	_____
Other: _____	_____
Other: _____	_____
Total annual estimated living expenses =	$ _____
I will need the following annual salary to meet these expenses:	$ _____
I will need the following hourly salary to meet these expenses:	$ _____
(divide annual salary needed by 2080 hours to determine hourly salary needed)	

This form is not meant to be a substitute for guidance provided by a financial counselor or tax advisor.
Scholarships or sign-on bonuses are not included in salary because they are one-time payments, not hourly salary.
Taxes could be reduced with personal exemptions, deductions, credits, etc. Consider these factors when calculating actual tax liability.

Figure 10-1 Annual living expenses.

Rationale: Some individuals work in this field because they truly love working with people and assisting with the diagnosis of their conditions. Others prefer working with complex electronic and computerized equipment and would rather not be involved in direct patient care. There is room for both types in this profession. Identifying the aspects of the field that excite you will help with your career planning.

Perhaps you wish to continue providing direct patient care. Maybe you would rather work in areas involving significant use of equipment, such as in quality control, medical physics, or the sale and service of equipment. Nothing will cause you to become more dissatisfied with your career choice than to be working in an area of radiologic technology to which you are not suited. Develop an awareness now of what you most enjoy doing. There is no right or wrong answer, and your choice does not make you "good" or "bad." Most important, be honest with yourself. You will have much to contribute to this field if you work where you are happiest and most productive.

Take some time and write in the space that follows your honest preferences based on your experiences so far. Remember, you are not setting a goal at this point, and your answer may change over time.

High tech versus high touch—my preference and why:

_____

_____

_____

_____

_____

12. Do I enjoy learning all that I can about this field, or do I want to learn only what I need to graduate?

Rationale: Your answer to this question is very important. The field you have chosen changes rapidly. You must be honest with yourself about your desire to study and learn. The equipment currently used in clinical education did not even exist just a few years ago. You will use equipment a few years after you graduate that does not exist today! If you are content to learn only what you need to graduate, you will soon possess skills that are outdated. You should also consider whether you truly enjoy learning or tend to regard it as a burden. Your education in this field will have barely begun by the time you graduate. Be aware that you will need to set a course for lifelong learning. Understanding this reality now will assist you in developing your professional attitude and planning for continuing education. Realizing the importance of a commitment to learning may also serve to motivate you through the remainder of your educational program.

Take time to assess your motivation for learning. In the space that follows, describe your honest feelings and attitudes about the enjoyment of learning for its own sake as opposed to learning just enough to perform your job.

I want to learn all that I can or just enough to get by. Here are my reasons and motivations:

_____

_____

_____

_____

_____

13. Which aspect(s) of the specialty of radiography do I enjoy the most (e.g., general, fluoroscopy, mobile, surgical, trauma, pediatric)?
14. Have I particularly enjoyed any other radiologic specialties (e.g., angiography, mammography, computed tomography, magnetic resonance imaging, sonography, nuclear medicine, radiation therapy, quality control)?

Rationale: You may not yet realize that radiography is a specialty within which are areas of further specialization (e.g., general, fluoroscopy, mobile). You are probably already familiar with the other specialties listed in question 14. By being aware of what you enjoy, you will have little difficulty later setting goals for employment or education. If you have not yet had the opportunity to spend clinical time in some of the mentioned areas, you may need to postpone answering this question. However, when such an opportunity arises, prepare yourself for the clinical experience by reading about the specialty area in your textbook and taking careful notes about your experiences. This field has countless opportunities for you in the practice of radiography or any of the other special imaging or therapy modalities.

Use the space that follows to list the areas in which you are particularly interested, and describe why you have enjoyed them. Also list the areas that you look forward to visiting, and explain why they are important to you.

I particularly enjoy working in the following area(s):

_____

_____

_____

I want to explore the following areas further:

_____

_____

_____

15. Are there any special projects that I have done that brought me satisfaction (e.g., research papers, exhibits, in-class presentations, participation in radiography college bowls)?
16. Am I interested in pursuing positions of leadership or membership in local, state, or national radiologic technology organizations?

Rationale: This profession needs you. It needs what you have to offer. It needs your fresh ideas and observations. It needs your leadership, motivation, talents, and abilities. By considering the issues raised in questions 15 and 16, you will be able to set goals for your postgraduation involvement.

Perhaps you have already written a research paper, constructed an exhibit, or participated in college bowl competition. Do not stop now. You have momentum working in your favor. Consider how these projects may have brought you satisfaction and served to motivate you further. Think about how you may set goals for doing additional projects as a radiographer for state or national presentations.

Local, state, and national professional organizations in radiologic technology need the involvement of motivated, committed professionals. Gauge your interest in becoming involved. Do not let fear of the unknown deter you. Remember that those who are currently active were at one time attending their first meeting, serving on a committee for the first time, or holding their first office. Think about how such involvement may add to your career and personal satisfaction.

In the space provided, write your thoughts and feelings about pursuing these activities. Describe how you would feel if you became involved at this level of the profession.

The special projects that brought me the most satisfaction were:

_____

_____

_____

I wish to become involved in the following organization(s) in this capacity:

_____

_____

_____

17. Do I believe I will have an interest in working with students when I am employed?

Rationale: You will need to assess your interest in working with students. Many of us truly enjoy helping students acquire skills, whereas others would prefer to avoid educating others. If you believe you would enjoy teaching, then seeking employment in an academic environment is a reasonable goal. If you would prefer not to work with students, it would be better for you and for the students to seek employment in another setting. Many otherwise excellent radiographers find frustration on the job because they are not suited to the clinical teaching role. Do not take this issue lightly. Having a student assigned to you every day of work can be exhilarating or burdensome, depending on your professional preferences.

In the space provided, state whether you prefer to work with students or to find employment in a nonteaching institution.

I would or would not like to work with students after graduation. Here are my reasons:

_____

_____

_____

_____

_____

18. In what type of clinical setting am I most comfortable (e.g., hospital, small clinic, physician's office, urgent care)?

Rationale: Health care assumes many forms, depending in part on the environment in which it is delivered. If you have had the opportunity to spend clinical time in more than one of the settings mentioned, decide which you enjoyed most. If you have not had this opportunity, check with your program director about the availability of clinical rotations. If none are available in the program, consider spending time outside of school in one or more of these clinical settings to get some idea of how they operate and to observe the radiographer at work.

Each clinical setting has qualities that will appeal to you as a radiographer and others that make it a less attractive choice. You may also be guided by a strong personal preference about where you would like to work. Consider these factors carefully when setting goals for employment.

I have had experience in the following clinical settings. Here is what I liked and disliked:

_____

_____

_____

_____

_____

19. What particular talents do I possess about which I feel proud?

Rationale: Identify your talents and all that you have to offer a potential employer. Consider how you may use these talents to pursue your personal and professional goals. Think of how your strengths may benefit the patients you serve. Understand the impact you may have on co-workers. It is important to be proud of your talents and use them. It is not conceited to list them. You must concentrate on being the best you can be by developing your abilities and acquiring others. Use them to enhance your practice of radiography and your personal life.

My particular talents and positive attributes follow. Here is how I have used them and why I am excited about them:

_____

_____

_____

_____

_____

_____

GOAL SETTING

By carefully answering the previous questions, you should develop a fairly good idea of the things that motivate you in this field. The choice of a career is important, and you should be intent on doing those things you particularly enjoy.

Individuals who have been successful in the field of radiologic technology are those who have set goals for themselves and worked hard to achieve them. Goal setting is not an easy task, particularly because it is seldom taught in school. However, all of the great motivational speakers and career planners indicate that goal setting should be a priority, not only when beginning a career, but throughout your working lifetime.

Goals are not meant to be etched in granite and never changed or updated. Goal statements should be flexible and fluid. As mentioned previously, goals should be updated as needed and at least annually.

The wording of goal statements can be as important as setting the goals themselves. Phrases such as "I want to be a nuclear medicine technologist within three years" are not powerful enough. "I will be a registered nuclear medicine technologist by the end of (specify year)" is more specific. It is action-oriented. It says you will do something, and you will direct your energies toward achieving that goal within a specific time frame. It is more than a wish; it is a statement of a goal that you expect to realize.

Post your goals where you can see them daily, and share them with those who are significant in your life. Their encouragement and moral support can help you achieve your goals. It is well documented that shared goals are more likely to be met because of the increased sense of accountability to others who are aware of them.

Following is a series of questions to consider as you write your goal statements. Sample goal statements are provided. Note that they are specific, have time frames, and use the words "I will." You may be thinking that you lack some of the information needed to write your goal statements. However, recognize that by writing goals and planning your future, you are in the process of making that future a reality. This helps you direct your energies toward pursuing and accomplishing your goals.

Setting goals should not be taken lightly, but it should not be so arduous a task that it becomes a burden. Be excited about setting your goals and beginning to map out your future. Do not get discouraged if your goals seem simple at first. They are there to provide you with direction. It will be up to you to adjust them and to direct the course you plan to follow.

1. What deadline have I set for completion of my goal statements? In other words, how soon will I have thought about them and written them down?

GOAL   *I will list my goals along with a timetable by the following date:* _____

2. What kind of review schedule have I established to prepare for the radiography certification exam?

GOAL   *I will review the subjects included on the exam according to the following schedule:*

Radiation protection:

_____

Equipment operation and maintenance:

_____

Image production and evaluation:

_____

Radiographic procedures:

_____

Patient care and management:

_____

3. Do I want to pursue additional education in radiologic technology or seek an advanced degree?

GOAL   *I will write letters requesting information on baccalaureate degrees by the following date:* _____

GOAL   *I will take* _____ *number of credit hours per semester beginning on* _____ *so that I will complete my degree on* _____ .

GOAL   *I will write letters requesting information on educational programs in (sonography, nuclear medicine, radiation therapy) by* _____ .

GOAL   *I will attend an educational program in (sonography, nuclear medicine, radiation therapy) beginning* _____ *and will graduate from the program in* _____ .

4. Do my regular study habits need to be examined and fine tuned?

GOAL   *I will examine my current study habits on* _____ .

GOAL   *I am modifying my current study habits as follows:* _____

_____

GOAL   *I will begin my new study habits on* _____ .

5. Do I need to examine my lifestyle choices regarding diet, exercise, sleep requirements, etc.?

GOAL   *I will evaluate my lifestyle choices in diet, exercise, sleep, and recreation on* _____ .

GOAL   *I am modifying my diet as follows (be specific):*

_____

_____

_____

_____

GOAL   *I am modifying my exercise routine as follows (be specific):*

_____

_____

_____

_____

GOAL   *I am modifying my sleep routine as follows:*

_____

_____

GOAL   *I am taking time for recreation as follows:*

_____

_____

_____

6. Have I taken into account the needs of my family or significant others?

GOAL   *I will consult with my significant others regarding these goals on* _____ .

GOAL   *I will list here the needs of my significant others in view of the goals I have set on* _____ .

_____

_____

7. What do I want to accomplish in the next 30, 60, and 90 days related to my career?

GOAL   *By 30 days from now, on* _____ ,

I will have accomplished the following to advance my career goals:

_____

_____

_____

_____

GOAL   *By 60 days from now, on _____ ,
I will have accomplished the following to advance my career goals (built on my 30-day objectives):*

_____

_____

_____

_____

GOAL   *By 90 days from now, on _____ ,
I will have accomplished the following to advance my career goals (built on my 30- and 60-day objectives):*

_____

_____

_____

_____

8. To reinforce my positive attitude, I will need to obtain access to motivational materials.

GOAL   *By _____ , I will read the following motivational books:*

_____

_____

_____

_____

9. Postgraduation needs that I must consider:

GOAL   *I will begin work by _____ .*

GOAL   *I will make the following hourly salary to maintain the lifestyle I have chosen: _____*

GOAL   *I will live in the following type of house or apartment: _____*

GOAL   *I will live in the following city or geographic area: _____*

10. High-tech versus high-touch aspects of radiography:

GOAL   *I will work in the following direct patient care area of medical radiography: _____*

GOAL   *I will work in the following nonpatient care area:*

_____

_____

11. Continuing education in radiography:

GOAL   *I will follow this schedule for remaining current in my chosen field:*

Type of meetings or conferences I will attend regularly:

Local: _____

State: _____

National: _____

12. Other radiologic specialties:

GOAL   *I will do extra reading and clinical observation in the following radiologic specialties (e.g., angiography, mammography, computed tomography, magnetic resonance imaging, sonography, nuclear medicine, radiation therapy, quality control) by the dates I have listed:*

_____

_____

_____

_____

_____

13. Special projects to pursue after graduation:

GOAL   *I will write a research paper and submit it for competition at the state or national level on _____ . The possible subjects for this paper are:*

_____

_____

_____

GOAL   *I will prepare an exhibit for presentation at a state or national meeting on _____ . The possible subjects for this exhibit are:*

_____

_____

_____

GOAL   *I will assist with planning the following local or state meeting: _____ on _____ .*

GOAL   *I will run for the office of my local, state, or national professional organization on _____ .*

14. Working with students:

GOAL   *I will work in a department that (is/is not) in a teaching institution.*

15. Work setting:

GOAL   *I will work in the following type of institution: hospital, clinic, physician's office, urgent care.*

_____

16. Professional attributes:

GOAL   *I will work to maintain the attributes that I admire most in the professionals who have helped in clinical education. Those attributes are:*

_____

_____

_____

_____

17. Other goals I am setting for myself:

GOAL

_____

_____

_____

GOAL

_____

_____

GOAL

_____

_____

GOAL

_____

_____

GOAL

_____

_____

By now you have had considerable experience in describing the aspects of this field that you find motivating. You have also listed specific career goals that you have the ability to achieve. Performing this type of personal inventory has gotten you off to a great start. In addition to reading your goal statements daily, reexamine these goals at regular intervals over the coming months. There will be no stopping you now!

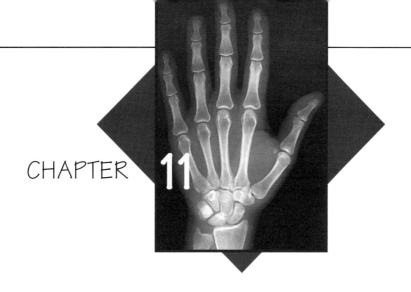

CHAPTER **11**

Writing a Professional Resume

PURPOSE OF A RESUME

Your resume is, in effect, your professional calling card. It is a summary of your academic and work history and relevant accomplishments and credentials. It should be brief (i.e., one or two pages). It is essentially a snapshot of your career to date. In addition to offering samples of resumes, this section also describes ways in which to use the resume and provides the rationale for including or excluding certain information.

There are probably as many different styles and formats for resumes as there are instructors attempting to describe them. You may wish to take advantage of your radiography instructor's expertise in this area. In addition, if you are enrolled in a collegiate radiography program, it may have a learning resource center, a writing center, or a career counseling center from which you can obtain additional guidance. A visit to a bookstore will reveal the many different books available on the subject of writing resumes. In addition, numerous software packages that provide guidance on writing resumes are available. With all of these resources to choose from, writing a resume can become a dizzying experience. However, the material presented in this chapter was developed for courses taught by a radiographer and has been used by students and graduates.

The resume may be used in three ways; it may be (1) sent as part of a mailing to prospective employers and followed with a telephone call, (2) left with an interviewer after an appointment, or (3) included with the job application form submitted to the human resources department.

Often, the student or graduate radiographer wishes to indicate availability to a large number of prospective employers in a certain geographic area. The resume, accompanied by a cover letter, may be mailed to the directors of radiology at all facilities in the area where the student is interested. Although this is the least effective method to use

in a job search, a well-constructed resume with an appropriate cover letter can produce results. Figure 11-1 shows a sample cover letter to accompany the resume in these situations. Such a mailing should always be followed by a personal telephone call to the radiology manager, as promised in the cover letter. Following up in this way can become time consuming, but it is one method to use when attempting to reach a large number of prospective employers.

In certain situations the student or graduate radiographer may actually have an informal interview with a radiology manager who is considering filling a position. This often occurs when students or graduates are told about a job opening. In these situations, there may be insufficient time to mail a resume in advance. When this occurs, the interviewee should take a copy of the resume and give it to the radiology manager at the interview. Similar to appropriate attire and grooming, a professional resume can make a powerful first impression during such an interview.

CONTENTS OF A RESUME

In addition to making certain that you have the appropriate writing tools available, it is also important to spend time thinking about what to include and exclude from the resume. Include all postsecondary (i.e., after high school) education. You should account for all of your time since high school. Be sure to enter all professional society memberships, credential numbers, awards, and accomplishments on the resume.

The resume should contain only information that is relevant to your accomplishments and goals as a professional. Information of a personal nature (beyond that presented in the next section) or data that could be used to discriminate should be excluded from the resume. Your

```
Date


Director of Radiology
XYZ Hospital
Main Street
Anytown, USA  01234


Dear Director:

Enclosed please find my professional resume outlin-
ing my education and work experiences. I am very
interested in being considered for employment in
your department of radiology in the position of
staff radiographer. I appreciate whatever time and
attention you are able to give to this inquiry.

I will call you in a few days to see what employ-
ment opportunities you may have available.

Sincerely,
```

Figure 11-1   Sample cover letter.

resume is an opportunity to advertise yourself in your absence. Construct it wisely.

WRITING THE RESUME

Figures 11-2 and 11-3 show two resumes that could have been written by student or graduate radiographers. The resumes present applicants with slightly different backgrounds and therefore include different information. Your resume is likely to be a variant of these. Keep in mind that brevity is the rule when constructing your resume. However, do not use abbreviations for state names, organizations, and formal titles. Keep your resume polished and proper.

Personal Data

The first section should include your name, followed by the address and phone number at which you may be reached during your current job search. Be aware that if your address and phone number are going to change in the very near future, the prospective employer will be unable to contact you, possibly eliminating you as a candidate for the position. If you must change your address and phone number after submitting the resume, be sure to inform prospective employers in writing.

No additional personal information should be included on the resume. Specific items to be excluded are date of birth, gender, race, marital status, church affiliation, number of children, disabilities, and any other data that are irrelevant to your status as a job seeker. Although such information may not be used by a prospective employer, including it on your resume places you in the position of having raised it as an issue.

Goal Statement

As shown in the examples, the next section of the resume should include your goal statement. The goal statement can be as simple as "To obtain a position as an entry-level radiographer," or it may include your desire to cross-train in another specialty, such as "To obtain a position as an entry-level radiographer; desire to cross-train in computed tomography." Careful consideration should be given to the goal statement. If the wording suggests that you absolutely must have the opportunity to cross-train in other modalities, you will be eliminated from consideration if the prospective employer is looking for a staff radiographer only. Wording such as "To obtain a position as an entry-level radiographer; willing to be cross-trained in other modalities" indicates your desire to expand your horizons but without the sense of urgency conveyed by the previous statement.

The goal statement may also be altered depending on where you are seeking employment. If you know the prospective employer is seeking radiographers who definitely want to cross-train, then that interest should be included in your goal statement. In addition, if one of your goals is to cross-train and you are unwilling to accept a position that does not offer that opportunity, then you should definitely include it in your goal statement, realizing that you may be excluded from consideration if such a position is not available. Words in the goal statement that identify the strength of your interest are "desire to cross-train" or "willing to cross-train."

As you prepare to write your resume and begin setting your professional goals, give them serious consideration. The goal statement may include you in the final group of candidates for a position, or it may exclude you immediately, depending on how it is worded. As a final example, consider the goal statement of an applicant to a clinic or urgent care setting. Many times the responsibilities in these positions are multifaceted. A goal statement such as "To obtain a position as a radiographer; willing to perform venipuncture, simple laboratory procedures, and electrocardiograms and take patient histories and vital signs" indicates not only a willingness to learn new procedures but an ability to be flexible and work as a team member in a small clinic setting. Conversely, if you have no desire to perform these other functions, you should not include such places in your job search.

Employment Experiences

Beginning with your most recent employment and working backward, you should list all employment experiences

Personal Data
    Applicant Name
    Applicant Address
    City, State, Zip Code
    Telephone Number

Goal
    To obtain a position as an entry-level radiographer

Employment Experience
    December 20__-Present
    Darkroom Assistant and Transporter
    Department of Radiology
    XYZ Area Hospital
    This Town, State
    Process films; clean processor; transport patients to and from radiology department

    May 20__-October 20__
    Nursing Assistant
    Elderly Manor
    This Town, State
    Answered residents' call lights; served meals; assisted with bathing; assisted with meals

Education
    20__-Present
    School of Radiography
    ABC Memorial Hospital
    That City, State
    Accredited program in medical radiography
    Will graduate June 20__

    19__-20__
    Liberal Arts Coursework
    Black Hawk Community College
    This Town, State
    Took 36 semester hours

Professional Accomplishments, Associations, and Credentials
    • Registry eligible—Taking exam in May 20__
    • Student member, American Society of Radiologic Technologists
    • Student member, This State Society of Radiologic Technologists
    • Awarded Second Place for presentation of research paper entitled "Crohn's Disease" at State Society
      Annual Conference

References available upon request.

Figure 11-2 Sample resume.

related either to health care or working with the public. Indicate the month and year that each position began and ended, the name of the employer, the location of the employer, and a simple phrase describing your responsibilities. It is not necessary to list the names of supervisors or the salary you received. It is also not necessary to account for every job held since high school. Remember, the resume is your statement of professional experience. Include those positions that demonstrate your ability to work with people.

Education

Your resume should include all of the formal education you have acquired since high school, listed in reverse chronologic order (i.e., beginning with the most recent). It is not necessary to provide a detailed list of the courses studied. Rather, you may wish to indicate a broad area of study (e.g., liberal arts and sciences). Some entries in this section will be self-explanatory. A radiology manager will not require explanation of an entry such as "School of Radiography." In

Personal Data

Applicant Name
Applicant Address
City, State, Zip Code
Telephone Number

Goal

To obtain a position as an entry-level radiographer; willing to cross-train in angiography or mammography

Employment Experience

September 20__-Present

Front Office Clerk
Imaging Department
City Memorial Hospital
This Town, State
Greet patients; enter computer record; file radiographs

November 19__-July 20__
Serving Line Worker
Dietary Department
Saints Hospital
Our Town, State
Greeted employees and visitors in cafeteria serving line; served their choice of food; ran cash register on weekends

Education

June 20__-May 20__
Associate Degree Radiography Program
Our Community College
This City, State
Accredited program in medical radiography
Graduated May 20__; awarded Associate in Applied Sciences Degree

19__-20__
Radiography program prerequisites
Our Community College
This Town, State
Took 48 semester hours in liberal arts and sciences

Professional Accomplishments, Associations, and Credentials

- Certified by the American Registry of Radiologic Technologists, #987654
- Licensed by State of __, # 123-45-6789-1-1.
- Active member, American Society of Radiologic Technologists
- Active member, This State Society of Radiologic Technologists
- Awarded Second Place for presentation of research paper entitled "Crohn's disease" at State Society Student Conference
- Member of student team competing in annual Radiography College Bowl sponsored by State Society of Radiologic Technologists

References available upon request.

Figure 11-3   Sample resume.

each of your educational experience entries, indicate whether you graduated or received some form of certificate or diploma. The dates in this section, along with those accompanying your employment history, should account for most of your time since high school.

Professional Accomplishments, Associations, and Credentials

In this section, you should list all professional organizations to which you belong. Be sure to include any offices or other positions of responsibility you have held, such as being a member or head of a committee. Examples of information for this section include membership in local, state, or national professional societies; membership in student radiographer associations; and any professional licenses already held. Awards for academic excellence should be included, as well as participation in competitions, such as research paper writing, scientific exhibits, and college bowls. You may also wish to include a list of your attendance at state or national professional society meetings.

If you have not yet taken the ARRT exam, you should describe your status as "Registry Eligible—Taking exam in May 20__." If you have taken the exam but have not yet received your results, describe your status as "Registry Eligible—Took exam in August 20__; waiting for results." Radiology managers encounter this situation routinely and are not dissuaded from considering your application because of your transitional status. If you have received your results, you should indicate your ARRT number and expiration date. Do not include your test score.

References

References are not listed on the professional resume. The prospective employer will provide space on the job application form for listing both work and personal references. For the resume itself, the statement "References available upon request" will suffice. Be sure you have obtained the permission of those individuals you wish to use as references so that they will be expecting inquiries from prospective employers.

THE COVER LETTER

If mailed, the resume should always be accompanied by a brief and concise cover letter. Figure 11-4 shows a sample of a cover letter that you can adapt for your use.

APPEARANCE OF THE RESUME AND COVER LETTER

One of the most valuable tools that can be used to write the resume is a computer or word processor. You will be able to

Date

Director of Radiology
XYZ Hospital
Main Street
Anytown, USA 01234

Dear Director:

It was with great interest that I read your hospital's advertisement for the position of staff radiographer. Enclosed please find my professional resume outlining the experiences and education that I believe qualify me for this position.

I wish to notify you of my interest in being employed in your department. I am also completing an application for employment in your Department of Human Resources and am including a copy of my resume with it. I look forward to hearing from you regarding a personal interview so that we may discuss our mutual needs and interests.

Sincerely,

Figure 11-4 Sample cover letter.

work through a rough draft and refine the resume as required fairly easily. Be certain to take advantage of the "spell check" if your computer is equipped with this feature. Handwritten and even typewritten resumes are no longer acceptable. For the most professional-looking resume, you should print your documents using a laser or ink-jet printer.

Be aware that others who are competing with you for the same positions are preparing and printing their resumes with modern writing equipment. If you do not own such equipment, computers and word processors are available in college writing centers and in many copy shop retail stores. Use of these facilities and equipment, which typically are available at a modest price, is a wise investment.

There are as many different types of paper available as there are resume formats. The resume and cover letter should be printed on 60- to 75-lb text paper that is preferably white or ivory, which will provide a positive image for your resume. Because this paper has a heavier weight, it should not be folded. Therefore you should use a large manilla envelope so that the resume and cover letter are flat and unfolded. If you are unfamiliar with paper types and weights, your writing center or retail copy shop will be happy to provide you with information.

Avoid using copier or typewriter paper; it is an inexpensive grade of paper and does not make a positive impression on the reader. In addition, many papers of this type will produce a poorer printed image when used with a laser printer.

JOB APPLICATION FORM

Students are often dismayed that after investing much time and effort into writing a resume, they must still complete a job application form. This is a standard practice for many employers. Regardless of whether you are applying at several radiology facilities or just one, you should always bring a copy of the resume and make sure it is attached to the job application form. You should never indicate on the application form that the resume is attached; however, by bringing the resume to the human resources office, you will have most of the information you need to fill in the job application form.

Figure 11-5 shows a typical job application form for a community hospital. Note the information that you will need to completely fill out a form of this type. Make certain you bring all of the information with you (e.g., names and addresses of former employers; names, addresses, and telephone numbers of references), especially if it is not included on the resume.

Be aware that you may request former employers not be contacted. In addition, a detailed employment and reference check cannot be conducted without your signed authorization. Be certain to carefully read the statement you are signing at the bottom of the application form. Remember, although you have provided all of the information requested on the application form, it is still important to attach the resume.

Proper preparation of a professional resume is a task not to be taken lightly. Spend the time needed to carefully construct your resume, and be aware of its impact on potential employers. Your resume is a statement of your professionalism that speaks about you in your absence.

EMPLOYMENT APPLICATION

Last Name	First	Middle	Social Security Number
Present address	City	State Zip	Telephone Number
Position applied for	Date		Salary desired

How were you referred to this facility?	Are you available for: ☐ Full-time ☐ Part-time
Do you have relatives or friends employed in this facility? ☐ Yes ☐ No Department:	☐ Regular ☐ Temporary Date available:

Have you ever been employed by this facility? ☐ Yes ☐ No When:	Are you under 18? ☐ Yes ☐ No	Would you consider working: Weekends & holidays ☐ Yes ☐ No
Long-range occupational goals:		Rotating shifts ☐ Yes ☐ No On call ☐ Yes ☐ No Any shift ☐ Yes ☐ No
Are you a United States citizen or an alien legally authorized to work in the United States? ☐ Yes ☐ No		Shift preference:
Have you been convicted of a felony? ☐ Yes ☐ No If yes, explain:		☐ Days ☐ Evenings ☐ Nights ☐ 8-hour shift ☐ 12-hour shift

After reviewing the essential functions of the job for which you are applying, are you able to perform them? ☐ Yes ☐ No If no, please explain.

School	Name & Address of School	Course of study	Did you graduate?	Diploma or degree
High				
College				
College				

Other: Business college, Other Special Courses (Include Special Military Training)

Ares of Specialization or Major Interest:	Typing: Approx. WPM _____ Shorthand: Approx. WPM _____

List health care, business, or industrial equipment operated:

Professional Licenses and/or Certifications

Are you currently: ☐ Registered ☐ Licensed ☐ Certified
    Eligible for: ☐ Registration ☐ Licensure ☐ Certification

	Type	State Issued	Date	Number
If Licensed, Registered, or Certified	Type	State Issued	Date	Number
	Type	State Issued	Date	Number

Figure 11-5 Sample job application form. *Continued*

List previous employers with most recent first	From	To	Immediate Supervisor	Last Salary
Job Title				

Employer Name _____ Phone _____
Address_____
Duties _____
Reason for leaving_____

	From	To	Immediate Supervisor	Last Salary
Job Title				

Employer Name _____ Phone _____
Address_____
Duties _____
Reason for leaving_____

	From	To	Immediate Supervisor	Last Salary
Job Title				

Employer Name _____ Phone _____
Address_____
Duties _____
Reason for leaving_____

State if you do not want us to contact any of the above listed former employers and the reasons you do not want each contacted.

Can we run a detailed employment check, including, but not limited to, a check with your previous employers? ☐ Yes ☐ No
Please sign here to authorize reference check _____

List references who are not relatives or employers:

Name	Company and Address	Present Title	Telephone #

Carefully read this section prior to providing signatures below.

I consent to any medical examination required by the facility at any time to determine my ability to perform the duties of my job or other jobs with the facility and I understand that my employment may be conditioned upon satisfactorily passing a physical examination.

I understand that my employment can be terminated at any time and for any reason, at the option of either the facility or myself. I understand that no one has any authority to enter into any agreement for employment for any specified period of time or to make any agreement contrary to the foregoing, except for a written employment agreement signed by the Chief Executive Officer of this facility.

I hereby affirm that the information provided on this application (and accompanying resume, if any) is true and complete. I understand that any false or misleading representations or omissions may disqualify me from further consideration for employment and may result in discharge even if discovered at a later date.

I hereby authorize persons, schools, my current employer (if applicable) and previous employers and organizations named in this application (and accompanying resume, if any) to provide this facility and all affiliates with any relevant information regarding an employment decision, and I release all such persons from any and all liability regarding the provision or use of such information.

Date _____   Signature _____

Figure 11-5, cont'd   Sample job application form.

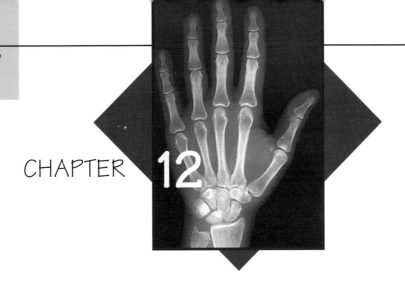

CHAPTER 12

Interviewing Techniques

PURPOSE OF AN INTERVIEW

If your resume is your detailed calling card, then your personal interview is your house call. It is your only opportunity to make a strong, lasting first impression with your possible future employer. Because of the many legal changes surrounding the issue of discrimination, the personal interview may not be as detailed as it has been in the past. However, this does not diminish its significance or the importance of proper preparation.

The employer can use the personal interview to verify information submitted on the resume or job application. It can serve as an opportunity for the employer to show you the facilities in which you may be working, familiarize you with the equipment, and determine your experience with such equipment. The interviewer may also be interested in your career goals and plans for establishing a career.

Keep in mind that another purpose of an interview is for you to become acquainted with your prospective employer. It is also a time for you to decide whether you want to work for that department or organization if offered a job. As you prepare for the interview, always remember that it is a two-way street.

PERSONAL APPEARANCE

There is no substitute for making a strong first impression with the person or persons who will be conducting your interview. Like it or not, we are a very visual society, and your physical appearance during your initial contact with the interviewers will have a profound effect on their perception of you as a potential employee.

How you choose to present yourself for your interview says a lot about your professional self-image. Regardless of where you work, you represent that department or organization to the patient or customer. Appropriate professional attire begins with the interview and continues every day once the job begins.

Dressing for social occasions varies by age group and geographic region of the country. However, dressing for a professional job interview is fairly standard regardless of age or location. What you choose not to wear is as important as what you do wear. For the interview, do not wear your professional uniform. Casual attire and trendy clothing, such as blue jeans, T-shirts, and athletic shoes, are also inappropriate.

By taking the time to prepare your personal appearance and dress professionally, you are telling the interviewers that you appreciate their serious consideration of you as a job candidate. You are also making a statement about how you believe a professional should appear, not only to potential employers but to your peers. It will be assumed that although you would be wearing a professional uniform at work, you would appear as neat and clean when caring for patients, as your appearance during the interview suggests.

Pay attention to details. It does little good to wear a clean, pressed business suit only to have the interviewer see dirty fingernails. Similarly, proper grooming loses its impact when your cologne precedes you to the interview by 5 minutes. Because you will undoubtedly be nervous, your mouth will probably be dry. Use a breath mint until the interview begins to keep your mouth moist and your breath fresh. Gum chewing is never acceptable in a professional setting.

Conservative clothing is a must. Men should always wear a business suit or sport coat, tie, and dress slacks. Female applicants should wear either a business suit or a dress. Clothing must be free of wrinkles and clean. Shoes (polished), socks, and belts should complement the clothing. Hose must be free of runs. Hair should be neatly styled and pulled back if shoulder length or longer. Jewelry should be conservative and kept to a minimum.

As your attire varies from these suggestions, the likelihood of a favorable impression on the interviewer decreases. Under no circumstances should you wear casual slacks, jeans, shorts, walking or running shoes, and so forth. Applying for a professional position requires that you dress professionally.

PREPARING FOR THE INTERVIEW

To prepare for the interview, you should attempt to find out as much about your potential employer as possible. If this information cannot be ascertained ahead of time, you may ask those questions during the interview. Information you may want to find out may include why the current position is available; whether there is a very high rate of turnover in the particular department you are considering; the value that this organization places on its employees; whether there is harmony among the employees in the department; whether patients and employees speak highly of the department; the kind of advancement opportunities that are available, including cross-training in other imaging modalities; whether the organization provides continuing education, in-service programs, or tuition reimbursement; the financial security of the organization; an examination of the organization's most recent annual report (which can be obtained from the office of public relations at the institution); and the organization's reputation in the community. The overall reputation in the community and the financial stability of your prospective employer are factors that you should consider before accepting a job offer.

It should not be necessary to bring anything to the interview unless you have not previously submitted your resume to the interviewer; if you have not, bring a clean copy inside a manilla folder. All of the facts pertaining to your professional preparation are on the resume. If documentation is required for any item, it may be submitted at a later time to the department of human resources. Similarly, your list of references is probably already entered on the job application form. If not, these may also be furnished later to human resources. In most cases, individual department heads do not perform reference checks because of the legalities involved.

If you are not exactly sure where the interview will be held, you should find the building and the office several days ahead of time. You do not want to be searching for the site on the day the interview is scheduled. You should allow plenty of time to get to your destination. If you arrive early, there is always a waiting area. Arriving late for an interview is inexcusable.

When you arrive at the interview site, you may want to visit the restroom. Anxiety about the interview may make this necessary, but it will also give you the opportunity to make sure your hair and attire are presentable. When arriving at the appropriate office, greet everyone as if they were going to conduct the interview. Many radiology managers ask receptionists and secretaries their impressions of the individual who is being interviewed.

It is normal to feel nervous and apprehensive about an interview, especially if it is for a position you greatly desire. Try to convert your nervous energy into enthusiasm when speaking with others throughout the course of the interview.

THE INTERVIEW PROCESS

When the interviewer approaches, stand and shake hands firmly. A smile and an enthusiastic (although not excessively demonstrative) attitude will create a positive first impression. As the interview begins, try to appear as calm, comfortable, and professional as possible. Maintain appropriate eye contact and smile. Maintain good posture and remain alert. Be pleasant, avoid joking, and be attentive. Speak distinctly and use appropriate terminology. Be a good listener. You may wish to bring up your career goals as summarized in the goal statement on your resume. Carefully indicate how you may be an asset to the department without sounding as though you are bossy or demanding. Remember to answer the interviewer's questions clearly, avoiding very short or very long answers.

There have been numerous legal challenges in recent years to what are alleged to be discriminatory interview questions and techniques. Although the emphasis of such legal rulings has been to require the interviewer to ask only questions that reveal your job qualifications, it is wise for you to know what can and cannot be asked in a job interview. This will assist you in preparing for the interview. It will also make you aware of your rights so that you may recognize potentially discriminatory situations.

Following is a list of topics that may be addressed during your interview. They are relevant to the job and are therefore legitimate areas of inquiry. You may wish to write out your answers ahead of time in anticipation of the interview. Other interview questions not included in this list may also be appropriate and within current legal guidelines.

Questions about the following *are* appropriate:
- Any information you entered on the application form
- Why you left your last job
- How your former employers view you
- What your duties were in your last job or a summary of your clinical rotations if you are a new graduate
- What you liked or disliked about your previous jobs or your favorite or least favorite experiences as a student
- What job duties interest you

- The days or hours you are (or are not) available to work
- The size of the facility in which you previously worked
- What you thought of your previous supervisors or instructors (e.g., whether you got along, what kind of persons they were, whether they were strict or easy-going)
- The kind of supervisor you prefer
- How employee or student problems and complaints were solved at your previous job or clinical site and whether you thought it was a good procedure
- How you would prefer to have employee problems and complaints handled if hired for this job
- What wages you received at your previous job
- How frequently pay raises were given at your previous job and on what were they based (e.g., productivity, merit)
- Whether pay raises were given in fixed amounts or percentages of pay
- How many pay raises you received if they were based on merit
- Whether you were promoted and on what criteria the promotion was based (e.g., merit, length of service)
- Whether you received a shift differential, how much it was, and whether it was a fixed amount or a percentage
- Which benefits you received at your previous job, including whether you paid part of your insurance coverage and whether the cost was deducted from your paycheck
- How you were notified about your benefits (e.g., booklets, memos, handbooks, bulletin board notices)
- How much you expect an employer to communicate with you and to keep you involved in workplace activities
- Which mode of communication you prefer

The interviewer will probably provide you with information about the salary structure, benefits package, sick leave, vacation time allowed, and so forth. Although this information is important to you, try to wait until the interviewer brings it up. In this way, you will not appear to be interested only in money and benefits.

In any interviewing situation, you should be aware of the types of questions that may *not* be asked. This is important so that you do not answer irrelevant questions that may harm your chances for securing the job. If a series of improper questions is asked, you may not wish to continue pursuing the position. If blatant harassment or violation of ethical interviewing guidelines occurs, you must ask yourself whether you wish to work in such an environment. If either of these situations develops, you may decide to conclude the interview with a statement such as, "Thank you for your time, but I feel you are asking irrelevant questions in violation of my rights. Please remove my name from consideration for this position," or you may opt to finish the inter-

view and remove your name from consideration in a follow-up letter.

Be careful not to answer questions such as those that follow. You are not required to answer them and should not be put in a position of volunteering such information. If you believe you have been discriminated against based on questionable interview practices, you may wish to seek legal counsel as a last resort. Recommendations concerning legal issues that may arise during the interview are beyond the scope of this text. Your personal attorney is best equipped to answer such questions.

Questions about the following are *not* appropriate:
- Your age
- Your birth date
- How long you have resided at your present address
- Your previous address
- The church you choose to attend (if any) or the name of your priest, minister, or rabbi
- Your father's surname
- Your maiden name if you are female
- Whether you are married, divorced, separated, widowed, or single
- Who lives with you
- How many children you have or intend to have
- The ages of your children
- Who will care for your children while you are working
- How you will get to work (unless owning a car is a job requirement)
- Where a spouse or parent works or lives
- Whether you own or rent your place of residence
- The name of your bank or any information concerning outstanding loan amounts
- Whether you have ever had your wages garnished or filed bankruptcy
- Whether you have ever been arrested
- Whether you have ever served in the armed forces of another country
- How you spend your spare time or to which clubs or organizations you belong
- Which foreign languages you can speak, read, or write (unless it is a job requirement)
- Your position on labor unions or whether you have ever been a member of a union
- The nationality of your name

In addition, beware of other phrases, attitudes, or questions that may discriminate against you on the basis of gender. For example, you may not be referred to as "sweetie," "honey," "hunk," and so forth. Flirtatious behavior is not to be tolerated. Do not allow the interviewer to take advantage of your friendly nature to ask questions that should not be asked or pry into personal aspects of your life. This is not a conversation between friends; it is a professional job interview. If you conduct yourself professionally, a competent interviewer will respect you and your position.

INTERVIEW OUTCOMES AND FOLLOW-UP

Even after a good interview, you may not be hired or take the job offer. Following are some of the appropriate reasons:

1. You are unable to work the required hours.
2. You choose to reject the job offer because you are not interested in the position available.
3. You are not qualified for the position available, or other candidates were better qualified or had more experience.
4. You were obviously under the influence of drugs or alcohol during the interview, or you did not pass the drug screening portion of the physical exam.
5. Inconsistent, inaccurate, or fraudulent statements were made on your application form.
6. You are physically unable to perform the job duties; however, the Americans with Disabilities Act guidelines must be considered.

The last impression can be as important as the first. At the conclusion of the interview, be sure to shake hands and thank the interviewer for the time spent with you. The interviewer will probably give some indication of when the hiring decision will be made based on the number of applicants and the date by which the position must be filled. As you leave, be sure to say good-bye to secretaries or receptionists you pass.

Immediately send a follow-up letter to the interviewer. A sample of such correspondence is shown in Figure 12-1. Be sure it is printed on good-quality paper and reinforces the positive impression you have sought to make. Keep in mind that this is basically a thank-you letter and not meant to provide additional information about yourself. Most

Radiology Manager's Name
Imaging Center
Shepherd Road
My Town, VA 12345-9876

Date

Dear Radiology Manager's Name:

Thank you for the opportunity to interview for the position of staff radiographer. I appreciate the time you spent with me yesterday. It was a pleasure meeting you and seeing your radiology department.

I look forward to hearing from you regarding this position.

Sincerely,

Applicant, R.T. (R)

Figure 12-1   Sample interview follow-up letter.

important, be sure to send it. Many individuals fail to follow up with a letter, and consequently, you will stand out from the rest!

Following the guidelines and suggestions in this chapter will not guarantee employment. However, it will guarantee that you will present yourself as the true professional you have worked so hard to become.

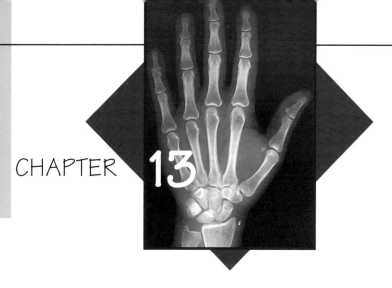

CHAPTER 13

Employer Expectations

ENTERING THE HEALTH CARE WORKFORCE

As you enter the workforce in medical radiography, those in charge of the facility in which you will work will have expectations of you as a professional. From their standpoint, it is reasonable to expect that you will be able to fulfill the requirements of your job description. You are being hired because you have the abilities to function as an entry-level radiographer. Of course, ultimately, the most important expectations that you must exceed are those of the patient.

The task inventory conducted by the American Registry of Radiologic Technologists (ARRT) lists the skills expected of an entry-level radiographer. Although these should coincide with the terminal competencies of your educational program, you should also be aware that your new employer will have these expectations regardless of where you attended school. The task inventory is provided here so that you can understand the technical skills expected of you as you enter the workforce.

TASK INVENTORY*

Completion of your educational program should enable you to carry out the following tasks:

1. Evaluate the need for and use of protective shielding.
2. Take appropriate precautions to minimize radiation exposure to patients.
3. Restrict beam to limit exposure area, improve image quality, and reduce radiation dose.
4. Set kVp, mA, and time or automated exposure system

to achieve optimum image quality, safe operating conditions, and minimum radiation dose.
5. Prevent all unnecessary persons from remaining in the area during x-ray exposure.
6. Take appropriate precautions to minimize occupational radiation exposure.
7. Wear a personnel monitoring device while on duty.
8. Review and evaluate individual occupational exposure charts.
9. Warm-up x-ray tube according to manufacturer's recommendations.
10. Prepare and adjust radiographic unit and accessories.
11. Prepare and adjust fluoroscopic unit and accessories.
12. Recognize and report malfunctions in the radiographic and fluoroscopic unit and ancillary accessories.
13. Perform basic evaluations of radiographic equipment and accessories (e.g., lead aprons, collimator accuracy).
14. Inspect and clean screens and cassettes.
15. Perform start-up or shutdown procedures on automatic processor.
16. Recognize and report malfunctions in the automatic processor.
17. Process exposed film.
18. Process digital/electronic images.
19. Reload cassettes by selecting film of proper size and type.
20. Store film/cassette in a manner that will reduce the possibility of artifact production.
21. Select appropriate film-screen combination.
22. Determine appropriate exposure factors using calipers and technique charts.
23. Modify exposure factors for circumstances such as involuntary motion, casts and splints, pathologic conditions, or patient's inability to cooperate.

*From Content specifications for the examination in radiography, St Paul, 2001, American Registry of Radiologic Technologists.

24. Use radiopaque markers to indicate anatomic side, position, or other relevant information (e.g., time upright, decubitus, postvoid).
25. Evaluate patient for appropriateness of examination.
26. Evaluate radiographs for diagnostic quality.
27. Determine corrective measures if radiograph is not of diagnostic quality, and take appropriate action.
28. Select equipment and accessories (e.g., grid, compensating filters, shielding) for the examination requested.
29. Remove all radiopaque materials from patient or table that could interfere with the radiographic image.
30. Explain breathing instructions before making the exposure.
31. Position patient to demonstrate the desired anatomy using body landmarks.
32. Explain and confirm patient preparation (e.g., diet restrictions, preparatory medications) before radiographic/fluoroscopic examinations.
33. Properly sequence radiographic procedures to avoid residual contrast material affecting future exams.
34. Examine radiographic requisition to verify accuracy and completeness of information (e.g., patient history, clinical diagnosis).
35. Utilize standard (universal) precautions.
36. Confirm patient's identity.
37. Question female patients of childbearing age about possible pregnancy and document response.
38. Verify/obtain patient consent form.
39. Explain procedure and postprocedural instructions to patient or patient's family.
40. Evaluate patient's ability to comply with positioning requirements for the requested exam.
41. Observe, monitor, and document vital signs.
42. Use proper body mechanics and/or mechanical transfer devices when assisting patients.
43. Provide for patient safety, comfort, and modesty.
44. Select immobilization devices when indicated to prevent patient movement and/or ensure patient safety.
45. Verify accuracy of patient identification on radiograph.
46. Maintain confidentiality of patient information.
47. Use sterile or aseptic technique when indicated.
48. Confirm type and prepare contrast media for administration.
49. Before administration of contrast agent, gather information to determine appropriate dosage and whether the patient is at increased risk of adverse reaction.
50. Observe patient after administration of contrast media to detect adverse reactions.
51. Recognize need for prompt medical attention, and administer emergency care.
52. Document required information on patient's medical record.
53. Clean, disinfect, or sterilize facilities and equipment, and dispose of contaminated items in preparation for next examination.
54. Follow appropriate procedures when in contact with patient in reverse/protective isolation.
55. Monitor medical equipment attached to the patient (e.g., IVs, oxygen) during the radiographic procedure.
56-117. Position patient, x-ray tube, and image receptor to produce radiographs of the following.

Thorax

56. Chest, routine
57. Chest, obliques, apical lordotic, decubitus
58. Ribs
59. Sternum

Extremities

60. Toes
61. Foot
62. Os calcis
63. Ankle
64. Tibia, fibula
65. Knee
66. Patella
67. Femur
68. Fingers
69. Hand
70. Wrist
71. Forearm
72. Elbow
73. Humerus
74. Shoulder
75. Scapula
76. Clavicle
77. Acromioclavicular joints
78. Bone survey
79. Long bone measurement/scanogram
80. Bone age
81. Soft tissue/foreign bodies

Head and Neck

82. Skull
83. Facial bones
84. Mandible
85. Zygoma and arches
86. Temporomandibular joints
87. Nasal bones
88. Orbits
89. Paranasal sinuses

Spine and Pelvis

90. Cervical spine
91. Thoracic spine
92. Scoliosis series
93. Lumbosacral spine

94. Sacrum
95. Sacroiliac joints
96. Coccyx
97. Pelvis
98. Hip

Abdomen and Gastrointestinal (GI) Tract

99. Esophagram
100. Swallowing dysfunction study (video)
101. Abdomen
102. Upper GI series
103. Small bowel series
104. Endoscopic retrograde cholangiopancreatography
105. Barium enema
106. Operative cholangiography
107. T-tube cholangiogram
108. Cholecystogram

Other

109. Venogram
110. Myelogram
111. Arthrogram
112. Conventional tomogram
113. Cystogram
114. Cystourethrogram
115. Intravenous urogram
116. Retrograde pyelogram
117. Retrograde urethrogram

ORGANIZATIONAL STRUCTURE AND YOUR PROFESSIONAL RESPONSIBILITY

The employer has a right to expect you to use your knowledge and abilities in radiography efficiently and provide high-quality service to the patient. In return, you have a right to expect the salary and benefits to which you and your employer agreed. You should also expect to perform your job in an environment that is in compliance with safety and public health requirements and free of all forms of harassment.

You are entering a dynamic and fluid sector of the national economy. Health care advances in diagnosis, treatment, and delivery are in a constant state of flux. This is the nature of the industry in which you have chosen to work and build a career. You should expect to stay abreast of changes in the delivery of health care and remain alert to how such changes affect your employer. Remember that issues affecting your employer will also affect you and your co-workers.

Your employer will expect you to function as part of a team, all of the members of which will be dedicated to cost-effectively providing efficient, accurate care to the patient. At the same time the employer is the coach of the team and has an obligation to maintain the provision of quality service to patients and proper accountability to payers. An examination of the expectations of your employer will reveal that your job responsibilities actually fall into three distinct sets.

Expectations of Administrators

The administrators of the facility in which you are about to be employed expect that you are going to fulfill the job description associated with an entry-level radiographer. They expect you to be honest and straightforward with them while providing excellent care and service to the patient/customer. High-quality customer service is paramount to your success. It is vitally important that the patient know that true professionals are providing care.

Administrators trust that you will speak highly of the facility and be supportive of its efforts to provide quality patient care. You are expected to arrive for work on time and keep absenteeism to an absolute minimum. There may be times when you are expected to work extra hours, such as when another employee is on vacation or is sick. Administrators are looking for employees who are willing to be strong, supportive team players.

The administrators also expect that you will be willing to contribute new ideas for more efficient operation. They assume that you will work in harmony with other departments in the facility. They may request that you serve on committees or perform other tasks not directly related to radiography. Be the type of employee who exceeds the expectations of administration, and you will be well on your way toward establishing the type of reputation that will ensure your success.

Expectations of Physicians

Physicians are customers too. The physicians with whom you will be working, both radiologists and referring physicians, have their own particular set of expectations. Referring physicians expect that their orders for radiologic examinations will be carried out as written. They expect that quality radiographs will be made by the radiographers and properly interpreted by the radiologists. Although your interactions with these physicians may be minimal, they are nevertheless important.

Referring physicians often come to the radiology department to view radiographs themselves or consult with the radiologist. They may be unfamiliar with the department and where supplies are kept. They may be there to perform a procedure. They expect to be treated as professionals. They expect to be shown where supplies are kept and be assisted as needed. As a professional radiographer, it will be your responsibility to meet or exceed those expectations and provide high-quality service to the physician as well as the patient.

The physicians with whom you will interact most frequently are the radiologists, and most of this exchange will occur during fluoroscopy. The radiologists expect to receive the highest quality radiographs you are capable of producing. They will be providing the diagnosis from your radiographs. Radiologists do not expect to have to ask you to retake a film that you already know is unacceptable. They do not want to hear excuses for poor radiographs. Radiologists insist that you keep them informed about variations from protocol. They expect you to take an adequate but concise patient history for their use during the interpretation of the radiographs.

As a student, there may have been radiographers to facilitate your interactions with the radiologists. As a new, entry-level radiographer, it is now your responsibility to be straightforward and professional during interactions with the radiologists. This includes not only providing the highest quality radiographs that you can but also demonstrating a willingness to resolve personality and work-related conflicts.

It is important to determine ahead of time how you wish to be regarded by the physicians. You have a right to be treated respectfully and should take immediate steps to rectify a situation in which you are being mistreated. At the same time the physicians have a right to expect that you will reciprocate in your professional conduct.

Expectations of the Radiology Manager

The person who is hiring you, the radiology manager, also has a particular set of expectations. It is this individual who is directly responsible for your on-the-job performance and overall value to the patient/customer and administration. In research I conducted, radiology managers from across the United States responded to a survey regarding their expectations of new radiography graduates. Of particular interest are the traits that the radiology managers considered most important in an applicant and the areas in which radiology managers have had the most difficulty with employees once they were hired.

Not surprisingly, 43% of radiology managers said that knowledge of the technical aspects of radiography was the most important factor they considered when hiring a new graduate radiographer. This is a given because the new employee must be able to perform the job. However, 33% responded that customer service skills and interpersonal communication skills were the factors they most considered when hiring a recent graduate. These individuals are assuming you know how to perform the job and expect that you will provide excellent service to the patient while performing it. This research shows that radiology managers have high expectations of you. They expect you to know the practice of radiography, deliver quality service to patients, and be capable of establishing positive relationships with your co-workers.

A second question inquired about problems radiology managers encountered with radiographers on the job.

Thirty-seven percent identified poor communication skills as the most significant problem and usual cause for a reprimand or termination. Thirty-six percent cited lack of knowledge of the technical aspects of the job as the primary reason for a reprimand or termination. In handwritten comments on the survey forms, many radiology managers mentioned attendance problems, tardiness, lack of dependability, and substance abuse as problems in the workplace that led to reprimands and terminations. Once again, the need for balance between the high-touch and high-tech aspects of radiography is evident. It is no surprise that radiology managers have high expectations of new employees. Be certain that you are prepared to exceed those expectations.

Another survey question asked the managers which areas should be most strongly emphasized with student radiographers as they prepare to enter the workforce. Handwritten comments stressed the following:
1. Ongoing technical training
2. Knowledge of basic nursing skills, such as using IV pumps, taking vital signs, and performing venipuncture
3. Ability to work alone without constant supervision
4. Awareness of the customer's/patient's viewpoint
5. Strong communication skills
6. Provision of quality service with a smile
7. Professionalism in dealing with the public
8. Loyalty to the employer
9. Maintenance of clinical skills

Because you are about ready to enter the workforce, you must determine how many of these traits are present in your practice already and which ones need additional attention. The managers have carefully described what they need and expect. Are you prepared to enter their workplace?

The radiology managers were then asked to rank the factors they considered to positively affect customer service the most in their department. Not surprisingly, the most important factor (according to 60% of the respondents) was a pleasant and courteous staff.

Like the administrators to whom they report, radiology managers expect you to be ready to begin work on time and to keep absenteeism to a minimum. They are counting on you to show up and provide the highest quality patient care each day you are assigned to work.

The radiology manager also expects that you will conduct yourself as a professional in your dealings with the patient/customer, the physicians, and your co-workers. You are expected to be a reliable member of the radiology team. You must be flexible and have a positive attitude about handling all of the different assignments that you may be given in a typical work day.

Other areas of concern raised by the radiology managers included bringing personal problems to work, substance abuse by employees, and overall lack of initiative. These are all problems you should keep out of your radiography practice. Should any of these issues become matters of personal concern for you, seek counseling immediately so that you can bring such problems under control. Your employer and your patients deserve no less.

Your radiology manager will expect you to remain busy throughout the day. In addition to performing your primary job duties, you may be asked to complete assignments that do not involve patient care. Quality control and cleaning of the automatic processor or x-ray equipment may be requested. You may be assigned to assist with filing, patient transportation, or the cleaning of radiographic and fluoroscopic rooms; to stock supplies; to clean cassettes, intensifying screens, and lead aprons; and to perform other housekeeping chores around the radiology department.

Expectations of Students under Your Supervision

Your new employer may have students present as part of an educational program in radiologic technology. The employer may be the sponsor of the program or may serve as a clinical site for a program sponsored by another institution.

It may seem ironic that while you are probably reading this as a student still in school, it is already time to consider the aspect of future student expectations. Should you choose to work in an imaging department that serves as a clinical site, you will be working with students shortly after graduation. This is an awesome responsibility, especially because you will still be in learning mode yourself, learning the requirements of a staff radiographer in your new position.

Working with students is a task to be taken seriously. As you already know from your experiences, the students will expect you to share with them your knowledge of the art and science of imaging, patient care, and procedures. They will want fair and honest evaluations of their performance. They will want to be treated with the respect due an adult in college, not as another worker, inexpensive laborer, or someone to perform menial tasks. The students under your supervision will rely on you to help them through the learning process.

Whether or not it is part of the orientation to your new job, be sure to seek out the clinical instructor for students in your department. Find out what is expected of you from the educational program. Become thoroughly familiar with the evaluation forms and competency testing forms that you may be expected to use. Being a new graduate yourself, determine whether there is a limit to what role you can play. Learn the specific requirements of direct and indirect supervision of students performing examinations and repeat radiographs. Consider carefully the legal ramifications of following such supervision requirements.

As you work with students, remember that you are shaping the next generation of radiographers. These individuals will be your co-workers upon their graduation. This is a key role to play as you become acclimated to the role of radiographer as well. You have the ability to be a strong influence on future professionals in your field. Take the

responsibility seriously, and take pride in the impact you will have on these radiographers who will follow you into the field.

Expectations of Your New Co-Workers

At the same time that you are orienting to a new job, possibly working with students, taking and passing the credentialing exam, and learning your new employer's expectations, there will be another very important set of expectations to consider. This area includes your employer's expectations of your relationship with your new co-workers.

As a new graduate, you will, in some respects, be like a new student all over again. Learning the technical aspects of a new job, even in your chosen field, will take much time and energy. At the same time, becoming part of a work group such as a department of radiology, urgent care center, cardiac catheterization laboratory, or physician's office will probably take more energy than you might expect. Establishing your professional relationships will make a world of difference in the satisfaction you receive from your work and your ability to provide the level of care you expect of yourself.

Approach your new position as a learner, eager to find out all you can regarding routines, protocols, professional relationships within the work setting, and how the group functions together. Determine everyone's level of responsibility and where you fit in. Your new employer expects that you will establish professional working relationships and conduct yourself with everyone as a member of a tight work unit. You will be expected to avoid gossip, cliques, and any other behavior that inhibits the delivery of high-quality patient care and service. Your employer will expect that you are ready to learn all you can from your co-workers regarding the technical aspects of imaging, as well as operation of the imaging department and/or clinic. Personal problems with co-workers will need to be worked out as professionals and not allowed to enter the flow of the workplace.

Your co-workers will expect you to come up to speed quickly and to ask questions when necessary. They will expect that you conduct yourself as a new graduate, still in learning mode but ready to assume a high level of responsibility taking on your share of patient care. They will expect that you establish a positive, uplifting relationship with them. They can assist you as you enter the field as a professional. Use their experience and knowledge to your benefit as you deliver patient care. Respond to their help by working with them cooperatively, as a new colleague, as a professional who is eager to assume a key role in their work unit. Exceed your new employer's expectations by working cooperatively and learning all you can from your new co-workers.

If you think of your work area as an integral part of your practice, that sense of ownership will motivate you to care for it. Slow periods at work may be few and far between; you should take advantage of them whenever they occur. Your attitude toward the aspects of your work that do not involve patient care may determine whether the radiology manager gives you other assignments you prefer. If you consider lounge areas off limits and keep busy throughout the day, you will find great fulfillment in your work and will likely exceed the radiology manager's expectations.

In a field that changes as rapidly as radiologic technology, your radiology manager will expect you to be knowledgeable about the newest types of equipment and advances in imaging techniques. You are also expected to keep your skills at a level that allows you to perform all of the different types of radiologic procedures required in your radiology department. On a regular basis, you should review your favorite radiographic positioning and procedures text to refresh your memory and maintain your skills.

You have become accustomed to studying, and throughout the course of your radiography program, you have had to learn how to learn. This process does not end with graduation or passing the certification exam. It is important to keep abreast of events in the field by reading the latest radiologic technology journals and textbooks. Textbooks are not written solely for students. As a practicing radiographer, you will want to keep your personal library updated with the best resources available.

Another way to be aware of current developments in the field and exceed your manager's expectations is to become an active member of your national and state professional organizations. Both have publications that will bring you the latest news in the profession. In addition, these organizations need your talents to be successful. As a student, you have acquired a store of information and have developed skill in communicating this knowledge. Take advantage of that momentum, and continue to do research in the field.

Most radiology managers will expect you to give something back to your profession, which will increase your level of knowledge. Present research papers at state or national meetings, hold an office in one of the organizations, or offer to help out in the planning and conducting of a continuing education meeting. Organizing and conducting an in-service education program for your department is a great place to begin. If you have never taken part in such activities, this is a perfect time to begin. It does not matter whether you are sure about what you are doing; just offer to help or do that first research paper as a graduate.

Meeting and exceeding the radiology manager's expectations are sure ways to set a course for success in your chosen field. Those who follow this path derive the most satisfaction from their job and are held in the highest esteem by their employers. Most important, a commitment to excellence in your profession results in healthy self-esteem, which is reflected in the care and service provided to the patients.

PART III

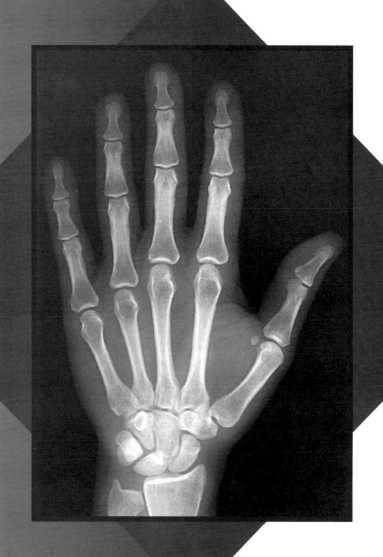

Continuing Education Opportunities

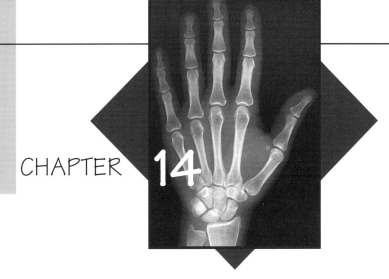

The quality of a person's life is in direct proportion to their commitment to excellence regardless of their chosen field of endeavor.

VINCE LOMBARDI

CHAPTER 14

Continuing Education Requirements

MEETING PROFESSIONAL AND GOVERNMENTAL REQUIREMENTS

The purpose of certification is to assure the public that you are competent to practice in your chosen field. However, even though you pass a certification exam to enter the profession, there is no assurance that you will remain competent. It is of the utmost importance that you have the most current knowledge and skills needed to practice radiologic technology.

Mandatory continuing education has been established in an attempt to ensure the continued competence of clinicians. Even though research indicates that mandatory continuing education in any field of study is not necessarily a guarantee of competence, it is the route that has been chosen for many of the health professions, including radiologic technology.

After you receive your initial registration on successful completion of the certification exam, the American Registry of Radiologic Technologists (ARRT) requires documentation of continuing education for you to renew it. Participating in continuing education and documenting your participation are your responsibility as a registered technologist. Although acquiring continuing education credits is not difficult for the vast majority of technologists, knowledge of the applicable rules and regulations is of paramount importance.

In addition to certification, many states require those practicing medical radiography to hold licensure or accreditation issued by the state. Because legislation regulating state licensure may be subject to the addition or revision of statutes at any time, a list of the requirements specific to each state is not included here. Most states accept the ARRT certification as proof of the applicant's competency. In those states, you will need to apply to the appropriate agency, supply a copy of your ARRT credentials, and pay the proper fee. Be sure to obtain the rules and regulations pertaining to licensure in the state or states in which you will be employed. Such rules will advise you of the application process, any testing or fees involved, and continuing education requirements. Educators or radiology managers should be consulted for the name and address of the specific state agency responsible for such credentialing.

It is important to keep in mind that state and national continuing education requirements may differ. Once again, it is the individual technologist's responsibility to keep abreast of the current requirements for continuing education. Neither the state nor the national agencies accept a lack of knowledge of the rules and regulations as an excuse for failure to meet the requirements. An insufficient number of continuing education credits may result in the issuance of probationary status, the levy of fines by the state, or loss of the ability to work.

Be sure to take time to review the following ARRT continuing education requirements. Your instructors will be happy to answer any questions you may have. You may also contact the ARRT office at 651-687-0048.

ARRT CONTINUING EDUCATION REQUIREMENTS

Although you will renew your certification with the ARRT each year, you will need to submit proof of continuing education activities every 2 years. There are three ways to satisfy the requirement of 24 hours of continuing education for that 2-year period. The first is to attend 24 hours of continuing education courses that have met the criteria established by the ARRT. The second is to pass an entry-level exam in an area of radiologic technology in which you were not previously credentialed (e.g., radiation therapy, nuclear medicine, sonography). Finally, you may pass one of the advanced-level exams offered by the ARRT. These advanced-level exams are described in Chapter 15.

You must begin to comply with the rules governing continuing education beginning with your first birth month after you pass the radiography examination.

Continuing education activities must be organized to expand the knowledge and skills needed by a radiologic technologist in clinical practice. In attempting to meet the requirement by attending 24 hours of continuing education, you should be aware that the ARRT organizes such activities into two categories.

Category A credits are awarded for classes or programs that have been approved by a recognized continuing education evaluation mechanism (RCEEM). Examples of RCEEMs are the American Society of Radiologic Technologists (ASRT), the Society of Diagnostic Medical Sonographers, and the Society of Nuclear Medicine—Technologist Section. In addition, the ARRT will award Category A credits for programs approved by the American Medical Association as Category 1 and by the American Nurses Association if they pertain to the radiologic sciences. These are some of the approval mechanisms that you will want to look for on program advertisements before you register for the program.

Category A credits are awarded without RCEEM approval for cardiopulmonary resuscitation (CPR) certification and approved postsecondary academic courses (e.g., biologic, physical, radiologic, medical, or social science courses; communications, math, computers, management, or education courses). For these two types of activities, the ARRT will accept a CPR card or college transcript as proof of attendance.

The ARRT will also accept continuing education credits that have been approved by the licensing agencies in certain states. Be sure to check with your state to determine whether it is one of the approved continuing education providers.

Category B credits are continuing education activities that do not meet the Category A criteria and consequently must be individually approved. Of the 24 credits that you must earn every 2 years to meet ARRT requirements, at least 12 must be from Category A. The remaining 12 may be Category A or Category B credits.

The coordinator of a continuing education program will be happy to answer questions concerning the approval of the event. As a technologist, you are not responsible for submitting a program for approval to obtain credit. The sponsor of the event seeks approval before the date of the presentation.

Credits are awarded on the basis of a contact hour. A contact hour is 50 to 60 minutes in length and is awarded one continuing education credit. Programs 30 to 49 minutes long are awarded a half credit. Approved academic courses are awarded 16 continuing education credits for each semester credit. (A grade of C or above must be earned.) CPR is awarded three Category A credits for each area of certification, with no more than six credits allowed during each 2-year cycle.

You may also receive credit for conducting a presentation. If the presentation has been approved as a Category A activity, you may be awarded three continuing education credits for the preparation and one continuing education credit per hour of the presentation. No more than 12 such credits may be accumulated during a 2-year period.

The ARRT will place technologists who fail to meet the continuing education requirements on probationary status. Inquiries submitted to the ARRT by employers will receive a response that includes a notation of probationary status and may result in your rejection as a job applicant or loss of employment.

CONTINUING EDUCATION OPPORTUNITIES

There are multiple opportunities to obtain continuing education credits. The primary mission of your professional societies is continuing education. Be certain that you are an active member of the ASRT. Through its annual conference and numerous home study programs, as well as its directed readings in the journal *Radiologic Technology,* you can obtain a considerable portion of your continuing education credits. The ASRT may be contacted at 15000 Central Avenue SE, Albuquerque, NM 87123-3917, 505-298-4500, www.asrt.org.

The various state affiliate societies of the ASRT provide many continuing education opportunities every year. Ask your instructors or the radiologic technologists in clinical settings for membership information. As part of the state society, your local professional society probably has monthly or quarterly meetings that stress continuing education. Be certain to take advantage of these meetings.

If you choose a career in any of the radiologic specialties, education, or management, there are a number of other professional organizations to which you may belong. Each organization offers approved continuing education as part of its mission. Being an active member of a professional society will help ensure that you are informed about the continuing education programs that will contribute most to your skill development.

As a registered technologist, it is your responsibility to know whether the continuing education program you are attending has been approved and to obtain the necessary documentation proving your participation in the activity. At the end of each 2-year period, you must submit proof that you have satisfied the requirement. Be sure to keep the original attendance documents for at least a year beyond the 2-year period. The ARRT will conduct random audits to verify such documentation. The documentation will need to show the date of the program, title and content, number of contact hours, and signature of an individual associated with the program, such as the speaker, instructor, or coordinator. The documentation should also include (if applicable) a continuing education reference number provided by the RCEEM. It would be wise to set up your own file for continuing education before you graduate so that it will be in place and ready for immediate use as soon as you are registered. Be certain to keep copies of all documents for audit purposes.

For information about continuing education opportunities, visit the website www.asrt.org. For the latest continuing education guidelines, visit the website www.arrt.org.

It is your responsibility to learn about modifications to the continuing education requirements. Be sure to read all of the information sent to you from the ARRT, particularly the *Annual Report to Technologists*, published every spring. You should also remain alert for changes to such requirements in your state.

Continuing education is a vital part of your medical radiography practice. View it as an opportunity to learn and enhance your skills rather than as an imposed obligation. Attend programs that you know will help you become a better technologist. Take an active part in these events, both as an attendee and as a coordinator. Conduct your own presentation for a more complete learning experience. You will find that such activities enhance your professional image and gain the respect and admiration of your colleagues.

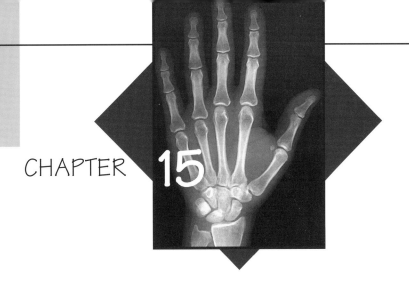

CHAPTER 15

Radiologic Specialties

PREPARING FOR MULTICREDENTIALING

As demand increases for radiologic technologists with multispecialty capabilities, many radiography students, graduates, and practicing technologists are considering furthering their education. It is often a difficult and tedious process to obtain all of the information needed to make a decision regarding such a career-enhancing move. This chapter is provided so that you may get some idea of what is involved in studying in each of the areas. Currently, the radiologic specialties requiring advanced-level education are diagnostic medical sonography, nuclear medicine technology, and radiation therapy technology. This section addresses the educational opportunities available in those areas.

Other radiologic specialties such as computed tomography, angiography, magnetic resonance imaging, quality management, cardiovascular-interventional technology, mammography, and bone densitometry do not have specific additional educational requirements for credentialing. In addition, education programs offered in those areas do not undergo approval by the usual accrediting organizations. However, information concerning advanced-level examinations is available in these areas, and such information is included in this chapter. The reader should be aware that requirements for all specialty areas could change at any time; therefore the appropriate credentialing agencies listed in this chapter should be contacted when pursuing such a career.

Information about each of the three major specialties presented in this chapter includes a brief summary of the educational program and the content specifications for the exam. The names, addresses, and websites of the professional organizations associated with that specialty are then provided. This enables the reader to access the most current and accurate listing of all educational programs in the

country accredited by that organization. Because certification requirements and educational programs are subject to change for a variety of reasons, the interested professional should use the websites for such information. You should also be aware that there are many sonography programs that do not carry Joint Review Committee on Education in Diagnostic Medical Sonography (JRCDMS) accreditation. Lack of programmatic accreditation at that level means there is no guarantee regarding curriculum content.

When writing to one of the programs in which you are interested for information, keep the letter brief. Program directors receive countless requests for informational brochures, so being concise is extremely helpful. It is recommended that you write at the beginning of your second year of radiography studies if you are planning to enroll in a specialty program immediately after graduation. The quickest way to obtain the desired information may be the institution's website. You may wish to use the sample letter shown in Figure 15-1.

For each exam and specialty listed in this chapter, it is important to contact the certifying organization for details regarding specific clinical requirements that may need to be documented as part of the application process. This chapter is meant to be informational only and does not attempt to take the place of the formal and comprehensive handbooks published by the respective organizations.

DIAGNOSTIC MEDICAL SONOGRAPHY

Educational programs in sonography may be 1½, 2, or 4 years in length, depending on the inclusion of earned credit hours from an academic degree. The course of study will involve biology, sectional anatomy, patient care, physics and

Program Director
Radiation Therapy Program
Community Hospital
Your Town, New York 10021

Date

Dear Program Director:

I am a second-year radiography student interested in pursuing additional education in radiation therapy technology. Please send a copy of your program's informational brochure/catalog along with an application form to me at the address below.

Thank you for your attention to my request.

Sincerely,

Student Radiographer
123 Main Street
My Town, Illinois 62650

Figure 15-1 Sample request for specialty program informational brochure.

equipment of ultrasound, diagnostic procedures, imaging, and image evaluation. Clinical education will also constitute a major portion of the program.

The education program will prepare the student to take the certification exam, which includes the subject matter that follows.

Content Specifications for the Examination in Ultrasound Physics and Instrumentation Administered by the American Registry of Diagnostic Medical Sonographers

I. Elementary Principles
II. Propagation of Ultrasound Through Tissues
III. Ultrasound Transducers
IV. Pulse Echo Instruments
V. Principles of Pulse Echo Imaging
VI. Image, Storage, and Display
VII. Hemodynamics, Doppler, Color Flow, and Color Power Imaging
VIII. Artifacts
IX. Quality Assurance of Ultrasound Instruments
X. Bioeffects and Safety

Content Specifications for the Examination in Obstetrics and Gynecology Administered by the American Registry of Diagnostic Medical Sonographers

I. Obstetrics
II. Gynecology
III. Patient Care Preparation/Technique

Content Specifications for the Examination in Abdomen Administered by the American Registry of Diagnostic Medical Sonographers

I. Liver
II. Biliary Tree
III. Pancreas
IV. Urinary Tract
V. Scrotum
VI. Prostate
VII. Spleen
VIII. Retroperitoneum
IX. Abdominal Vasculature (including Doppler)
X. GI Tract
XI. Neck
XII. Superficial Structures (Breast, Musculoskeletal, Non-cardiac Chest) Instrumentation

Content Specifications for the Examination in Adult Echocardiography Administered by the American Registry of Diagnostic Medical Sonographers

I. Anatomy and Physiology
II. Technique
III. Valvular Heart Disease
IV. Pericardial Disease
V. Systemic and Pulmonary Hypertensive Heart Disease
VI. Cardiomyopathies
VII. Ventricular Function
VIII. Cardiac Tumors
IX. Miscellaneous
X. Congenital Heart Disease in the Adult
XI. Diseases of the Aorta
XII. Doppler
XIII. Stress Echo

Content Specifications for the Examination in Breast Administered by the American Registry of Diagnostic Medical Sonographers

 I. Breast Instrumentation and Technique
 II. Normal Anatomy
 III. Benign vs. Malignant Features
 IV. Specific Lesions—Benign
 V. Specific Lesions—Malignant
 VI. Other
 VII. Invasive Procedures

Content Specifications for the Examination in Cardiovascular Principles and Instrumentation, Physics Administered by the American Registry of Diagnostic Medical Sonographers

 I. Anatomy of the Heart (Review)
 II. Basic Embryology
 III. Congenital Defects
 IV. Cardiac Physiology
 V. Cardiac Evaluation Methods
 VI. Principles of Cardiac Hemodynamics
 VII. Elementary Principles
 VIII. Propagation of Ultrasound Through Tissues
 IX. Ultrasound Transducers
 X. Pulse Echo Instruments
 XI. Principles of Pulse Echo Imaging
 XII. Images, Storage, and Display
 XIII. Doppler
 XIV. Image Features and Artifacts
 XV. Quality Assurance of Ultrasound Instruments
 XVI. Bioeffects and Safety

Content Specifications for the Examination in Neurosonology Administered by the American Registry of Diagnostic Medical Sonographers

 I. Physics and Instrumentation
 II. Technique in Neurosonography
 III. Anatomy and Physiology
 IV. Recognition of Pathology and Differential Diagnosis
 V. Medical Care of the Neonate During Scanning

Content Specifications for the Examination in Ophthalmic Biometry Administered by the American Registry of Diagnostic Medical Sonographers

 I. Keratometry
 II. Physics
 III. Biometry Instrumentation

 IV. Instrument Settings for Biometry
 V. Examination Techniques for Biometry
 VI. Sources of Error in Biometry
 VII. Intraocular Lens Power Calculation

Content Specifications for the Examination in Ophthalmology Administered by the American Registry of Diagnostic Medical Sonographers

 I. Physics
 II. Instrumentation
 III. Exam Techniques
 IV. Biometry
 V. Anatomy and Physiology
 VI. Pathology

Content Specifications for the Examination in Pediatric Echocardiography Administered by the American Registry of Diagnostic Medical Sonographers

 I. Instrumentation
 II. Phases of the Cardiac Cycle
 III. Normal Anatomy
 IV. Hemodynamics
 V. Scanning Technique
 VI. Functional Assessment
 VII. Congenital Pathology
 VIII. Acquired Pathology
 IX. Surgically Repaired Congenital Heart Disease
 X. Fetal Echocardiography

Content Specifications for the Examination in Vascular Physical Principles and Instrumentation Administered by the American Registry of Diagnostic Medical Sonographers

 I. Ultrasound Physics
 II. Ultrasonic Imaging
 III. Physiology and Fluid Dynamic
 IV. Physical Principles
 V. Ultrasound Safety and Quality Assurance

Content Specifications for the Examination in Vascular Technology Administered by the American Registry of Diagnostic Medical Sonographers

 I. Cerebrovascular
 II. Venous
 III. Peripheral Arterial
 IV. Abdomen/Visceral
 V. Miscellaneous Conditions/Tests
 VI. Quality Assurance

Content Specifications for the Examination in Diagnostic Medical Sonography Administered by the American Registry of Radiologic Technologists

A. Patient Care   10
B. Equipment Operation and Maintenance   35
C. Image Production and Evaluation   35
D. Sonographic Procedures   <u>130</u>
TOTAL   210 questions

Content Specifications for the Examination in Vascular Sonography Administered by the American Registry of Radiologic Technologists

A. Physics and Instrumentation   40
B. Image Production and Evaluation   35
C. Vascular Sonographic Procedures   <u>85</u>
TOTAL   160 questions

Professional Organizations

For information on a career as a diagnostic medical sonographer, contact the following organization:

Society of Diagnostic Medical Sonographers
12770 Coit Road, Suite 508
Dallas, TX 75251
972-239-7367
www.sdms.org

For information on acquiring registration as a diagnostic medical sonographer, contact the following organization:

American Registry of Diagnostic Medical Sonographers
600 Jefferson Plaza, Suite 360
Rockville, MD 20852-1150
301-738-8401

American Registry of Radiologic Technologists
1255 Northland Drive
St. Paul, MN 55120-1155
651-687-0048
www.arrt.org

immunology, radionuclide therapy, and statistics. Diagnostic procedures, imaging, and image evaluation, including extensive clinical education, will also constitute a major portion of the program.

Test Specifications

The education program will prepare the student to take the certification exam, which includes the following content categories:

A. Radiation Protection   20
B. Radionuclides and Radiopharmaceuticals   20
C. Instrumentation Quality Control   26
D. Diagnostic Procedures   118
E. Patient Care and Management   <u>16</u>
TOTAL   200 questions

Professional Organizations

For information on a career as a nuclear medicine technologist, contact the following organizations:

American Society of Radiologic Technologists
15000 Central Avenue, Southeast
Albuquerque, NM 87123
505-298-4500
www.asrt.org

Society of Nuclear Medicine—Technologist Section
136 Madison Avenue
New York, NY 10016
www.snm.org

For information on acquiring registration as a nuclear medicine technologist, contact the following organizations:

American Registry of Radiologic Technologists
1255 Northland Drive
St. Paul, MN 55120-1155
651-687-0048
www.arrt.org

Nuclear Medicine Technology Certification Board
2970 Clairmont Road, Suite 935
Atlanta, GA 30329-4421
404-315-1739

NUCLEAR MEDICINE

Educational programs in nuclear medicine technology may be 1, 2, or 4 years in length, depending on whether credits from an academic degree are included. The course of study will involve biology, anatomy, patient care, nuclear physics and instrumentation, computer technology, biochemistry, radiopharmacology, radiation biology and health physics,

RADIATION THERAPY TECHNOLOGY

Educational programs in radiation therapy technology may be 1, 2, or 4 years in length, depending on the inclusion of earned credit hours from an academic degree. The course of study will involve biology, radiation oncology, pathology, radiation biology, physics and equipment of radiation therapy, dosimetry, computer technology, hyperthermia, and quality assurance.

Test Specifications

The educational program will prepare the student for the certification exam in radiation therapy technology, which includes the following content categories:

A. Radiation Protection and Quality
   Assurance 40
B. Treatment Planning and Delivery 130
C. Patient Care, Management, and
   Education .... <u>30</u>
TOTAL .... 200 questions

Professional Organizations

For information on a career as a radiation therapist, contact the following organization:

American Society of Radiologic Technologists
15000 Central Avenue, Southeast
Albuquerque, NM 87123
505-298-4500
🌐 www.asrt.org

For information on acquiring registration as a radiation therapist, contact the following organization:

American Registry of Radiologic Technologists
1255 Northland Drive
St. Paul, MN 55120-1155
651-687-0048
🌐 www.arrt.org

ADVANCED-LEVEL EXAMINATIONS

The American Registry of Radiologic Technologists offers examinations leading to certificates of advanced qualifications in the radiologic specialties of computed tomography, magnetic resonance imaging, cardiovascular-interventional technology, mammography, quality management, and bone densitometry. These examinations do not lead to certification because there are as yet no formal educational requirements to enter these specialties.

In the following section, content specifications for each exam are listed to give you an idea of the knowledge base that is tested. For full details concerning advanced-level examinations, contact the following organization:

The American Registry of Radiologic Technologists
1255 Northland Drive
St. Paul, MN 55120-1155
651-687-0048
🌐 www.arrt.org

Computed Tomography

Content specifications for the computed tomography exam are as follows:

A. Patient Care 30
B. Imaging Procedures 75
C. Physics and Instrumentation .... <u>45</u>
TOTAL .... 150 questions

Magnetic Resonance Imaging

For information regarding the Section for Magnetic Resonance Technologists of the International Society for Magnetic Resonance in Medicine, visit the following website:

🌐 www.ismrm.org/smrt/

Content specifications for the magnetic resonance imaging are as follows:

A. Patient Care and MRI Safety 17
B. Imaging Procedures 53
C. Data Acquisition and Processing 62
D. Physical Principles of Image Formation <u>43</u>
TOTAL .... 175 questions

Cardiovascular-Interventional Technology

For information about the Association of Vascular and Interventional Radiographers, visit the following website:

🌐 www.rsna.org/about/orgs/avir.html

Content specifications for the cardiovascular-interventional exam are as follows:

A. Equipment and Instrumentation 23
B. Patient Care 37
C. Specific Procedural Studies
   1. Neurologic 12
   2. Genitourinary 18
   3. Gastrointestinal 26
   4. Peripheral 29
   5. Cardiopulmonary 20
   6. Miscellaneous Studies .... <u>5</u>
TOTAL .... 170 questions

Mammography

Content specifications for the mammography exam are as follows:

A. Patient Education and Assessment 15
B. Instrumentation and Quality Assurance 23
C. Anatomy, Physiology, and Pathology
   of the Breast 19
D. Mammographic Techniques 20
E. Positioning and Image Evaluation .... <u>23</u>
TOTAL .... 100 questions

Quality Management

Content specifications for the quality management exam are as follows:

A. Radiographic and Mammographic
   Quality Control   77
B. Quality Improvement   42
C. Program Standards and Guidelines   _21_
TOTAL   140 questions

Bone Densitometry

Content specifications for the bone densitometry exam are as follows:

A. Osteoporosis and Bone Health   15
B. Equipment Operation and Quality
   Control   16
C. Patient Preparation and Safety   4
D. DXA Scanning of Lumbar Spine   16
E. DXA Scanning of Proximal Femur   16
F. DXA Scanning of Forearm   _8_
TOTAL   75 questions

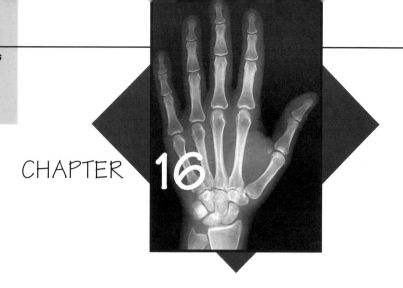

CHAPTER **16**

Advanced Academic Degrees

FACTORS INFLUENCING DEGREE PROGRAM SELECTION

An increasing number of radiography students and technologists are interested in pursuing higher-level academic degrees. This is particularly true for individuals seeking a career in radiology management or education. Master's degrees are required of radiography program directors. Baccalaureate degrees are required of clinical coordinators. Others would like to pursue degrees because they enjoy learning or will find the achievement fulfilling. Some hope to expand their earning potential or raise the level of their professional status. The baccalaureate degree is considered the professional level for radiologic technologists.

The U.S. Departments of Education and Labor have ample data to support the contention that earnings and employment opportunities are greater for those with higher levels of education. Regardless of the motivation, such career planning and goal setting must be based on accurate information.

This section provides a list of postsecondary institutions offering degrees or completion degrees in radiologic technology at the baccalaureate, master's, and doctoral levels. The list is current as of the date of publication; however, college and university enrollment statistics and governing board decisions exert a constant influence on degree availability. Those interested in pursuing such degrees should request the latest edition of the college or university catalog (or visit that institution's website) to determine that the curriculum is offered. Information available on the Internet will also provide listings of degree programs as they become available.

As with many other health professions an advanced degree in radiologic technology is not required for career advancement. However, baccalaureate and master's degrees in business, management, and education have become increasingly important. You should carefully define your career goals and pursue advanced education opportunities that are specific enough to provide skills in certain areas but broad enough to allow for flexibility.

If your career goals include teaching in radiologic technology, you should plan to pursue successive baccalaureate and master's degrees in education. If you plan to become a director of radiology, pursue a baccalaureate degree in health care administration or business and then a master's degree in health care administration or business administration. Rising to higher levels of responsibility in radiologic technology no longer depends entirely on moving up through the ranks; a solid college education is required.

If an advanced degree is among your career goals, begin planning now. Keep in mind that requests for information take time to process and be mailed. The use of websites greatly expedites the process. The sooner you acquire the needed information, the sooner you will be able to establish your plans for further education and achieve your desired goals. Figure 16-1 shows a sample letter that may be used to request a college or university catalog from the department of admissions and registration of any of the institutions listed in this chapter, should you go that route rather than by Internet.

As mentioned previously, the program list that follows may change at any time. Be sure to enlist the help of your reference librarian or career guidance office at a local community college or university for updates to the listing. This listing does not include the many off-campus degree completion programs available to health care professionals. Such programs are often advertised in monthly, bimonthly, or quarterly journals in radiologic technology.

Today's Date

Office of Registration and Admissions
State University
College Town, IL 65432

Please forward one copy of the latest undergraduate (graduate) catalog. I am particularly interested in pursuing a major in (subject area) and would appreciate any additional degree information or program brochures that my be available in that area.

Thank you in advance for this information.

Sincerely,

Interested Technologist
123 Main St
My Town, IL 61265

Figure 16-1 Sample catalog request letter.

Be sure to interview radiologic technologists at your clinical sites who are currently enrolled in degree completion programs. They can provide you with helpful information about the college or university in which they are enrolled.

ADVANCED DEGREE PROGRAMS

Baccalaureate Degree Programs or Degree Completion Programs in Radiologic Technology (Radiography, Nuclear Medicine, Radiation Therapy)

ALABAMA
University of Alabama—Birmingham
University Station—University Center
Birmingham, AL 35294
800-421-8743
🌐 www.uab.edu

University of South Alabama
307 University Boulevard
Mobile, AL 36688
800-872-5247
🌐 www.southalabama.edu

ARKANSAS
Arkansas State University
P.O. Box 790
State University, AR 72467
800-382-3030 (in state), 800-643-0080 (out of state)
🌐 www.astate.edu

University of the Ozarks
415 College Avenue
Clarksville, AR 72830
800-264-8636
🌐 www.ozarks.edu

University of Central Arkansas
Conway, AR 72032
501-450-3128, 800-243-8245 (in state only)
🌐 www.uca.edu

University of Arkansas for Medical Sciences
College of Pharmacy
4301 West Markham
Little Rock, AR 72205
501-686-5454
🌐 www.uams.edu

CALIFORNIA
California State University—Northridge
18111 Nordhoff Street
Northridge, CA 91330
818-677-1200
🌐 www.csun.edu

California State University at Long Beach
1250 Bellflower Boulevard
Long Beach, CA 90840
562-985-5471
🌐 www.csulb.edu

Loma Linda University
Loma Linda, CA 92350
909-558-4467
🌐 www.llu.edu

CONNECTICUT
Quinnipiac College
Mt. Carmel Avenue
Hamden, CT 06518
800-462-1944
🌐 www.quinnipiac.edu

University of Hartford
200 Bloomfield Avenue
West Hartford, CT 06117
800-947-4303
🌐 www.hartford.edu

DISTRICT OF COLUMBIA
George Washington University
2121 I Street, Northwest, Suite 201
Washington, DC 20052
800-447-3765
🌐 www.gwu.edu

Howard University
2400 Sixth Street, Northwest
Washington, DC 20059
800-822-6363
⊕ www.howard.edu

FLORIDA
University of Central Florida
P.O. Box 25000
Orlando, FL 32816
407-823-3000
⊕ www.ucf.edu

GEORGIA
Medical College of Georgia
1120 Fifteenth Street
Augusta, GA 30912
706-721-2725
⊕ www.mcg.edu

IDAHO
Boise State University
1910 University Drive
Boise, ID 83725
800-632-6586 (in state), 800-824-7017 (out of state)
⊕ www.boisestate.edu

Idaho State University
Campus Box 8368
Pocatello, ID 83209
800-888-4781
⊕ www.isu.edu

ILLINOIS
National-Louis University
2840 Sheridan Road
Evanston, IL 60201
800-443-5522

Roosevelt University
430 South Michigan Avenue
Chicago, IL 60605
312-341-3515
⊕ www.roosevelt.edu

Southern Illinois University—Carbondale
Carbondale, IL 62901
618-536-4405
⊕ www.siu.edu

INDIANA
Indiana University Northwest
3400 Broadway
Gary, IN 46408
800-437-5409
⊕ www.iun.edu

Indiana University—Purdue University at Indianapolis
425 University Boulevard
Indianapolis, IN 46202-5143
317-274-4591
⊕ www.iupui.edu

Marian College
3200 Cold Spring Road
Indianapolis, IN 46222
317-929-0123, 800-772-7264 (in state only)
⊕ www.marian.edu

IOWA
Briar Cliff College
3303 Rebecca Street
Sioux City, IA 51104-2100
800-662-3303
⊕ www.briar-cliff.edu

KANSAS
Fort Hays State University
600 Park Street
Hays, KS 67601
800-432-0248
⊕ www.fhsu.edu

KENTUCKY
Northern Kentucky University
Nunn Drive
Highland Heights, KY 41099
800-637-9948
⊕ www.nku.edu

LOUISIANA
Loyola University New Orleans
6363 St. Charles Avenue
New Orleans, LA 70118
800-456-9652
⊕ www.loyno.edu

McNeese State University
4205 Ryan Street
Lake Charles, LA 70609
337-475-5000, 800-622-3352 (in state only)
⊕ www.mcneese.edu

Northeast Louisiana University
700 University Avenue
Monroe, LA 71209
318-342-5252
⊕ www.nlu.edu

Northwestern State University of Louisiana
209 Roy Hall
Natchitoches, LA 71497
800-426-3754 (in state), 800-327-1903 (out of state)
⊕ www.nsula.edu

MAINE
St. Joseph's College
278 Whites Bridge Road
Standish, ME 04084
800-338-7057
⊕ www.sjcme.edu

MASSACHUSETTS
Massachusetts College of Pharmacy and Allied Health
  Sciences
179 Longwood Avenue
Boston, MA 02115
617-732-2850, 800-225-5506 (out of state only)
🌐 www.mcp.edu

MICHIGAN
Andrews University
Berrien Springs, MI 49104
616-471-3303
🌐 www.cs.andrews.edu

Madonna University
36600 Schoolcraft Road
Livonia, MI 48150
800-852-4951
http://madonna2.siteobjects.com

St. Mary's College
3535 Indian Trail
Orchard Lake, MI 48324
877-252-3131
🌐 www.stmarys.ols.edu

Wayne State University
100 Antoinette, Room 165
Detroit, MI 48202
313-577-3577
🌐 www.wayne.edu

MISSISSIPPI
William Carey College
489 Tuscan Avenue
Hattiesburg, MS 39401
800-962-5991
🌐 www.wllmcarey.edu

MISSOURI
Avila College
11901 Wornall Road
Kansas City, MO 64145
800-462-8452
🌐 www.Avila.edu

Southwest Missouri State University
901 South National
Springfield, MO 65804
800-492-7900
🌐 www.smsu.edu

University of Missouri—Columbia
130 Jesse Hall
Columbia, MO 65211
573-882-2456, 800-225-6075 (in state only)
🌐 www.missouri.edu/mu/

NEBRASKA
Clarkson College
101 South 42nd Street
Omaha, NE 68131
800-647-5500
🌐 www.clarksoncollege.edu

Nebraska Methodist College of Nursing and Allied Health
8501 West Dodge Road
Omaha, NE 68114
800-335-5510
🌐 www.methodistcollege.edu

NEVADA
University of Nevada—Las Vegas
4505 Maryland Parkway
Las Vegas, NV 89154
800-334-8658
🌐 www.unlv.edu

NEW JERSEY
Thomas Edison State College
101 West State Street
Trenton, NJ 08608-1176
800-981-2092
🌐 www.tesc.edu

NEW YORK
Long Island University—C.W. Post Campus
Northern Boulevard, College Hall
Greenvale, NY 11548
800-548-7526
🌐 www.liunet.edu

SUNY Health Science Center—Syracuse
155 Elizabeth Blackwell Street
Syracuse, NY 13210
315-464-4570
🌐 www.upstate.edu

SUNY Health Center—Brooklyn
450 Clarkson Avenue
Brooklyn, NY 11203
718-270-2446
🌐 www.hscbklyn.edu

NORTH CAROLINA
Queens College
1900 Selwyn Avenue
Charlotte, NC 28274
800-849-0202
🌐 www.queens.edu

University of North Carolina—Chapel Hill
210 Pittsboro Street, Campus Box 6210
Chapel Hill, NC 27599
919-966-3621
🌐 www.unc.edu

NORTH DAKOTA
Jamestown College
6081 College Lane
Jamestown, ND 58405
800-336-2554
🌐 www.jc.edu

Minot State University
500 University Avenue West
Minot, ND 58707
800-777-0750
🌐 www.misu.nodak.edu

University of Mary
7500 University Drive
Bismark, ND 58504
800-288-6279
🌐 www.umary.edu

OHIO
Ohio State University—Columbus
1800 Cannon Drive, 1210 Lincoln Tower
Columbus, OH 43210
614-292-3980
🌐 www.osu.edu

OKLAHOMA
University of Oklahoma—Health Science Center
P.O. Box 26901
Oklahoma City, OK 73190
405-271-2359
🌐 www.ou.edu

OREGON
Oregon Institute of Technology
3201 Campus Drive
Klamath Falls, OR 97601
800-422-2017
🌐 www.oit.edu

PENNSYLVANIA
Bloomsburg University
400 East 2nd Street
Bloomsburg, PA 17815
717-389-4316
🌐 www.bloomu.edu

College Misericordia
301 Lake Street
Dallas, PA 18612
800-852-7675
🌐 www.misericordia.edu

LaRoche College
9000 Babcock Boulevard
Pittsburgh, PA 15237
412-367-9241
🌐 www.laroche.edu

RHODE ISLAND
Rhode Island College
The Forman Center
Providence, RI 02908
800-669-5760
🌐 www.ric.edu

SOUTH CAROLINA
Medical University of South Carolina
171 Ashley Avenue
Charleston, SC 29425
803-792-3281
🌐 www.musc.edu

TEXAS
Midwestern State University
3400 Taft Boulevard
Wichita Falls, TX 76308
800-842-1922
🌐 www.mwsu.edu

University of Texas Medical Branch—Galveston
301 University Boulevard
Galveston, TX 77555-1305
409-772-1215
🌐 www.utmb.edu

UTAH
Weber State University
3750 Harrison Boulevard
Ogden, UT 84408
800-634-6568
🌐 www.weber.edu

VERMONT
Champlain College
P.O. Box 670
Burlington, VT 05402
800-570-5858
🌐 www.champlain.edu

University of Vermont
194 South Prospect Street
Burlington, VT 05401-3596
802-656-3370
🌐 www.uvm.edu

WEST VIRGINIA
Alderson-Broaddus College
College Hill
Philippi, WV 26416
304-457-1700
🌐 www.blue.ab.edu

University of Charleston
2300 MacCorkle Avenue, Southeast
Charleston, WV 25304
800-995-4682
🌐 www.uchaswv.edu

WISCONSIN
Concordia University
12800 North Lakeshore Drive
Mequon, WI 53092
414-243-4300
⊕ www.cuw.edu

Marian College of Fond Du Lac
45 South National Avenue
Fond Du Lac, WI 54935
800-262-7426
⊕ www.marian-coll.edu

Master's Degree Programs in Radiologic Technology

CALIFORNIA
University of California—Irvine
UCI College of Medicine
Medical Sciences I-E112
Irvine, CA 92717
714-824-5011

DISTRICT OF COLUMBIA
Georgetown University
303 Maguire Hall
37th and O Street, Northwest
Washington, DC 20057
202-687-3600
⊕ www.georgetown.edu

TEXAS
Midwestern State University
3400 Taft Boulevard
Wichita Falls, TX 76308
800-842-1922
⊕ www.mwsu.edu

Doctoral Programs in Radiologic Technology

CALIFORNIA
University of California—Irvine
UCI College of Medicine
Medical Sciences I-E112
Irvine, CA 92717
714-824-5011

DISTRICT OF COLUMBIA
George Washington University
2121 I Street, Northwest, Suite 089
Washington, DC 20052
800-447-3765
⊕ www.gwu.edu

For additional college and university information, visit the following websites:

Chronicle Guidance Publications
⊕ www.chronicleguidance.com (requires purchase of *Chronicle Four-Year College Databook*; excellent source of information)

College Net
⊕ www.collegenet.com

College Edge
⊕ www.collegeedge.com

College View
⊕ www.collegeview.com

Peterson's Education and Career Center
⊕ www.petersons.com/ugrad/

Princeton Review
⊕ www.princetonreview.com

U.S. News College and Careers Center
⊕ www.usnews.com

In addition, use all major search engines, typing in keywords such as radiologic technology, radiography, radiologic technology degree, and so forth.

For additional financial aid information, visit the following websites:

Federal Student Aid
⊕ www.fafsa.ed.gov

Financial Aid Information Page
⊕ www.finaid.org

FastWEB
⊕ www.fastweb.com

As you begin planning for an advanced degree, be sure to inquire about advanced standing or credit for previous radiologic technology education. Many institutions will award 2 full years of college credit, whereas others are more selective. Your program director may have advice about writing a portfolio of educational and work experiences to help you receive additional college credit for what you already know and have accomplished.

The work environment of the twenty-first century requires that you have as much knowledge and as many credentials as possible to advance in your career. Now is a good time to begin planning and setting goals for a lifetime of learning and achievement!

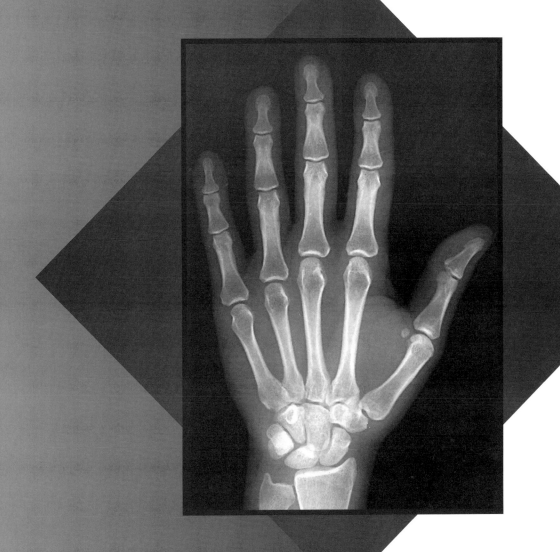

Appendix

Answers to Review Questions

CHAPTER 2

1. C
2. D
3. D
4. D
5. C
6. B
7. B
8. D
9. D
10. B
11. E
12. D
13. A
14. B
15. C
16. E
17. A
18. C
19. D
20. A
21. B
22. A
23. The correct answer is D. Choice B is incorrect. In fact, rem = rad multiplied by a quality factor. Choice C is a good answer, but choice D is more complete, making it the best answer.
24. The correct answer is C. Choice B is correct, but choice C expands on the information. Choice D is incorrect because the amount of radiation received by the patient would be measured in rads and the unit reported on film badge reports is rem.
25. The correct answer is B. Choices C and D are both very good answers, but their total amount of information is combined in choice B, the correct answer.
26. The correct answer is A. Choice B is correct, but choice A expands on it. Choice C is incorrect because particulate radiations deposit more energy than wave radiations. Choice D is incorrect because a quality factor is used when calculating absorbed dose equivalent.
27. C
28. A
29. The correct answer is D. Choice A is not as complete. Choices B and C are incorrect because they imply that there is no risk of damage to the individual.
30. D
31. E
32. B
33. A
34. B
35. C
36. D
37. B
38. B
39. D
40. E
41. A
42. B
43. C
44. C
45. B
46. A
47. The correct answer is D. The quality factor takes into account the source of exposure that may be wave or particulate and the actual amount of energy deposited per unit length of tissue—the LET.
48. The correct answer is A. The amount of energy deposited in tissues is directly responsible for any biologic damage that may occur.
49. C
50. The correct answer is D. Remember that the cellular life cycle always begins with interphase. The reason D is the correct answer is that the three steps in interphase are listed in their proper order. This makes D a better answer than choice B.
51. The correct answer is D. Choice A defines cell division for somatic cells only.
52. C
53. B
54. D
55. A
56. A
57. E
58. A
59. C
60. A
61. The correct answer is D. Because the cellular cytoplasm is so much larger than a cell's nucleus, it is more likely to be struck by an incoming x-ray photon. Therefore, statistically speaking, more damage will occur to cells because of indirect effect rather than the statistically less probable occurrence of direct effect.
62. A
63. C
64. A
65. The correct answer is D. Although the numerical portion of this answer, 25, is correct, the unit of measurement must also be correct.
66. A
67. B
68. A
69. The correct answer is C. It is important to remember that most somatic effects of exposure to ionizing radiation cannot occur at doses used during diagnostic procedures. However, it is still important to practice ALARA.
70. A
71. D
72. D
73. The correct answer is D. The percentages indicated under choices B and C are reversed. Choice A is incorrect because gonadal shielding would not need to be used on patients beyond childbearing age.
74. The correct answer is B. Use of low-mAs, high-kVp techniques always result in a lower patient dose. In this case, it is coupled with a 400-speed film-screen combination. Choice A would result in a higher dose because it is a high-mAs, low-kVp technique. Choices C and D have slower speed-film screen combinations. Focal spot size is not related to patient dose.
75. The correct answer is A. This answer takes into account that collimation and use of high-speed film-screen combinations will reduce dose to the patient. Choice D is not part of the answer because the use of grids requires an increase in mAs, which results in an increased patient dose.
76. C
77. D
78. B
79. B
80. C
81. E
82. A
83. C
84. A
85. B
86. The correct answer is C, mean marrow dose.
87. The correct answer is A, genetically significant dose.

88. The correct answer is D. Choice A is incorrect because the timer must sound an alarm after 300 seconds, or 5 minutes. Choice B is incorrect because the purpose of the alarm is to sound an alert. Choice C is incorrect because the alarm sounds after 5 minutes.

89. D

90. The correct answer is B. This problem is different from many you have been asked in that it is giving you the new dose and asking you to figure out what the new distance should be. You should not need to use an equation on paper or a calculator to solve this problem. The question wants you to reduce your dose to ¼ the amount you receive at a distance of 2 feet. Keeping in mind the inverse square law, you may recall that doubling distance causes the dose to drop to ¼. Therefore the correct answer would be to step back to a distance of 4 feet from the table. Choice A implies that you need to quadruple your distance from the table to reduce the dose to ¼. Choice D would result in a decrease in dose because of shielding but not the specific reduction in dose mentioned in the problem.

91. A

92. The correct answer is C. Choice A is incorrect because holding patients should never be routine. Choice B is incorrect because a radiographer should be the last choice to hold the patient. Choice D is incorrect because routinely using student radiographers is unacceptable in practice.

93. D

94. B

95. The correct answer is A. Film badges are sensitive to a reading as low as 10 mrem.

96. The correct answer is B. The highest dose that can be read with a pocket ionization chamber is 200 mR. If the needle on the indicator is resting on the number 200, it may mean 200 mR or more than 200 mR had been received. Choice C is incorrect because it indicates millirads. Choice A is incorrect because pocket ionization chambers read in mR.

97. C

98. B

99. D

100. The correct answer is D. Choices A, B, and C are all reasons filtration is used; however, filtration should never be adjusted by the radiographer. A qualified radiation physicist should be the only individual adjusting x-ray beam filtration.

CHAPTER 3

1. The correct answer is C. Choice 1 is incorrect because there are no electrons in the atomic nucleus. Choice 3 is incorrect because kinetic energy is the energy of motion. Choices 5 and 6 are incorrect because some radiations in the electromagnetic spectrum are nonionizing, such as ultrasound invisible light.

2. A

3. C

4. D

5. A

6. B

7. A

8. D

9. C

10. The correct answer is D. The octet rule states that there can be no more than eight electrons in the outer shell. It does not stipulate that there must be eight electrons in the outer shell.

11. B

12. A

13. C

14. A

15. The correct answer is D. Spelling counts.

16. The correct answer is D. Wavelength can be measured from crest to crest or trough to trough.

17. C

18. C

19. B

20. A

21. The correct answer is C. Choice B cannot be the answer because the distance has not been squared. Choice D cannot be the answer because the equation in the answer is actually the density maintenance formula, not the inverse square law.

22. D

23. The correct answer is B. Choice 2 cannot be the answer because the movement of electrons from one object to another is called *electrification*. Choice 3 cannot be the answer because like charges repel and unlike charges attract. Choice 5 cannot be the answer because friction, contact, and induction are methods of electrification.

24. The correct answer is A. Keep in mind that the question asks for which statements are false. Choice 4 is false because the ampere is the unit of electric current. Choice 6 is false because the volt is the unit of electromotive force, and choice 9 is false because Ohm's law is calculated using the equation V = IR.

25. The correct answer is C. Electromagnetic induction does not require that two conductors touch one another.

26. D

27. B

28. C

29. The correct answer is D. A motor converts electrical energy to mechanical energy.

30. B

31. A

32. C

33. D

34. B

35. A

36. C

37. The correct answer is D. Older x-ray machines require the line voltage compensator to be adjusted manually, whereas most newer equipment lets the machine do the adjustment itself.

38. A

39. C

40. E

41. A

42. D

43. B

44. C

45. B

46. D

47. B

48. B

49. A

50. D

51. A

52. E

53. C

54. D

55. A

56. C

57. B

58. The correct answer is D. All x-ray equipment must be warmed up before use. This is especially true for equipment that is being used for the first time during a workday, but the warm-up procedure should also be performed on most equipment if the equipment has not been in use 1 to 2 hours. Failure to properly warm the anode before making exposures may cause tube failure because of the extreme amount of heat imparted on a cool anode. Choice B is false because the warm-up technique is not high kVp or high mAs but is in fact a low heat-producing technique. Choice C is incorrect because merely turning on the x-ray equipment does not actually warm up the anode.

59. The correct answer is C. Most first-year students experience this activity. Choice B is incorrect because merely activating the rotor does not produce ionizing radiation. Choice D is incorrect because unnecessarily heating the filament actually reduces x-ray tube life.

60. The correct answer is A. Choice B is incorrect because the electronics in x-ray equipment prevent an exposure from being made until the filament is properly heated and the anode is spinning at full speed. Choice C is incorrect because merely choosing an mA station does not cause the filament to begin heating. Choice D is incorrect because the anode does need to be at full speed and the machine will not let an exposure be made until it is so.

61. The correct answer is D. Choice B is also correct but not as complete as choice D, which explains why the focusing cup is negative. Choice C is incorrect because thermionic emission occurs at the filament wire itself.

62. The correct answer is B. Choice A is partly correct by stating that most of the energy is converted to heat.

63. C

64. D

65. The correct answer is C. Choice A is also correct, but choice C describes the type of x rays produced.

66. A

67. The correct answer is B. Choice 1 is incorrect because x rays do not carry electrical charges. Choice 5 is incorrect because the speed of light is 186,000 miles per second. Choice 6 is incorrect because the wavelengths of x rays are between 0.1 and 0.5 angstroms. Choice 9 is incorrect because x rays cannot be focused by any means. Collimation merely restricts the area being irradiated.

68. The correct answer is D. Choice A is correct in stating that the x-ray beam is heterogeneous, but the second half of choice A is incorrect.

69. C

70. The correct answer is A. Choice B is incorrect because soft rays have long wavelengths. Choice C is true, but it is not the primary purpose of filtration. Choice D is incorrect because long-wavelength rays are called *soft rays*.

71. B

72. D

73. D

74. The correct answer is D. These charts are almost never used in modern radiography because for more than 20 years, x-ray machines have been able to regulate themselves by not allowing an exposure that would cause damage to the anode.

75. The correct answer is A. These charts are seldom used in modern radiography because many x-ray machines automatically shut off when the amount of heat produced approaches a predetermined percentage of the heat storage capacity of the x-ray tube.

76. A

77. B

78. C

79. A

80. D

81. A

82. B

83. The correct answer is D. This is why the formula for heat units for three-phase, six-pulse equipment is multiplied by 1.35.

84. The correct answer is B. This is why the formula for calculating heat units for three-phase, twelve-pulse equipment is multiplied by 1.41.

85. C

86. D

87. C

88. A

89. D

90. B

91. D

92. The correct answer is C. Keep in mind that because the current never falls to zero when using three-phase equipment, a spinning top test will not show dots but will show arcs. A 1-second exposure would be expected to produce a full circle, which would be an arc of 360 degrees. A timer setting of $1/60$ second would be expected to produce a $1/60$-degree arc, which is a 6-degree arc. Choices A and B would be incorrect because they indicate dots. Choice D is incorrect.

93. D

94. A

95. D

96. C

97. D

98. The correct answer is B. Note that this question is asking the amount of mAs actually used and not the actual setting of the mAs on the control panel.

99. The correct answer is C. Choices A, B, and D are also marks on the focal track, but they are caused by a malfunction.

100. A

CHAPTER 4

1. The correct answer is D. Choices B and C define density. Choice A actually defines contrast.

2. D

3. B

4. D

5. C

6. D

7. The correct answer is D. Choice A is incorrect because kVp controls the energy of the beam. Choice B is incorrect because x rays are not produced at the cathode. Choice C is incorrect because mAs controls the quantity but not the quality of x rays; kVp controls the quality of the x rays.

8. D

9. The correct answer is D. Choice A is incorrect because mAs controls the quantity of x rays produced. Choice B is incorrect because kVp controls the quality of x rays produced. Choice C is incorrect because focal spot size has nothing to do with contrast.

10. The correct answer is B. The relationship between kVp and density is governed by the 15% rule.

11. The correct answer is D. The correct statements are choices A and C.

12. The correct answer is A. Choice 3 is incorrect because as kVp decreases, wavelength increases. Choice 5 is incorrect because changes in kVp do affect density.

13. The correct answer is D. The correct choices are B, which has a 15% increase in kVp, and choice C, which has a doubling of the mAs. Choice A has a doubling of mAs and an increase of almost 15% kVp, which would quadruple the density.

14. The correct answer is C. Be careful: Choice D appears correct but does not have the distances squared.

15. The correct answer is D. This is another way of asking about the inverse square law.

16. The correct answer is A. This is another way of asking about the inverse square law.

17. C

18. A

19. C

20. The correct answer is B. Choice A is incorrect because grids do not always reduce density if the mAs is adjusted to compensate for their use. Choice C is partially correct in that density may be decreased by absorbing scatter radiation, but compensation in technique usually occurs. Choice D is incorrect because a higher grid ratio will cause a decrease in density if mAs is not adjusted.
21. The correct answer is D. Choice A is incorrect because short wavelengths are not absorbed by filtration. Choice B is incorrect because high-energy x rays are not absorbed by filtration. Choice C is incorrect because there is little effect on density from using filtration.
22. The correct answer is C. If the x-ray beam is restricted even tighter, density will decrease. Choice B is incorrect because x rays cannot be focused.
23. D
24. C
25. B
26. D
27. A
28. D
29. The correct answer is B. High kVp allows for more uniform penetration of the anatomic part being radiographed. It also is responsible for increasing the number of Compton's interactions.
30. The correct answer is A. A lower kVp x-ray beam is less penetrating and causes an increase in the number of photoelectric interactions.
31. B
32. D
33. The correct answer is C. Choice A is incorrect because the x-ray beam cannot be focused. Choice B is incorrect because the use of beam restriction necessitates an increase in mAs used.
34. The correct answer is D. Choice A is incorrect because nothing has been done to the x-ray beam to change the wavelength. Choice B is incorrect because beam restriction does not change the wavelength of the beam. Choice C is incorrect because mAs should be increased, and there will already be a decrease in the number of Compton's interactions taking place.
35. The correct answer is D. Choice B is also correct but does not explain why.

36. The correct answer is C. Contrast will decrease because the x-ray beam is harder. Choice D is misleading because it includes the fact that the beam is harder; however, it indicates the contrast increases, which is incorrect.
37. D
38. D
39. A
40. C
41. D
42. The correct answer is A. Choices B, C, and D are all examples of distortion. Choice A takes them all into account.
43. The correct answer is B. Choice D is incorrect because it would cause magnification.
44. D
45. D
46. A
47. D
48. D
49. B
50. C
51. A
52. D
53. D
54. A
55. D
56. A
57. D
58. A
59. A
60. D
61. D
62. A
63. D
64. D
65. C
66. B
67. C
68. D
69. A
70. B
71. D
72. C
73. The correct answer is B. Choice A is incorrect because decreased density in the middle would not be caused by using an inverted parallel grid. Choice C is incorrect because density would decrease in the middle of this radiograph. Choice D is incorrect because density could decrease across the entire radiograph, depending on how the grid has been positioned.
74. The correct answer is A. The grid conversion factor or Bucky factor for a 12:1 grid is 5 times the original mass.
75. D

76. The correct answer is D. The correct choices are B and C. Choice A is incorrect because AECs are not used for some examinations (notably, those of the extremities).
77. The correct answer is D. Automatic exposure controls are set to terminate the exposure after a certain amount of radiation has passed through the ionization chamber. Consequently, changes in kVp will have no effect on density. There may be some effect on contrast if the change in kVp is substantial.
78. D
79. C
80. A
81. B
82. The correct answer is D. The fixing agent does not clear all silver halide crystals, it only removes the unexposed crystals. Water is merely used as the solvent. The fixer solution is acidic.
83. The correct answer is C. Developer solution is generally kept at 90° to 95° F. The hardener in the developer solution does control the swelling of the emulsion; however, silver halide crystals could not escape in this solution.
84. D
85. A
86. B
87. C
88. The correct answer is D. Choice A is incorrect because the temperature setting is approximately 120° F. Choice B is a good answer but is incomplete.
89. The correct answer is D. The entire processor does not need to be cleaned weekly. The developer tank does not need to be cleaned daily. Starter solution is added only to developer, not to the fixer.
90. B
91. A
92. C
93. D
94. D
95. A
96. The correct answer is D. Inadequate drying would have little, if any, effect on density or contrast.
97. A
98. D
99. The correct answer is A. Chemical contamination would cause a rapid increase in density because of chemical fog.
100. D

CHAPTER 5

1. D
2. A
3. D
4. C
5. B
6. A
7. D
8. A
9. B
10. The correct answer is C. Although choices A and B are certainly valid, choice C takes precedence over all the others. Choice D is incorrect because the radiographer may take additional projections as needed.
11. The correct answer is D. Choice A is incorrect because it does not mention that a physician has approved such removal. Choice B is incorrect because it is not necessary for a radiologist to provide the order. Choice C is incorrect because the patient's attending physician may direct the collar to be removed.
12. A
13. C
14. A
15. B
16. D
17. A
18. A
19. C
20. D
21. B
22. B
23. The correct answer is B. AP and lateral projections are not required. AP and AP with internal rotation films may suffice. Choice 3 is incorrect because deep veins can be imaged. Choice 5 is incorrect because automatic film changers are not required for imaging.
24. A
25. The correct choice is D. Choice 1 is incorrect when performing a cervical myelogram. Choice 2 is incorrect because contrast agents used in myelography are water soluble. Choice 4 is incorrect because gravity is used to distribute the contrast medium. Choice 5 is incorrect when performing lumbar myelography.
26. C
27. B
28. The correct answer is D. The correct choices are A and C. Choice B is incorrect because the ulnar surface is in contact with the film.

29. The correct answer is C. Choice 2 is incorrect because the thumb should be up. Choice 4 is incorrect because the elbow should be flexed 90 degrees. Choice 5 is incorrect because the central ray should be directed to the midpoint of the forearm.
30. The correct answer is B. Choice 1 is incorrect because the forearm and humerus should be in the same plane. Choice 4 is incorrect because the hand must be supinated.
31. The correct answer is A. Choice 1 is incorrect because the hand is not pronated. Choice 4 is incorrect because the arm may be slightly abducted.
32. The correct answer is C. Choice 2 is incorrect because no angle is put on the central ray. Choice 4 is incorrect because respiration should be suspended.
33. The correct answer is B. Choice A is incorrect because it would not be appropriate to double-expose the film. Choice C is incorrect because both joints may not necessarily be placed on the same film. Choice D is incorrect because the patient should be standing, if possible, and respiration must be suspended.
34. The correct answer is D. Choice 1 is incorrect because the clavicle is commonly radiographed using an AP projection. Choice 2 is incorrect because the direction of tube angle in the PA axial projection should be caudad.
35. The correct answer is A. Choice 2 is incorrect because the affected scapula should be centered to the cassette.
36. D
37. A
38. C
39. B
40. C
41. The correct answer is D. Choice 1 is incorrect because a trough filter is used for chest radiography. A wedge filter would be used for the foot. Choice 2 is incorrect because the plantar surface rests on the cassette. Choice 3 is incorrect because the central ray would be directed toward the heel. Choice 4 is incorrect because the central ray is directed at the base of the third metatarsal.
42. The correct answer is A. Choice 2 is incorrect because the plantar surface of the foot should be perpendicular to the cassette. Choice 4 is incorrect because the central ray enters the foot at the base of the fifth metatarsal.

43. The correct answer is B. Choice 2 is incorrect because this rotates the ankle too far. Choice 3 is incorrect because rotation should be adjusted 15 to 20 degrees. Choice 4 is incorrect because rotation should be at 45 degrees.
44. The correct answer is D. Choice 3 is incorrect because the patient should be rolled toward the affected side. Choice 6 is incorrect because the fibula should appear posterior to the tibia on the radiograph.
45. The correct answer is C. Choice 3 is incorrect because the patella must be perpendicular to the film. Choice 4 is incorrect because the central ray should be directed 5 degrees cephalad.
46. A
47. D
48. D
49. B
50. B
51. D
52. C
53. A
54. The correct answer is B. Choice 4 is incorrect because the lateral projection of the cervical spine is always taken with the cervical collar in place until the finished radiograph has been cleared by a physician. Choice 5 is incorrect because it would distort the image.
55. The correct answer is C. Choice 2 is incorrect because no angulation is placed on the central ray.
56. The correct answer is D. Choice 2 is incorrect because the hips and knees should be flexed.
57. C
58. A
59. The correct answer is D. Emphysema is a condition in which air is trapped in the alveoli, which hyperinflates the lungs and makes them much easier for x rays to penetrate.
60. A
61. D
62. The correct answer is D. Because emphysema makes the lungs so easy to penetrate, automatic exposure controls sometimes cannot shut off fast enough, which causes the film to be too dense.
63. B
64. The correct answer is C. These letters stand for *chronic obstructive pulmonary disease.*

65. The correct answer is A. Choice 2 is incorrect because the shoulders should be rotated anteriorly, moving the scapulae out of the field of the ribs. Choice 4 is incorrect because respiration should be on full inspiration.

66. The correct answer is C. Choice A is incorrect because the body should be rotated only 15 to 20 degrees. Choice B is incorrect because this is an anterior oblique. Choice D is incorrect because breathing causes a blurring of lung detail. A falling load generator should not be used because it inhibits the ability to use long exposure times that run several seconds.

67. The correct answer is B. Choice A is incorrect because a PA projection causes superimposition of the spine and a lateral projection is not possible. Choice C is incorrect because respiration should be suspended. Choice D is incorrect because an AP projection would increase magnification.

68. D
69. B
70. C
71. A
72. C
73. The correct answer is D.
74. B
75. The correct answer is D. Choice A is incorrect because it describes the wrong three-point landing. Choice B is incorrect because it describes angulation from the perpendicular. Choice C is incorrect because the central ray exits the affected orbit.

76. The correct answer is C. Choice B is incorrect because of the degree of angulation. Choice D is incorrect because it indicates the head is resting on the nose.

77. The correct answer is A. Read choices B, C, and D carefully and note that only one or two words are different from those in the correct answer.

78. D
79. The correct answer is C. Whereas the Waters also shows all of the paranasal sinuses, the upright projection will best indicate fluid levels.

80. C
81. D
82. B
83. D
84. A
85. C
86. D
87. A
88. C

89. B
90. B
91. D
92. C
93. The correct answer is A. Choices B and D can immediately be eliminated because it places the patient prone. A lateral decubitus position requires the patient to be lying on the side.

94. C
95. D
96. C
97. A
98. C
99. B
100. C

CHAPTER 6

1. D
2. C
3. D
4. D
5. B
6. B
7. D
8. D
9. The correct answer is A. Keep in mind that assault does not have to involve touching the patient at all.

10. The correct answer is B. Notice that the question asks which item is false concerning invasion of privacy. Choice B could be considered false imprisonment.

11. A
12. B
13. D
14. The correct answer is C. Choice B actually involves loss of life or limb; gross negligence does not have to involve an actual loss.

15. D
16. D
17. The correct answer is A. Choice 2 is incorrect because a brochure does not have to be given to the patient. Choice 5 is incorrect because it is not possible that patients completely understand all of the aspects of a procedure.

18. The correct answer is B. Choice A is incorrect because a patient who is ambulatory would not be on a cart. Choice C is incorrect because patient care must never be compromised because of short staffing. Choice D is incorrect because safety is of paramount importance.

19. D
20. C
21. A
22. B
23. A

24. C
25. B
26. A
27. A
28. D
29. C
30. A
31. B
32. C
33. A
34. B
35. C
36. A
37. B
38. D
39. D
40. B
41. D
42. D
43. B
44. E
45. A
46. C
47. B
48. C
49. B
50. E
51. D
52. The correct answer is D. Choice A is incorrect because it indicates normal body temperature in degrees Centigrade. Choice B is incorrect because it indicates a range of normal temperature in degrees Centigrade.

53. A
54. B
55. C
56. D
57. C
58. C
59. A
60. C
61. E
62. A
63. D
64. B
65. A
66. D
67. B
68. The correct answer is C. Choice 2 is incorrect because the patient should never be left alone under any circumstances. Choice 3 is incorrect because of potentially devastating consequences; a spinal injury should always be assumed.

69. D
70. E
71. The correct answer is A. Nosocomial infections are those acquired in the health care setting. Most of these infections are the result of the use of the urinary catheter.

72. B
73. C

74. D
75. The correct answer is A. Choice 1 is incorrect because air is a negative contrast agent. Choice 3 is incorrect because barium should be mixed with warm water. Choice 4 is incorrect because nonionic contrast media do contain iodine.
76. The correct answer is D. Choice A is incorrect because pharmaceutical companies are unable to prove a link between seafood allergies and contrast agent sensitivity.
77. A
78. D
79. A
80. B
81. D
82. A
83. B
84. D
85. C
86. A
87. D
88. C
89. D
90. A
91. B
92. C
93. B
94. A
95. B
96. B
97. A
98. B
99. B
100. B

CHAPTER 7
Answers to Challenge Test #1

1-30. See Figure A-1 (p. 276) and the following selected answers:
Across
4. GSD (genetically significant dose)
12. Filters. The intensity of the radiation is measured by the film.
13. Roentgen. This is the traditional unit of in-air exposure. Although SI units are not asked on the ARRT exam, you should also remember that the SI unit of in-air exposure is the coulomb per kilogram.
20. Five rem. The annual effective absorbed dose equivalent limit for radiographers is also commonly expressed as 5000 millirem.
24. One hundred mR. Milliroentgens are used because this is in-air exposure.
28. The intensity of scatter at a 90-degree angle from the patient 1 meter away is only ¹/₁₀₀₀ the intensity of the primary beam.
Down
2. Rem. This is the traditional unit of dose equivalency. Although SI units

are not asked on the ARRT exam, you should also remember that the SI unit of dose equivalency is the sievert.
7. Rad. This is the traditional unit of absorbed dose. Although SI units are not asked on the ARRT exam, you should also remember that the SI unit of absorbed dose is the gray.
11. RBE (relative biologic effectiveness)
17. MMD (mean marrow dose)
21. Millirem. The annual effective absorbed dose equivalent limit for the general public is also commonly expressed as 0.5 rem.

31-60. See Figure A-2 (p. 277) and the following answers:
31. Alternating current
32. Anode
33. Anode cooling curve
34. Atomic number
35. Autotransformer
36. Bremsstrahlung
37. Cathode
38. Characteristic
39. Circuit
40. Falling load
41. Focusing cup
42. Four kVp
43. Frequency
44. Half-value layer
45. Heat
46. Input phosphor
47. Ionization chamber
48. kVp times mAs
49. Linearity
50. One millisecond
51. Output phosphor
52. Photocathode
53. Rectifier
54. Reproducibility
55. Step-up transformer
56. Thermionic emission
57. Three-phase
58. Tube rating chart
59. Two percent of SID
60. Wavelength
61. D
62. W
63. A
64. R
65. K
66. H
67. J
68. L
69. E
70. F
71. C
72. O
73. V
74. XX
75. X
76. S
77. U
78. M
79. Q

80. P
81. G
82. N
83. I
84. B
85. T
86. BB
87. UU
88. Y
89. PP
90. II
91. FF
92. HH
93. JJ
94. CC
95. DD
96. AA
97. MM
98. TT
99. VV
100. QQ
101. SS
102. KK
103. OO
104. NN
105. EE
106. LL
107. GG
108. Z
109. RR
110. WW
111. Minor calyces
112. Major calyces
113. Renal pelvis
114. Ascending colon
115. Hepatic flexure
116. Transverse colon
117. Descending colon
118. Incisura angularis
119. Pylorus
120. Rugae
121. Fundus
122. Spinous process
123. Lamina
124. Pedicle
125. Transverse process
126. Intervertebral foramen
127. Pedicle
128. Lesser trochanter
129. Greater trochanter
130. Ischial tuberosity
131. Lateral epicondyle
132. Lateral condyle
133. Tibial plateau
134. Medial condyle
135. First carpometacarpal joint
136. Second metacarpophalangeal joint
137. Second proximal interphalangeal joint
138. Second distal interphalangeal joint
139. Scaphoid
140. Lunate
141. Triquetral
142. Pisiform
143. Trapezium

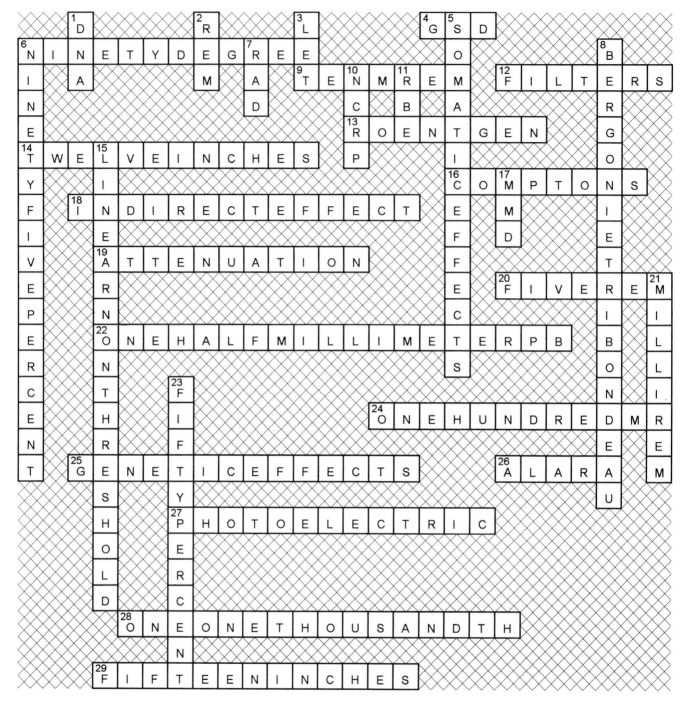

Figure A-1

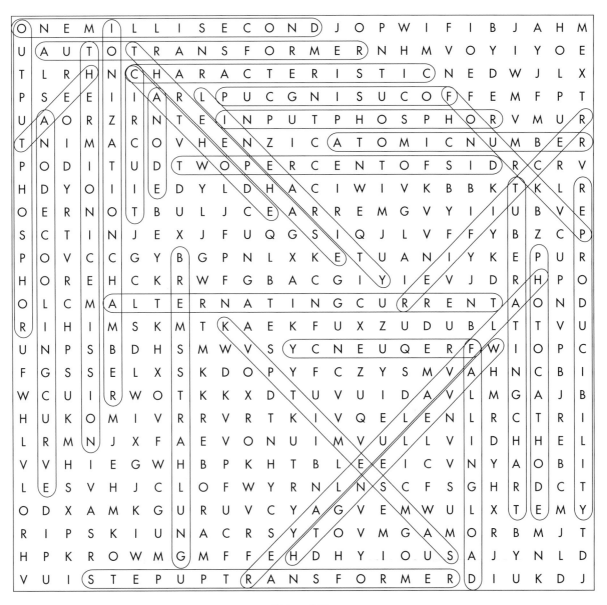

Figure A-2

Answers to Challenge Test #2

1. D. This is a more complete answer than A because it defines each factor.
2. The correct answer is C. Choice A is incorrect because it is expressed as aluminum equivalency.
3. A
4. The correct answer is B. Choice A is incorrect because it is expressed in lead equivalency.
5. A
6. The correct answer is A. Choices B and D are incorrect because they have the wrong unit of measurement.
7. C

8. C. Although A is also a correct answer, choice C indicates a more thorough understanding of lead apron thickness needs.
9. The correct answer is C. Choice D is incorrect because it has the wrong unit of measurement.
10. B. Choice C has the correct radiation measurement but is incomplete because it does not specify the distance from the tube.
11. The correct answer is A. Remember that the question is referring to mobile.
12. C

13. B. Choice A is close, but dilithium crystals are used only in science fiction.
14. D
15. C
16. D. All are examples of radiation effects on the individual being exposed.
17. The correct answer is D. Choices B and C are correct. Choice A is incorrect because photoelectric interaction produces contrast.
18. The correct answer is D. The correct equation would be rads multiplied by a quality factor equals rem.

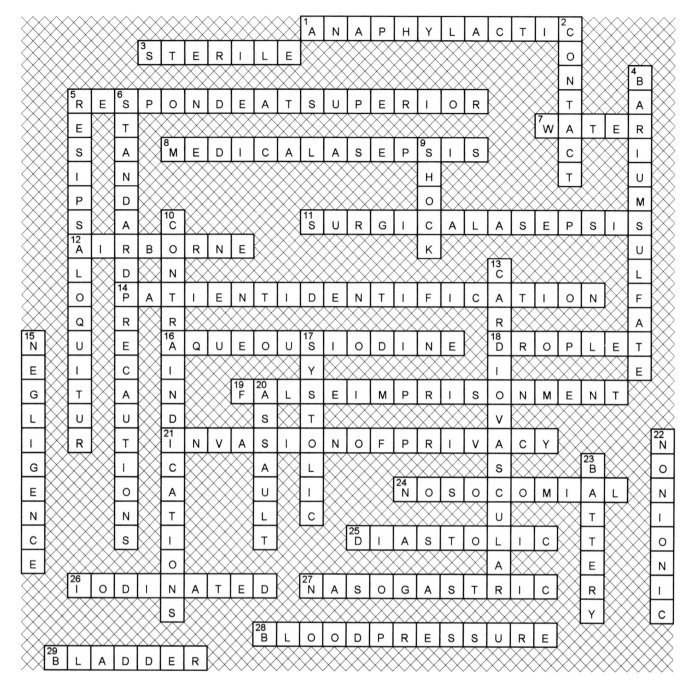

Figure A-3

19. The correct answer is A. Choice B is incorrect because no level of radiation is considered completely safe. Choice C is incorrect because no such immunity has been proven. Choice D is incorrect because the effective absorbed dose equivalent limit for the general public is 500 mrem per year.

20. B. High-LET radiation is depositing a lot of energy in the tissues, causing much ionization.

21. C

22. B

23. The correct answer is D. Because the cellular cytoplasm is substantially larger than the cellular nucleus, it is more likely to be struck by incoming x-ray photons. Thus most of the cellular response to radiation is indirect. The direct effect results from x-ray photons directly striking the cellular nucleus.

24. The correct answer is A. Indirect effect occurs when radiation strikes the cytoplasm of the cell. Target theory states there is a master molecule that governs cellular activities, that is, DNA.
25. B
26. C
27. B
28. A
29. The correct answer is A. Choices B and D refer to electrons and brems radiation, which apply to action inside the x-ray tube; the photoelectric effect is a photon-tissue interaction.
30. C
31. A
32. D
33. C
34. The correct answer is A. This question asks which of the choices does not define matter. According to Einstein, matter cannot travel at or beyond the speed of light.
35. A step-up transformer steps up voltage and steps down current.
36. D
37. The correct answer is D. Choice B looks tempting, but silicone is a substance that is sometimes used in plastic surgery.
38. The correct answer is D. Choice A is false because the octet rule states that no more than eight electrons may occupy the outer shell at any time. Choice B is false because falling load generators cannot produce the long exposure times required for breathing techniques. Choice C is false because electrons are not contained in the nucleus of an atom.
39. C. Hence, the use of the constant 1.41 when calculating heat units for this type of equipment.
40. D
41. B
42. A
43. D
44. E
45. A
46. B
47. C
48. D
49. The correct answer is B. This is one of the electron-focusing lenses.
50. The correct answer is D. This is the photocathode, which releases electrons wherever it is struck by visible light.
51. The correct answer is A. This is the output phosphor, which releases visible light wherever it is struck by electrons.

52. The correct answer is C. This is the input phosphor, which releases visible light wherever it is struck by x rays.
53. D
54. D
55. A
56. A
57. The correct answer is B. The accuracy of collimation must be within 2% of the SID.
58. The correct answer is C. The accuracy of kVp must be within 4 kVp.
59. D
60. D
61. D
62. A
63. C
64. The correct answer is D. The correct choices are A and B. Choice C is unacceptable because the dose to the patient actually increases when using a grid.
65. The correct answer is D. Choice A is also correct, but choice D includes tooth enamel.
66. B
67. D
68. The correct answer is C. Choice A is incorrect because reducing SID by half would quadruple the density. Choice B is incorrect because doubling the SID would cause a drop in density to a quarter of the original. Choice D is incorrect because changing technique one "step" in time is highly inaccurate; adjacent steps on a timer switch are not necessarily the same percentage of change.
69. B
70. D
71. B
72. E
73. A
74. C
75. A
76. B
77. B
78. B
79. A
80. A
81. B
82. A
83. A
84. B
85. The correct answer is D. This curve represents the fastest film, which would have the largest silver bromide crystals.
86. The correct answer is D. This is the fastest film, so it would have the highest contrast.

87. The correct answer is D. This is the fastest film, so it would be most sensitive to radiation, thereby exposing the patient to less radiation.
88. The correct answer is A. This is the slowest film, so it would be able to provide the highest resolution, which is measured in line pairs per millimeter.
89. The correct answer is A. This is the slowest film, so it would be least sensitive to x rays and the light from the intensifying screens.
90. The correct answer is A. This is the slowest film, so it would have fewer sensitivity specks.
91. The correct answer is D. This is the fastest film, so it would demonstrate the fewest number of gray tones, which are represented by optical density numbers.
92. The correct answer is D. This is the fastest film, so it has the narrowest latitude.
93. A. A smaller effective focal spot is produced.
94. C. kVp is the controlling factor of contrast.
95. B. Density decreases as distance is increased, with no changes in exposure factors.
96. A. A decrease in OID results in less magnification of the image.
97. B. Lower developer temperature results in a less active solution and lower density.
98. B. Higher kVp results in more Compton's interactions and a more uniform penetration of the part.
99. A. A slower system speed has smaller silver halide crystals in the film and smaller phosphors or a thinner active layer in the screens.
100. A. The grid absorbs scatter radiation. In addition, because no compensation has been made in mAs, the absorption of image-forming rays will be quite noticeable.
101. A. A shorter SID will result in greater magnification.
102. C. There is no correlation between kVp and recorded detail. kVp does control visibility of detail.
103. B. This results in an increase in OID.
104. B. This results in magnification of the image.
105. C. Leaving the film in solution in the processor will have a dramatic effect on density, contrast, and visibility of detail, but not on recorded detail.
106. B. The beam wavelength becomes predominantly shorter, which makes it more penetrating.

107. B. As collimation is tightened without technique compensation, fewer rays strike the patient.
108. A. There is a decrease in the number of Compton's interactions as the area being irradiated is limited. This is true regardless of whether compensation is made by adjusting mAs.
109. C. Focal spot size controls recorded detail.
110. C. Changing kVp while using automatic exposure controls has no effect on density.
111. A
112. D
113. The correct answer is D. The Jefferson fracture is a comminuted fracture of the ring of the atlas.
114. The correct answer is C. A boxer's fracture is a transverse fracture of the neck of the fifth metacarpal.
115. The correct answer is B. A Colles' fracture is a transverse fracture through the distal radius.
116. The correct answer is A. *Talipes* is another term for clubfoot.
117. The correct answer is E. Ankylosing spondylitis is an inflammatory disease of the spine that causes fusion of the joints involved.
118. D
119. D
120. A
121. D
122. C
123. C
124. B
125. A
126. D
127. B
128. A
129. E
130. A
131. B
132. B
133. D
134. C
135. B
136. D
137. C
138. D
139. B
140. A
141. C
142. A
143. D
144. The correct answer is D. Choice A is incorrect because this is a radiograph of a lower leg. Choice B is incorrect because the tibia and fibula cannot be superimposed. Choice C is incorrect because both joints should be included.
145. D
146. B

147. C
148. A
149. B
150. D
151. B
152. D
153. C
154. The correct answer is C. Autotomography involves placing superimposing structures in motion while the x-ray tube and film remain stationary.
155. B
156. The correct answer is D. This is a PA axial projection of the clavicle, so the tube angulation is caudad. The tube angulation is cephalad for the AP axial projection.
157. C
158. The correct answer is D because the patient is prone.
159. B. Place the proximal femur (the thicker part of the thigh) under the cathode portion of the x-ray beam. A trough filter is used for chest radiography. Another form of compensating filter could be used on the femur.
160. A
161. The correct answer is D. If this were a PA oblique projection, choice B would be correct.
162. B. This is an AP oblique.
163. B. This is a PA oblique.
164. The correct answer is C. The second inspiration would be deeper than just a single inspiration.
165. A
166. The correct answer is B. Choice 3 is incorrect because the central ray exits at the nasion when examining the frontal bone. Choice 4 is incorrect because the MSP is perpendicular to the cassette.
167. The correct answer is D. This projection is also called the *Towne's projection.* Choice 1 is incorrect because the OML should be perpendicular to the cassette. Choice 2 is incorrect because the central ray should be directed 30 degrees caudal to the OML. Choice 3 is incorrect because the central ray should be directed 30 degrees to the OML. Choice 4 is incorrect because the MSP should be perpendicular to the plane of the film.
168. C
169. The correct answer is C. Another way of wording this answer would be "placing the MSP 53 degrees from the plane of the film."
170. The correct answer is A. Another correct answer would be "if the OML formed a 53-degree angle from the perpendicular."

171. D. The key word is *must,* although radiographers should be proficient in taking blood pressure also. As radiographers' scope of practice expands, so will the need to be proficient in the use of a wide range of medical instruments.
172. C
173. D
174. B. Retrograde flow of urine commonly causes bladder infections. The urinary system is the primary site of nosocomial infections.
175. A
176. The correct answer is B. This question asks which item is not required for valid consent. A consent form is not always used.
177. C. Hence, the need for proper body mechanics at all times.
178. D. The patient may not yet know the extent of the diagnosis.
179. A
180. A
181. B
182. C
183. D
184. A
185. D
186. B
187. D
188. The correct answer is C. Choice 2 is incorrect because this is beyond the radiographer's scope of practice. Choice 4 is incorrect because in a trauma situation, other health care workers need to be in the room.
189. D
190. D
191. B
192. E
193. C. You can never assume there will be no reactions. Choice B is incorrect because other contrast examinations could include barium studies, which would not have a risk of reaction.
194. D. The key word is *must.* Choice B is close, but *should* is not acceptable.
195. A. Palpating the vein one more time after cleansing contaminates the injection site.
196. B. Although informed consent is vital, some patients react because it has been suggested that a reaction may occur.
197. C
198. B
199. The correct answer is D. As a professional, you should know what your credentials mean.
200. D

Answers to Challenge Test #3

1. The correct answer is D, primary radiation. Remnant radiation exits the body (choice A); gamma radiation is not produced in the x-ray tube (choice B). Choice C, nonionizing radiation, is incorrect because x rays are ionizing radiation.

2. The correct answer is C, photoelectric. Choice A is incorrect because Compton's produces scatter radiation. Choice B is incorrect because coherent scatter is produced at extremely low kVp levels. Choice D is incorrect because pair production occurs only at levels above 1.02 MeV.

3. The correct answer is A. Choice B is incorrect because coherent scatter occurs at extremely low kVp levels and does not produce a recoil electron. Choice C is incorrect because the photoelectric effect does not scatter the photon. Choice D is incorrect because pair production does not occur in diagnostic radiography.

4. The correct answer is D. Choice A is incorrect because coulombs/kilogram is an SI unit. Choice B is incorrect because rem is the traditional unit of dose equivalency. Choice C is incorrect because becquerel is the SI unit of activity.

5. The correct answer is B. Choice A is incorrect because coulombs/kilogram is the SI unit of in-air exposure. Choice C is incorrect because the curie is the traditional unit of activity. Choice D is incorrect because LET (linear energy transfer) is the amount of energy deposited per unit length of tissue irradiated.

6. The correct answer is A. Choice B is incorrect because the gray is the SI unit of absorbed dose. Choice C is incorrect because quality factor is multiplied by the absorbed dose to calculate dose equivalency. Choice D is incorrect because LET (linear energy transfer) is the amount of energy deposited per unit length of tissue irradiated.

7. The correct answer is D. Choice A is incorrect because rem is the traditional unit of dose equivalency. Choice B is incorrect because the gray is the SI unit of absorbed dose. Choice C is incorrect because quality factor is multiplied by absorbed dose to calculate dose equivalency.

8. The correct answer is D. Choice A is incorrect because the becquerel is the SI unit of activity. Choice B is incorrect because the gray is the SI unit of absorbed dose. Choice C is incorrect because quality factor is multiplied by absorbed dose to calculate dose equivalency.

9. The correct answer is D.

10. The correct answer is C. Choice A is incorrect because *tissue exposure* is not a term used in radiology. Choice B is close, but this is not the standard term used. Choice D is incorrect because absorbed dose equivalent limit is 5000 mrem per year for occupational workers.

11. The correct answer is D. Choice A is incorrect. *Rads* multiplied by quality factor equals *rems*. Choice B is incorrect because roentgens is the traditional unit of in-air exposure. Choice C is incorrect because the gray is the SI unit of absorbed dose.

12. The correct answer is D. Choice A is incorrect because contrast is produced by photoelectric effect, not Compton's interaction. Choices B and C are incorrect because they provide part but not all of the answer.

13. The correct answer is B. The quality factor for x rays is 1.

14. The correct answer is D. Choice A is incorrect because none of the examples listed in the question would manifest in a short period of time. Choices B and C are incorrect: Genetic effects may express themselves in future generations as mutations.

15. The correct answer is A. The key words in this choice are *probably* and *appreciable*.

16. The correct answer is B, the National Council on Radiation Protection and Measurements. Choice A, the International Commission on Radiological Protection, is incorrect. Choice C is incorrect, but the Nuclear Regulatory Commission does have enforcement power. Choice D is incorrect because the American Society of Radiologic Technologists is the professional organization for radiation science professionals.

17. The correct answer is C. Choices A and D are incorrect because there is no threshold dose regarding radiation protection. Choice B is incorrect because we do not assume a nonlinear response for radiation protection.

18. The correct answer is B. Choice A is incorrect because the inverse square law states that the intensity of radiation is inversely proportional to the square of the distance from the source of radiation. Choice C is incorrect because the reciprocity law states that mAs = mAs. Choice D is incorrect because Ohm's law states that voltage is equal to current times resistance in a circuit.

19. The correct answer is D. Indirect effect occurs when radiation strikes the cytoplasm. This causes the formation of free radicals and hydrogen peroxide, which damage the cell. Choice B is incorrect because the law of Bergonié and Tribondeau describes the radiosensitivity of cells. Choice C is incorrect because target theory explains that DNA is the master molecule of the cell. Choice A is incorrect because direct effect causes only about 5% of the cellular response.

20. The correct answer is A. Direct effect occurs when radiation directly hits the cellular nucleus. Indirect effect occurs when radiation strikes the cytoplasm of the cell.

21. The correct answer is D. Choice A is incorrect because 500 mrem per year is the absorbed dose equivalent limit for the general public. Choice B is incorrect because 5 rem per year is the absorbed dose equivalent limit for radiation workers.

22. The correct answer is C. The effective absorbed dose equivalent limit for radiographers is 5000 mrem, or 5 rem, per year. Choice A is incorrect because there are no quarterly absorbed dose equivalent limits. Choice B is wrong because 500 mrem per year is the absorbed dose equivalent limit for the general public. Choice D is incorrect because there are no monthly absorbed dose equivalent limits for radiographers.

23. The correct answer is D. Cumulative occupational exposure is calculated by multiplying the worker's age in years times 1 rem. Choice A is incorrect because the unit is incorrect.

24. The correct answer is C. The annual effective dose equivalent for the general public is 0.5 rem, or 500 mrem.

25. The correct answer is D. Choice A is incorrect because this term is no longer used. Choice B is incorrect because *ALARA* stands for "as low as reasonably achievable."

26. The correct answer is D. Film badges are generally accurate down to the level of 10 mrem.
27. The correct answer is B. The exposure switch on a portable x-ray machine must be attached to a cord that is at least 6 feet long.
28. The correct answer is B. Under no circumstances should the radiographer be exposed to the primary beam.
29. The correct answer is D. For proper radiation protection, x-ray tubes operating above 70 kVp must have total filtration of at least 2.5-mm aluminum equivalent. Lead is not used as a filter material.
30. The correct answer is B. Choice A is incorrect because gonadal shielding may obstruct the area of interest in some projections. Choice C is incorrect because male patients must also be shielded. Choice D is incorrect because the gonads must be protected outside of pregnancy as well.
31. C
32. The correct answer is D. *Atomic number* refers to the number of protons, and in a stable atom, this would also be the number of electrons.
33. The correct answer is B. Choice A is incorrect because electrons are particles in orbit around the nucleus. Choice C is incorrect because ions are atoms that have had electrons added or removed. Choice D is incorrect because particulate radiations are not atoms.
34. C
35. The correct answer is D. Quanta are also referred to as *photons*, and both are waves. Choice A is incorrect because protons are particles in the nucleus of an atom. Choice B is incorrect because, at present, phasers exist only in science fiction. Choice C is incorrect because x rays are waves, not particles.
36. The correct answer is A. Choice B is incorrect because altitude is the height of an object above sea level. Choice C is incorrect because amplitude is the height of a sine wave. Choice D is incorrect because frequency is the number of sine waves passing a given point per unit time.
37. The correct answer is D. Choices A and B are incorrect because step-up and stepdown transformers use two coils of wire. Choice C is incorrect because even though transformers work on induction, there is no such thing as an induction transformer.

38. The correct answer is D. Choices A and B are incorrect because step-up and stepdown transformers cannot be varied.
39. A
40. The correct answer is C. Choice A is incorrect because the minimum response time is the minimum time that it takes the machine to respond and terminate exposure. Choice B is incorrect, although a falling load generator may be in use for the procedure. Choice D is incorrect because the ionization chamber is the sensing portion of automatic exposure control.
41. D
42. The correct answer is D. Choice A is incorrect because rectifiers change AC to DC. Choice B is incorrect because "generators" is an incomplete answer. Choice C is incorrect because timers determine the length of exposure.
43. The correct answer is C. Voltage is decreased but current is increased and sent to the filament during thermionic emission. Choice A is incorrect because a step-up transformer is not located in the high-voltage section. Choice B is incorrect even though mA going to the filament circuit is set at the autotransformer. Choice D is incorrect because a type of generator does not apply to this question.
44. C
45. D
46. D
47. The correct answer is C. Like charges repel, and this helps electrons leave the filament and travel to the anode.
48. D
49. B
50. C
51. D
52. A
53. D
54. The correct answer is A. An accurate timer should exhibit 120 dots for a 1-second exposure or 6 dots for a ½₀-second exposure.
55. C
56. The correct answer is A. Collimation must be accurate within ±2% of the SID.
57. C

58. The correct answer is C. Choice A is incorrect because the photocathode converts electron energy into light energy. Choice B is incorrect because the electron focusing lens helps restrict the electron beam toward the output phosphor. Choice D is incorrect because a vidicon tube is used to send an image to the TV.
59. A
60. The correct answer is B. The digital dosimeter has replaced many quality control test tools previously used.
61. The correct answer is C. Choice A is incorrect because contrast is the difference in densities on a radiograph. Choice B is incorrect because detail is the sharpness of the image. Choice D is incorrect because mAs controls density.
62. D
63. C
64. The correct answer is C. If one uses 40 mAs and 90 kVp, an image with 4 times the density will be produced. If one uses 30 mAs and 92 kVp, the density will more than double. If one uses 15 mAs and 92 kVp, an image with less than double the density will be produced.
65. The correct answer is C. The inverse square law governs the relationship between distance and density.
66. C
67. C
68. C
69. A
70. C
71. A
72. D
73. The correct answer is B. The speed step used during sensitometric testing is the one closest to a value density of 1. Choice A is incorrect because 0.25 is the toe of the curve. Choice D is incorrect because 2.0 is too close to the shoulder of the curve.
74. The correct answer is A. The developer solution is very sensitive to temperature and will become too active, resulting in dark films.
75. The correct answer is A. Choice B is correct because light films indicate that the film is not getting enough solution. Choice C is incorrect because milky films are caused by a fixer problem. Choice D is incorrect because greasy films are not caused by the developer.
76. The correct answer is D. Fog may add density to the entire film or to only a small portion of it.
77. C

78. The correct answer is D. This is a good reason why the tank should be drained daily.
79. D
80. D
81. The correct answer is B. Choice A is incorrect because the film is washed free of chemicals here. Choice C is incorrect because the developer converts exposed silver halide crystals to black metallic silver. Choice D is incorrect because no chemical reactions occur in the dryer.
82. The correct answer is D. The heat in the dryer helps seal the emulsion. Choice A is incorrect because the film is washed free of chemicals here. Choice B is incorrect because fixer removes unexposed silver halide crystals. Choice C is incorrect because the developer converts exposed silver halide crystals to black metallic silver.
83. C
84. A
85. B
86. C
87. B
88. D
89. C
90. The correct answer is B. *Grid ratio* is defined at the height of the lead strips divided by the distance between them. Choice A is incorrect because *H & D* refers to sensitometric curves. Choice C describes the reciprocity law. Choice D is incorrect because the 15% rule governs changes in technique involving kVp.
91. D
92. The correct answer is D. Wire mesh will blur in the area of poor contact. The phosphor layer, the reflective layer, and the protective layer cannot be tested, although the protective layer can be cleaned.
93. C
94. D
95. The correct answer is A. Contrast is primarily determined by the speed of the film. A faster-speed film-screen system will also exhibit a narrower latitude, poorer recorded detail, and increased density.
96. The correct answer is A. Contrast is primarily determined by the speed of the film. A slower-speed film-screen system will also exhibit a wider latitude, better recorded detail, and decreased density.
97. The correct answer is B. A faster film-screen system will exhibit a narrower latitude.

98. The correct answer is B. The section of an H & D curve that represents base plus fog is the toe. The shoulder represents unusable densities, and the body represents usable densities and contrast. The x-axis represents exposure.
99. The correct answer is A. The section of an H & D curve that represents D-max is the shoulder.
100. The correct answer is D. The section of an H & D curve on which exposure is plotted is the x-axis.
101. The correct answer is B. Blue tint may also act to enhance contrast.
102. D
103. D
104. The correct answer is D. The only factors listed that control recorded detail are SID and OID, and they are the same for each set of factors given.
105. The correct answer is A. Of all the factors listed, only kVp controls contrast. This set of factors has the lowest kVp and therefore exhibits the highest contrast.
106. The correct answer is C. Of all the factors listed, only SID and OID control magnification. This set of factors has the shortest SID.
107. The correct answer is A. Choice B would be correct *if* it included high kVp instead of low kVp. Choice C is incorrect because photoelectric interactions occur more often at lower kVp levels. Choice D is incorrect because Compton's interactions occur at higher kVp levels.
108. D
109. The correct answer is B. Subject contrast is controlled by kVp and the atomic number of the part being radiographed. Choice A is true to a degree, but there is a better answer. Choice C is incorrect because recorded detail is a geometric function. Choice D is incorrect because characteristic radiation is produced at the anode.
110. The correct answer is B. Contrast increases because less scatter radiation is produced as a result of fewer Compton's interactions. Choice A is incorrect because beam restriction reduces the number of Compton's interactions, thereby increasing contrast. Choice C is incorrect because beam restriction reduces the number of Compton's interactions, thereby shortening the scale of contrast.
111. D
112. C
113. B

114. A
115. B
116. D
117. C
118. A
119. D
120. B
121. D
122. D
123. A
124. D
125. C
126. A
127. B
128. D
129. B
130. C
131. B
132. D
133. D
134. D
135. D
136. C
137. D
138. D
139. C
140. A
141. B
142. D
143. D
144. B
145. C
146. A
147. A
148. D
149. D
150. D
151. B
152. A
153. D
154. D
155. D
156. B
157. A
158. D
159. A
160. D
161. C
162. B
163. C
164. D
165. D
166. D
167. D
168. C
169. D
170. C
171. D
172. C
173. C
174. D
175. B
176. A
177. C
178. D

179. B

180. C

181. The correct answer is D. Choice A is incorrect because hypovolemic shock is caused by a loss of fluids. Choice B is incorrect because septic shock follows massive infection. Choice C is incorrect because neurogenic shock causes blood to pool in peripheral vessels.

182. B

183. D

184. A

185. D

186. A

187. C

188. B

189. D

190. D

191. D

192. C

193. A

194. B

195. C

196. D

197. B

198. D

199. A

200. D

Bibliography

American Registry of Radiologic Technologists (ARRT): *Conventions specific to the radiography examination,* St Paul, Minn, May 1993 and December 1995, ARRT.

American Registry of Radiologic Technologists: *Content specifications for the examination in radiography,* St Paul, Minn, 2001, ARRT.

American Registry of Radiologic Technologists: *Continuing education requirements for renewal of registration,* St Paul, Minn, 2001, ARRT.

American Registry of Radiologic Technologists: *Examinee handbook: mammography, computed tomography, magnetic resonance imaging, cardiovascular-interventional technology, quality management, bone densitometry,* St Paul, Minn, 2001, ARRT.

American Registry of Radiologic Technologists: *Examinee handbook: radiography, nuclear medicine technology, radiation therapy technology,* St Paul, Minn, 2001, ARRT.

Anderson K, Anderson LE, Glanze WD: *Mosby's medical, nursing, & allied health dictionary,* ed 5, St Louis, 1998, Mosby.

Ballinger P: *Merrill's atlas of radiographic positions and radiologic procedures,* ed 9, St Louis, 1999, Mosby.

Ballinger P: *Pocket guide to radiography,* ed 4, St Louis, 1999, Mosby.

Bontrager K: *Textbook of radiographic anatomy and positioning,* ed 5, St Louis, 2001, Mosby.

Bushong S: *Radiologic science for technologists,* ed 7, St Louis, 2001, Mosby.

Callaway WJ: Graduate technologists and customer service: a 1991 survey, *Radiol Manage* 14:50, 1992.

Callaway WJ: *Associate degree radiography clinical handbook,* Springfield, Ill, 2002, Lincoln Land Community College.

Cullinan A, Cullinan J: *Producing quality radiographs,* ed 2, Philadelphia, 1994, Lippincott.

Darby M, Bushee E: *Mosby's comprehensive review of dental hygiene,* ed 2, St Louis, 1991, Mosby.

Dowd S, Tilson E: *Practical radiation protection and applied radiobiology,* ed 2, Philadelphia, 1999, WB Saunders.

Ehrlich R, McCloskey E, Daly J: *Patient care in radiography,* ed 5, St Louis, 1999, Mosby.

Eisenberg R, Dennis C: *Comprehensive radiographic pathology,* ed 2, St Louis, 1995, Mosby.

Fauber T: *Radiographic imaging & exposure,* St Louis, 2000, Mosby.

Gurley L, Callaway W: *Introduction to radiologic technology,* ed 5, St Louis, 2002, Mosby.

Hiss S: *Understanding radiography,* ed 3, Springfield, Ill, 1993, Charles C Thomas.

Jensen S, Peppers M: *Pharmacology and drug administration for imaging technologists,* St Louis, 1998, Mosby.

Laudicina P: *Applied pathology for radiographers,* Philadelphia, 1989, WB Saunders.

Mace J, Kowalczyk N: *Radiographic pathology for technologists,* ed 3, St Louis, 1998, Mosby.

Malott J, Fodor J: *The art and science of medical radiography,* ed 7, St Louis, 1993, Mosby.

Mitchell J, Haroun L: *Introduction to health care,* Albany, 2002, Delmar.

National Council on Radiation Protection and Measurements: *Quality assurance for diagnostic imaging,* NCRP Report No. 99, Bethesda, Md, 1988, NCRP.

National Council on Radiation Protection and Measurements: *Medical x-ray, electron beam and gamma-ray protection for energies up to MeV (equipment design, performance and use),* NCRP Report No. 102, Bethesda, Md, 1989, NCRP.

National Council on Radiation Protection and Measurements: *Radiation protection for medical and allied health personnel,* NCRP Report No. 105, Bethesda, Md, 1989, NCRP.

National Council on Radiation Protection and Measurements (NCRP): *Limitation of exposure to ionizing radiation,* NCRP Report No. 116, Bethesda, Md, 1993, NCRP.

Papp J: *Quality management in the imaging sciences,* St Louis, 1998, Mosby.

Saxton D: *Mosby's comprehensive review of nursing,* ed 16, St Louis, 1998, Mosby.

Selman J: *The fundamentals of x-ray and radium physics,* ed 9, Springfield, Ill, 2000, Charles C Thomas.

Thompson M: *Principles of imaging science and protection,* Philadelphia, 1994, WB Saunders.

Torres L: *Basic medical techniques and patient care in imaging technology,* ed 5, Philadelphia, 1997, Lippincott.

Illustration Credits

Figures 2-1, 2-2, 3-2, 3-3, 3-4, 4-1, 4-2, 4-3, 4-5 through 4-18—From Fauber TL: *Radiographic imaging & exposure,* St Louis, 2000, Mosby.

Figure 3-1—From Bushong SC: *Radiologic science for technologists: physics, biology and protection,* ed 7, St Louis, 2001, Mosby.

Figures 3-5 and 7-18—From Malott JC, Fodor J III: *The art and science of medical radiography,* ed 7, St Louis, 1993, Mosby.

Figure 4-4—From *Mosby's radiographic instructional series: radiographic imaging,* St Louis, 1998, Mosby.

Figures 5-19 through 5-63 and 7-20 through 7-30—From Ballinger P: *Merrill's atlas of radiographic positions and radiologic procedures,* ed 9, St Louis, 1999, Mosby.

Figures 6-1 and 6-2—From Jensen S, Peppers M: *Pharmacology and drug administration for imaging technologists,* St Louis, 1998, Mosby.

Figures 7-3 through 7-16—From Bontrager KL: *Textbook of radiographic positioning and related anatomy,* ed 5, St Louis, 2001, Mosby.

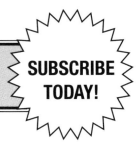
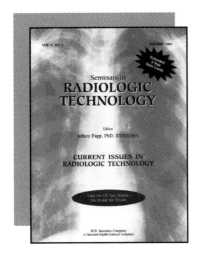

Seminars in Radiologic Technology

February 2002 — Select Topics in Radiography
May 2002 — Orthopaedic Radiography
August 2002 — Breast Imaging
November 2002 — Current Issues in Radiology

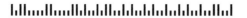